Global Pharmaceutical Policy

Zaheer-Ud-Din Babar
Editor

Global Pharmaceutical Policy

palgrave
macmillan

Editor
Zaheer-Ud-Din Babar
Centre for Pharmaceutical Policy and Practice Research
University of Huddersfield
Huddersfield, UK

ISBN 978-981-15-2723-4 ISBN 978-981-15-2724-1 (eBook)
https://doi.org/10.1007/978-981-15-2724-1

This Palgrave Macmillan imprint is published by the registered company Springer Nature Singapore Pte Ltd.
The registered company address is: 152 Beach Road, #21-01/04 Gateway East, Singapore 189721, Singapore

To Danyal

Preface

The pharmaceutical policy deals with access to safe, effective and "quality use of medicines". Around the globe, there are challenges in regard to access to innovative treatments and the affordability of expensive medicines. Also, "access to high-cost medicines", "innovative biologicals and vaccines" and the "issues related to medicines access, trade, and intellectual property rights" are central to any pharmaceutical policy. However, dealing with these issues and forming effective pharmaceutical policies has played a central role in improving access to medicines.

The pandemics like COVID-19 have again put a major emphasis on the need for newer innovative treatments and the availability of affordable vaccines. The national pharmaceutical policies have been effective in eradicating diseases and in improving patients' quality of life. However, forming these policies is a complex challenge and requires a number of capacity-building measures including good governance and legislation, trained workforce and human expertise as well as a viable local pharmaceutical industry.

This book documents a number of pharmaceutical policy issues in the form of synthesis, reviews, case studies as well as examples from a number of low-, middle- and high-income countries. The major themes include "medicines access", "medicines use" and "medicines safety".

"Access to medicines" being a major component of national medicine policies has been discussed in great detail in the book. There are a number of chapters covering pricing, access, generics, biosimilars, access to vaccine and immunization, public participation in access to medicines as well as access to cancer medicines. There are country case studies covering access to medicines in Mexico, Ukraine, Russia and Kyrgyzstan. Medicines pricing is the single most determining factor on access, and there is a chapter covering new medicine pricing models. Similarly, generic medicines play a vital role in promoting access and reducing costs. The chapter on generics discusses in detail the impact of generic medicines policies on global pharmaceutical policy.

There are also chapters on medicine safety, antibiotic use, antibiotics resistance as well as on the importance of the pharmaceutical supply chain. The book also includes chapters on pharmaceutical policy literature on Pakistan and China. There is also a series of editorials on "Medicines access, use, and pharmaceutical health system".

The book discusses global pharmaceutical policy from various angles, including key factors impacting it as well as challenges it faces. The book also narrates how different countries deal with it, and what makes a policy successful. I hope that the book would be useful for a wide range of readers including students, researchers, academics and policymakers in this field.

20 March 2020
Huddersfield, UK

Zaheer-Ud-Din Babar

Contents

List of Figures

List of Tables

1

Medicines Safety in the Globalized Context

Rabia Hussain, Mohamed Azmi Hassali and Zaheer-Ud-Din Babar

Abbeviations

ADR	Adverse drug reaction
DRAP	Drug Regulatory Authority of Pakistan
HCPs	Healthcare professionals
MNHSRC	Ministry of National Health Services and Regulation
NHS	National Health Service
NPC	National pharmacovigilance centre
PV	Pharmacovigilance
SADR	Spontaneous adverse drug reaction reporting
UMC	Uppsala Monitoring Centre
WHO	World Health Organization

R. Hussain (✉) • M. A. Hassali
School of Pharmaceutical Sciences, Universiti Sains Malaysia, Pulau Penang, Malaysia

Z. Babar
Centre for Pharmaceutical Policy and Practice Research, University of Huddersfield, Huddersfield, UK
e-mail: z.babar@hud.ac.uk

Z. Babar (ed.), *Global Pharmaceutical Policy*,
https://doi.org/10.1007/978-981-15-2724-1_1

Medicines Safety

Modern medicines have changed the way of management and control of disease; however, despite having beneficial effects, they contribute to adverse drug reactions (ADRs) (WHO 2014). In this context, the safe use of medicines is vital as it affects each member of the society (Edwards and Aronson 2000). Despite medicines' utility in the treatment and prevention of disease, it sometimes may result into undesirable or even fatal reactions, and in some countries ADRs are listed among the top ten causes of mortality (White et al. 1999).

The World Health Organization (WHO) defines an ADR as "a response to a drug that is noxious and un-intended and occurs at doses normally used in man for prophylaxis, diagnosis or therapy of disease, or for modification of physiological function" (WHO 2002). The risk of ADR is associated with the drug use including dose, administration frequency and pharmacodynamic and pharmacokinetic characteristics of population composed of paediatric and geriatric patients or those with hepatic and renal impairment (Sultana et al. 2013). Such conditions require special attention in regard to ADR monitoring, thus making ADRs to cause an additional economic burden on patients, caregivers and healthcare systems.

Hospital Admissions and Adverse Drug Reactions

Since the early 1980s, many studies have reported that the ADRs were the cause of hospital admissions with reporting rate of 2.9 to 6.0 percent. The hospital admissions due to ADRs incidents were found to be 1.5 to 20% and were higher than that to the total admissions to hospitals (Black and Somers 1984; Lazarou et al. 1998; Baker et al. 2004). A study by Classen et al. (1997) reported that during 1990–1993, the ADR incidence-related hospital admissions were 2.43 per 100 admissions (Classen et al. 1997). Similarly, Bates et al. (1995) found that ADR-related admissions were 6.5 ADRs out of 100 admissions (Bates et al. 1995). Pirmohamed et al. (2004)

conducted prospective analysis of 18,820 admissions in UK hospitals which accounted to the 1225 ADR-related admissions and found that there was a high burden of ADRs in terms of morbidity, mortality and cost to the National Health Service (NHS) (Pirmohamed et al. 2004). Wu et al. (2010) analysed a ten-year trend of hospital admissions related to ADR in England and found that 557,978 admissions were related to ADR, presenting 0.9% of total patient admissions due to an ADR. During this period, the number of ADR incidents increased from 42,453 to 75,076, and mortality rate also increased from 4.3% to 4.7% (Wu et al. 2010). A prospective study conducted in public hospitals of France in 2006–2007 showed that out of 2692 admissions, about 97 admissions were related to an ADR (Bénard-Laribière et al. 2015). Schneeweiss et al. (2002) conducted a longitudinal population-based study between 1997 and 2000 and found that among 10,000 hospital admissions, 9.4 admissions were drug related in Germany (Schneeweiss et al. 2002). Contrary to this, the data regarding ADR-related hospital admissions are scarce in developing countries (Ramesh et al. 2003).

Pharmacovigilance Systems

There is always a tradeoff between medicines' side effects and therapeutic benefits. However, evidence suggests that ADRs are very common and may lead to hospitalization and even deaths (WHO 2014). The thalidomide disaster, which took place half a century ago, is still perceived as a big tragedy in the history of healthcare, that has resulted in the foetus anomalies to thousands of pregnant mothers, who had used the drug to treat morning sickness problems (Nkeng et al. 2012). This incident marked the failure of medicines regulation, weak approval process as well as a hesitant approach by regulatory bodies to take action. It has also highlighted the lack of communication between the patients and the healthcare professionals (HCPs) (Caduff-Janosa 2017).

To address these issues, the WHO established a programme for monitoring of drug safety as a pilot project in 1968. Initially ten countries joined this project; however, as of June 2019, 166 countries are members of the WHO Programme for International Drug Monitoring (PIDM). Moreover,

136 countries are submitting ADR reports to the *VigiBase*, a WHO global database of ADRs (WHO 2019a, b). In 1971, WHO established its first pharmacovigilance centre in Uppsala, Sweden, known as the Uppsala Monitoring Centre (UMC) (WHO 2015). Now UMC has pharmacovigilance collaborating centres all over the world (UMC 2019a).

Pharmacovigilance (PV) is defined as "the science and the activities concerning the assessment, detection, understanding and the prevention of the harmful results or any adverse drug-related issues" (UMC 2018a). Many developed countries have successfully established strong pharmacovigilance systems in their countries. The system is meant to report suspected ADRs that are encountered by HCPs in their clinical practice. A pharmacovigilance centre collects spontaneous reports on possible drug-related issues to detect the ADRs in the post-marketing phase (Rolfes et al. 2014). This spontaneous reporting is considered as the most important feature of the PV system whereby the reports are submitted to the national reporting agency by healthcare professionals, general public and pharmaceutical manufacturers and are then further communicated to the WHO pharmacovigilance centre (UMC 2018b). The suspected ADR reports from member countries of the WHO Programme for International Drug Monitoring (PIDM) are sent to the WHO international database "*VigiBase*", which is managed by the WHO Uppsala Monitoring Centre (UMC). The reports are systematically reviewed and analysed and then the evidence-based recommendations are forwarded to the member countries (UMC 2017a).

Organization of Pharmacovigilance Activities

Pharmacovigilance activities in any country are carried out by the help of regional or local centres in these countries which collect ADR reports (serving as alarm signals), design surveys and other pharmacovigilance studies and provide additional information on drugs. Concerns about possible ADRs and requests for information about a drug are directed to the appropriate regional pharmacovigilance centre. In recent years, regional centres have expanded their pharmacoepidemiology activities such as finding associations between specific ADRs and factors such as age, gender, dosage, population phenotype, concomitant use of other medicines as well as environmental factors. The information is further communicated to the national pharmacovigilance centre, which then considers specific measures such as drug withdrawal from the market, modification in drug classification and restricting the approved uses of a drug, evaluation of risk-benefit ratio of medicines, sending additional information to physicians and then submitting the ADR reports to the UMC (Montastruc et al. 2006).

Apart from all the above-discussed pharmacovigilance activities, the main role of the pharmacovigilance system is associated with the signal detection which is a core activity of the UMC. This perhaps aims to find and describe medicines associated with the suspected harm to patients. Signal detection happens through the evidence provided by healthcare professionals in the form of spontaneous reporting of ADRs or reports submitted by pharmaceutical companies and patients. A signal is considered as a hypothesis of a risk associated with a medicine supported by arguments and the data (UMC 2019b). Globally, most of the pharmacovigilance systems depend upon the information about ADRs, which is communicated through the spontaneous reporting systems. The ADR reported from healthcare professionals is entered into the database and is regularly assessed for the signal generation (Edwards and Biriell 1994; Waller and Harrison-Woolrych 2010). During the post-marketing phase of an approved drug, spontaneous adverse drug reaction (SADR) reporting is used for the risk-benefit evaluation and the monitoring of new medicines (Lexchin 2006).

Pharmacovigilance Methods

Pharmacovigilance methods can be selected based on the situation, such as the product, the population, the indication and the problems to be addressed. The selection of method also depends upon the outcome, such as the need to identify the risk or missing information or to detect a signal or to demonstrate the medicines safety (EMA 2005).

There are several pharmacovigilance methods listed below:

Stimulated Reporting

The reporting of adverse events facilitates the reporting by HCPs, when a new product is introduced for a limited time exposure (Strom 2019). Such reporting includes online reporting and systematic evaluation of drug-related incidents based on a pre-designed method. Pharmaceutical manufacturers, during post-marketing, may also provide safety information of drugs and may encourage healthcare professionals to report any untoward effect towards the use of medicines. Stimulated reporting does not provide data to accurately generate incidence rates but can help in the estimation of reporting rates (EMA 2005).

Active Surveillance

Active surveillance seeks to collect the complete information about adverse events via a preorganized and continuous process. It can be done through a risk management programme, where a patient is followed up for a specific drug and may be asked to fill a survey form for future contact. The process of collecting ADR reports through active surveillance is better than passive surveillance as comprehensive data can be collected in this process (EMA 2005).

Passive Surveillance

The most common method used in pharmacovigilance is the passive surveillance which relies heavily on the spontaneous reporting of any suspected ADR experienced by the patients. The drawback of passive surveillance is that it may not generate large volumes of data, or accurate, complete or product-specific report of an ADR, such as in the case of spontaneous reporting of an ADR, thus limiting the scope of comparisons related to the target and subject-specific surveillance. However, passive surveillance may generate signals, which can be further taken up by active surveillance for further inquiry (USAID 2017).

Post-Marketing Surveillance and Spontaneous Reporting

Post-marketing surveillance is concerned with the techniques for the detection and measurement of incidence of ADRs (Inman 1986). It refers to the analysis of data collected for the purpose of detecting adverse effects after a drug receives marketing approval (Praus et al. 1993). It deals with the signal detection and evaluation as a result of spontaneous reporting of an ADR. Post-marketing surveillance was first introduced in the 1960s in response to the delayed recognition of the association between thalidomide use in pregnant females and congenital limb deformity (Stephens and Brynner 2009).

Spontaneous reporting is a type of passive surveillance referred to as an unsolicited communication by a patient, a healthcare professional or a consumer to a company, to a regulatory body or to other organizations (e.g. WHO, regional or national pharmacovigilance centres or poison control centres). In the report they describe the adverse drug reaction experienced by a patient, who was administered with one or more medicines, and this provides a real-life experience of medicine use (EMA 2003). It can report both known and unknown or undocumented adverse events whether serious in nature or not. Drug-related adverse events can happen due to problems related to drug quality (or medical devices), drug interactions and medication errors (USAID 2017).

The process of spontaneous ADR (SADR) reporting is inexpensive and simple, as reports are voluntarily submitted by HCPs, consumers and patients. The data obtained from these reports are entered into a database to detect any signal. Sometimes, the reporters for spontaneous ADR reporting can be contacted for follow-up of a report based on its importance and the extent of information collected (Waller 2006). Once a signal is identified, then all relevant available information from other sources is analysed (Waller and Lee 1999). As signal evaluation requires resources and due to generation of large number of signals from the database, the involvement of triage and impact analysis becomes a priority (Ståhl et al. 2004; Heeley et al. 2005; Waller et al. 2005). To complete the process of reporting, information must be conveyed to reporters through acknowledgement and through a bulletin describing the signals (Waller 2006). Since the late 1980s, the International Conference on Harmonisation (ICH) and the Council for International Organizations of Medical Sciences (CIOMS) have established international standards of reporting related to what, when, why and how an ADR should be reported (Bahri and Tsintis 2005).

Spontaneous reporting has a major contribution in the detection of safety signals in the post-marketing surveillance. It may help in the identification of rare adverse events, which remain unrecognized during clinical trials. It also provides help in the recognition of data which could be helpful for risk factors and clinical manifestations of known serious ADRs of the medicines (Faich 1996; Pinkston and Swain 1998; Hartmann et al. 1999).

Pharmacovigilance in the Developed World

The pharmacovigilance system and the current practices with reference to the developed countries, including Australia, Canada, European and Nordic countries, New Zealand, the UK and the USA, have been discussed in detail in the section below.

Pharmacovigilance System of Australia

In response to the thalidomide tragedy, Australia formally started pharmacovigilance in 1963 and formulated the Australian Drug Evaluation Committee. Since then, data is being continuously collected by the Advisory Committee on Medicines, a subcommittee of the Therapeutic Goods Administration (TGA) for pre- and post-marketing surveillance of medicines (Linger and Martin 2018). The clinicians report ADRs through an online reporting system, namely, the Australian Adverse Drug Reaction Reporting System, or may send reports through fax, email, telephone and post. ADR reporting by sponsor of both the listed and registered drugs is mandatory for sponsor, while this is not mandatory for clinicians and consumers (TGA 2017). In 2015, the TGA received 17,000 reports, 4% of which were from physicians, 15% from state health departments and 54% from sponsors (TGA 2015). All data on ADRs are entered into the online database and submitted to VigiBase to detect any signals on ADR. To improve the pharmacovigilance system, Australia is considering to introduce the Black Triangle Scheme to identify new drugs requiring more vigilance. However, underreporting remains an area of concern for the Australian pharmacovigilance system (Linger and Martin 2018).

Pharmacovigilance System of Canada

In 1965, Health Canada established the Canada Vigilance Program as the post-market surveillance programme to collect and assess reports of suspected ADRs. ADR reporting by healthcare professionals and patients is on a voluntary basis, and the information of ADRs collected can be accessed through the online database known as Canada Vigilance Online Database (Government of Canada 2018). The Canada Vigilance Program has seven regional offices providing a regional contact point for HCPs and consumers. The regional office collects the ADR reports and forwards them to the Canada Vigilance National Office. Similar to other countries, Health Canada primarily relies on voluntary ADR reporting after a marketing approval is sought. The passive system of reporting constitutes about 10% of ADRs in Canada. In one year Health Canada received 16,272 reports of suspected ADRs, whereby 11,596 reports highlighted ADRs related to pharmaceuticals and the rest covered radiopharmaceuticals, natural products and biotechnology products. Seventy percent of reported cases of ADRs are considered serious (Wiktorowicz et al. 2010). A study by Health Canada research found that 30% of healthcare professionals reported ADRs in their practice (Osborne 2010).

Pharmacovigilance System of European and Nordic Countries

Pharmacovigilance remains a major priority in European drug regulatory system, and spontaneous ADR reporting was introduced to generate signals regarding medicines (Waller et al. 1996). In the early 1990s, member states of the European Union (EU) proposed a more closely integrated system of drug regulation that led to the establishment of the European Agency for the Evaluation of Medicinal Products (EMEA), presently known as the European Medicines Agency (EMA) (EMA 2005).

In the EU, a new regulatory system is introduced that includes centralized authorization, multiple identical authorizations through mutual recognition and decentralized procedures. Although pharmacovigilance in EU member states is based on individual national system, however a central coordination is provided through the EMA and Pharmacovigilance Working Party (PhVWP). The collaboration involves the agreement on standards and procedures, and there is an exchange system for information and decision-making (Bahri et al. 2007).

The pharmacovigilance system in member states varies according to the development of national healthcare system (Bahri et al. 2007). Below are the details of pharmacovigilance systems developed by the member countries of the EU (Table 1.1).

Pharmacovigilance System of Japan

Japan started pharmacovigilance activities in 1967 from designated medical institutions, and in 1972 it became a WHO member state for drug monitoring (UMC 2019a). In 1984, pharmacies were also included to this programme, and since 1997 all pharmacies and institutes joined Japan's pharmacovigilance programme. The Pharmaceutical and Medical Devices Agency (PMDA) of Japan in collaboration with the Pharmaceutical Affairs Law provides legal basis to Japan's pharmacovigilance system through various communications issued by the Ministry of Health, Labour and Welfare (MHLW). It is mandatory for all healthcare professionals to report any ADR to MHLW as stipulated in the Pharmaceutical Affairs Act (PAA) of Japan (Biswas 2013).

Table 1.1 Pharmacovigilance activities in European and Nordic countries

Member state	Year of establishing NPC	Procedures of ADR report compilation	Way of safety information communication to HCPs
Austria	1979	Nationwide reporting to NPC	Press release in scientific journals, Email or fax-based system through regional health authority
Belgium	1976	Nationwide reporting to NPC	Press release, monthly bulletin for HCPs
Denmark	1968	Nationwide reporting to NPC	Press release in scientific journals, Website-based information
Finland	1966	Nationwide reporting to NPC; additional systems operated by hospitals communicate ADR reports to NPC	Press release, bimonthly drug bulletin
France	1973	Reporting by HCPs to regional centres (31 regional centres) and to NPC, Reporting by marketing authorization to NPC	Press release, bimonthly vigilance bulletin for HCPs
Germany	1978	Reporting by HCPs to drug commission and to NPC, Reporting by marketing authorization to NPC	Press release published in scientific journals
Ireland	1969	Nationwide reporting to NPC	Press release, Website-based information, through national prescribing guidance on a monthly basis
Italy	1980	Nationwide reporting to NPC	Press release, newsletter on agency website, Drug bulletin for HCPs, Free telephone-based information for public

(continued)

Table 1.1 (continued)

Member state	Year of establishing NPC	Procedures of ADR report compilation	Way of safety information communication to HCPs
Netherlands	1963	Nationwide reporting to NPC, five hospital-based regional centres linked to NPC	Press releases, Publications for HCPs, Website-based information
Spain	1983	17 regional centres collect reports and communicate to NPC	Press release, Biannual or quarterly bulletin for HCPs
Sweden	1965	Reporting to regional and NPC	Press release, Website-based information, Bimonthly drug bulletin for HCPs

Pharmacovigilance System of Singapore

Singapore established the Pharmacovigilance Unit, previously known as the Adverse Drug Reaction Monitoring Unit (ADRMU), in 1993 (Biswas 2013). Later in 1994, the Pharmacovigilance Unit joined the WHO programme for drug monitoring, and this now serves as the national centre for collection and review of ADRs (UMC 2019a). The Health Sciences Authority has formulated a Pharmacovigilance Advisory Committee (PVAC) of experts from medicine, pharmacy, forensic sciences and pharmacology to assess and improve drug safety (Biswas 2013).

Pharmacovigilance System of New Zealand

New Zealand (NZ) was among the founding members of the WHO initiative on PIDM in 1968 (UMC 2019a). In NZ, the New Zealand Pharmacovigilance Centre (NZPVC) has been established in the Department of Preventive and Social Medicine at the University of Otago and is responsible for monitoring of ADRs by reporting it to the Medicines and Medical Devices Safety Authority (Medsafe) (NZPVC 2019). It employed a three-approach system to ADR detection and management. The Centre for Adverse Reactions Monitoring (CARM) is established in 1965 as the national spontaneous reporting programme. In 1977, the Intensive Medicines Monitoring Programme (IMMP) was established for the monitoring of newly introduced medicines in the market, and in 2004 the Intensive Vaccine Monitoring Programme (IVMP) was started to monitor the safety of meningococcal B vaccine (Zhou et al. 2003; Kunac et al. 2008). The NZPhvC regularly reviews on safety and analyses data to identify any possibility of ADRs. Medsafe receives regular information from IMPP and CARM. The Medicines Adverse Reactions Committee (MARC) of NZ Health Ministry reviews unrecognized ADRs, signals from current literature as well as changes recommended for the product data sheet. The issues highlighted by MARC result in publication in the form of "Prescriber Update" bulletin (Kunac et al. 2008).

Though small as a country, NZ has a very good reporting culture with highest rate of spontaneous ADR reports per capita than other pharmacovigilance programmes in other parts of the world. NZPVC is perceived to be independent of drug regulation. NZPVC also contributes to global safety by sending anonymized data to the WHO database (Kunac et al. 2008).

Pharmacovigilance System of the United Kingdom (UK)

In the wake of the thalidomide crisis, the United Kingdom (UK), like many other countries started systematic collection of ADR reports by the establishment of the Committee on Safety of Medicines (CSM). At present, the Commission on Human Medicines collects and disseminates the ADR reports. To ensure medicines safety, in 1965, the chairman of CSM communicated to all dentists and doctors in the UK to report any untoward reaction of prescribed medicines and introduced the yellow card scheme (YCS) (Griffin and Weber 1992). In the UK, pharmaceutical industry has a statutory obligation to report suspected ADRs (Waller et al. 1996). In the UK, CHM and the Pharmacovigilance Expert

Advisory Group (PEAG) are responsible to collect all ADR reports which are usually collected through the YCS from all healthcare professionals (McLernon et al. 2010). The information is then conveyed to the Medicines and Healthcare Products Regulatory Agency (2019), formerly the Medicines Control Agency (MCA), and data are stored in ADR online information tracking database (ADROIT). This is to facilitate analysis of ADR reports and detection of any signals for drug safety (Light et al. 2006). Until 2002, five regional monitoring centres (RMCs) known as Yellow Card Centres (YCC) were introduced to support the YCS in the regions (Houghton et al. 1996). The new information on medicine's harm is communicated in the form of changes in product information and publication of Drug Safety Update or by direct communication to clinicians. MHRA also alerts and conveys information on ADRs to other information providers such as the British National Formulary or suppliers of clinical specialty software (MHRA 2019).

Pharmacovigilance System of the United States of America (USA)

The United States of America (USA) was among the pioneer members of PIDM established by the WHO in 1968 and revised the Food and Drug Administration (FDA) regulations to enhance the safety and efficacy of drugs before a medicine enters into the market (UMC 2019a).

As Americans mostly are the first to receive new medicines, thus challenge of early detection of drug safety issues has shifted to the post-marketing surveillance in the USA (Psaty et al. 2004). The system depends upon manufacturer's generation of FDA's immediate and summary of adverse event reports from the field. However, the system is considered slow, incomplete and expensive (Gottlieb 2005).

It is interesting to note that more than 80% of all spontaneous reports are from the pharmaceutical industry (Gibson et al. 2008). The United States (US) Department of Health and Human Services and FDA are managing pharmacovigilance system with the Center for Biologics Evaluation and Research (CBER) and Center for Drug Evaluation and Research (CDER) (FDA 2005). In the USA, ADR reporting is voluntary by healthcare professionals and is done through the MedWatch (FDA 2019). The ADRs are reported according to the post-marketing reporting to FDA, which then sends these reports to the FDA Adverse Event Reporting System (FAERS). The healthcare professionals, consumers, lawyers and regulated industries can report through 3500A or 3500B form to the FDA (2018). The ADR reports are evaluated by clinical reviewers from CBER and CDER. If FAERS acknowledges any safety concern, a supplementary evaluation is done, which may include studies using large databases, and the record is maintained for ten years (FDA 2018). Spontaneous reporting of ADR remains an important part of pharmacovigilance; however, it requires collaborative effort from the pharmaceutical industry, healthcare professionals, public, regulators and academia (Gibson et al. 2008).

Pharmacovigilance in Low- and Middle-Income Countries (LMICs)

The differences in data due to geographical settings, drug utilization patterns as well as prescription patterns make it difficult to extrapolate the data from a developed country in a developing country setting. Moreover, the drug use problems may vary across the countries due to varied and large population size. Moreover the lack of quality control and substandard medicines also contribute to the safety of medicines making it a critical challenge (Palaian 2018; McDowell et al. 2006). However increasingly, many developing countries have established their own national pharmacovigilance systems.

Pharmacovigilance System in Pakistan: A Case Study

There was no established pharmacovigilance system in the country until 2012. The active pharmacovigilance started when a locally manufactured cardiac drug (Isotab, 20 mg isosorbide mononitrate, batch number J093) caused the deaths of more than 200 patients and hospitalization of 1000 patients in Lahore, Pakistan (Government of Pakistan 2007; Government of Pakistan 2012; WHO 2013). As a result of this incident, the Drug Regulatory Authority of Pakistan established a national pharmacovigilance centre (NPC) (DRAP 2019). DRAP is one of the six divisions of the Ministry of National Health Services and Regulation (MNHSRC), which regulates the availability, quality and safety of therapeutic goods including medicines in the country (Atif et al. 2017). After the establishment of DRAP, the system for medicines safety started to get better. There are few tertiary care hospitals in the country where the pharmacovigilance system is in place; however, overall pharmacovigilance needs further improvement (Shamim et al. 2016).

The DRAP in collaboration with the international bodies including the US Pharmacopeia has developed a framework to carry out post-marketing surveillance of drugs in Pakistan (DRAP 2019). The DRAP is also planning to obtain access to WHO Uppsala Monitoring Centre's "*VigiFlow*", which is the global database system for pharmacovigilance reporting (UMC 2017b). The access to VigiFlow will help the medical professionals and drug regulators to stay updated with the latest safety information about the drugs (Wazir 2017).

Legal Basis for Pharmacovigilance in Pakistan

The DRAP Act of 2012 [XXI of 2012], Sects. 2 (xxvi) and 4 (1), governs the responsibility of pharmacovigilance activities in Pakistan. As per DRAP Act of 2012, the Division of Pharmacy Services is responsible to develop, mandate and regulate the pharmacovigilance activities in the country (DRAP 2019). In the National Health Vision 2016–2025, the establishment of a vibrant pharmacovigilance system at national level has also been planned and this is connected to provincial-level centres (Government of Pakistan 2016).

The pharmacovigilance programme in Pakistan evaluates and monitors the safety of therapeutic products and devices both in pre- and post-marketing phase. The programme also focusses on adverse events related to the medication errors, overdose, the use of substandard therapeutic products as well as the off-label or occupational exposure of medicines. The therapeutic goods covered under the Pakistan pharmacovigilance programme include allopathic, Chinese, biochemical, homeopathic, Ayurvedic and Unani products. Nutraceuticals, vaccines, biologics, medical devices and other related products are also covered under this programme. The aim of the pharmacovigilance programme in Pakistan is to detect ADR signals for Pakistan's pharmacovigilance database. This also seeks to make ADR reporting a mandatory requirement to be performed by healthcare professionals, to start active surveillance as well as to expand the scope of pharmacovigilance to all health units including the Basic Health Units (BHU) (DRAP 2019).

Pharmacovigilance: The Reporting of Mixed Methods and Intervention Study in Pakistani Setting

It is a fact that the success of any pharmacovigilance system lies in the participation of all healthcare experts especially pharmacists and physicians who are considered as the best experts to report activities related to pharmacovigilance.

Thus, a mixed method approach was employed to assess the knowledge, attitude and practices of healthcare professionals to evaluate pharmacovigilance activities in Lahore, Pakistan. The study was composed of two parts, of which qualitative phase was followed by the quantitative phase. In qualitative phase, physicians, pharmacists and nurses were interviewed, who were working in tertiary care public hospitals of Lahore, Pakistan. For qualitative study a total of 13 physicians, 10 pharmacists and 11 nurses participated, and 6 major themes emerged as the final outcome of interviews.

The findings from the qualitative study revealed six major themes that include familiarity with medicines safety and the ADR concept, current system of practice and reporting of ADR in hospital setting, willingness to accept the practice change, training needed to improve ADR reporting, barriers related to ADR reporting and recognition of the role as custodian of medicines safety and system change needs (Hussain et al. 2018).

The quantitative part of the study included a questionnaire-based survey evaluating knowledge, attitude and practices about pharmacovigilance from physicians, pharmacists and nurses working in tertiary care public hospitals of Lahore. The barriers involved in ADR reporting and facilitating factors that could improve reporting were also evaluated. In this study, the majority of the pharmacists showed better knowledge towards ADR reporting as compared to the physicians and nurses. This is similar to studies conducted by Li et al. (2004) and Su et al. (2010) where pharmacists were able to define ADR more appropriately than physicians (Su et al. 2010). This could be due to the different curricula of healthcare professionals (van Grootheest et al. 2004). Most of the pharmacists in the study had good knowledge about pharmacovigilance and were aware of the definition of pharmacovigilance, its purpose and location of the pharmacovigilance centres, while physicians and nurses did not. It was very similar to the studies done by Latif and Wahab (2015) and Almandil (2016) where pharmacists had a high level of awareness than physicians and nurses regarding the pharmacovigilance system (Almandil 2016; Abdel-Latif and Abdel-Wahab 2015).

The study explored the attitudes of all healthcare professionals towards pharmacovigilance activities and showed that overall all healthcare professionals had a positive attitude towards pharmacovigilance in general and ADR reporting in particular. Although the majority of the participants did not report ADRs in their work setting, they were motivated to perform such activities. Physicians, pharmacists and nurses considered ADR reporting as their professional responsibility. Similar to our study, the majority of the pharmacists (67.6%) reported an ADR and considered ADR reporting as their professional obligation when compared to the other healthcare professionals (van Grootheest et al. 2004; Li et al. 2004; Toklu and Uysal 2008).

It was found in this cross-sectional survey that physicians and nurses did not report any ADR in the last 12 months (only pharmacists reported an ADR); however, none of each category of healthcare professional kept the records of an ADR, and few of them ever sent any ADR report to DRAP or the drug manufacturer. Several studies have shown the similar trends in which majority of the healthcare professionals did not report any ADR, although they encountered many during their practice (Li et al. 2004; Bäckström et al. 2000; Oshikoya and Awobusuyi 2009).

The current study also identified barriers which the respondents experienced during the process of ADR reporting. Broadly, the barriers to ADR reporting can be classified into two categories, which are composed of healthcare system-related barriers and individual-related barriers (Hadi et al. 2017). The results of the study indicated a lack of knowledge if an ADR happened, a lack of confidence in discussing an ADR report among healthcare professionals and a lack of awareness about local settings and policies about the pharmacovigilance as significant barriers by many healthcare professionals.

Continuous medical or pharmacy education, training and seminars were identified as a key facilitator to overcome the problem of underreporting. Thus, to improve the reporting practices, the healthcare professionals also suggested that they would like to receive additional training regarding medicines safety and ADR reporting in the form of seminars or workshops as well as newsletters and reminders from national pharmacovigilance centres in Pakistan.

In the next and final phase of the study, a pilot study based on an educational intervention had evaluated the impact of education regarding improvement in knowledge of physicians in Lahore, Pakistan, and found that, after the educational intervention, physicians' knowledge about pharmacovigilance has improved. This has shown that educational programmes and training can improve the knowledge of healthcare professionals regarding pharmacovigilance (Hussain et al. 2019).

The barriers highlighted in both qualitative and quantitative studies included workload, time constraints to perform activities related to the ADR monitoring and reporting, lack of knowledge regarding pharmacovigilance and lack of support and coordination with other healthcare professionals as well as with the government drug safety bodies such as provincial healthcare system and DRAP on this issue.

The study has revealed that all healthcare professionals understand the role of pharmacist in the safe use of medicines and they were ready to make the change in the lead for the provision of medicines safety and inclined to perform the tasks associated with the reporting of ADRs and other pharmacovigilance activities.

Directions and Recommendations to Improve Medicines Safety

Medicines safety is emerging as a core issue affecting the healthcare system in both developed and developing countries; thus, appropriate reporting programmes and the ADR reporting mechanisms should be initiated; besides that, continuous professional development (CPD) and continuous pharmacy education (CPE) programmes for key healthcare personnel including physicians, nurses and pharmacists should also be initiated. Pharmacist, being the custodian of safe and effective use of medicines, should be responsible for the provision of the medicines safety issue and pharmacovigilance activities. Additionally, the universities and healthcare institutions should adopt a collaborative and integrated approach to train healthcare professionals for their role to improve the safe use of medicines.

The collaboration on medicines safety should be enhanced by encouraging the collaborative activities by the hospital management and between the other healthcare professionals, academia and regulatory bodies. Globally, the drug regulatory bodies should also promote the importance of pharmacovigilance as a priority.

References

Abdel-Latif, M. M. & Abdel-Wahab, B. A. (2015). Knowledge and awareness of adverse drug reactions and pharmacovigilance practices among healthcare professionals in Al-Madinah Al-Munawwarah, Kingdom of Saudi Arabia. *Saudi Pharmaceutical Journal*, 23, 154–161.

Almandil, N. B. (2016). Healthcare professionals' awareness and knowledge of adverse drug reactions and pharmacovigilance. *Saudi Medical Journal*, 37, 1359.

Atif. M, Ahmad. M, Saleem. Q, Curley. L, Zaman. M & Z., B. (2017). Pharmaceutical Policy in Pakistan. In: Z., B. (ed.) *Pharmaceutical Policy in Countries with Developing Healthcare Systems*. Springer International, pp 25–44.

Baker, G.R., Norton, P.G., Flintoft, V., Blais, R., Brown, A., Cox, J., Etchells, E., Ghali, W.A., Hébert, P., Majumdar, S.R. and O'Beirne, M. (2004). The Canadian Adverse Events Study: the incidence of adverse events among hospital patients in Canada. *Canadian Medical Association Journal*, 170(11), pp.1678–1686.

Bäckström, M., Mjorndal, T., Dahlqvist, R. & Nordkvist-Olsson, T. (2000). Attitudes to reporting adverse drug reactions in northern Sweden. *European Journal of Clinical Pharmacology*, 56, 729–732.
Bahri, P. & Tsintis, P. (2005). Pharmacovigilance-related topics at the level of the International Conference on Harmonisation (ICH). *Pharmacoepidemiology and Drug Safety*, 14, 377–387.
Bahri, P., Tsintis, P. & Waller, P. C. (2007). Regulatory Pharmacovigilance In The Eu. In: Mann, R. D. & Andrews, E. B. (eds.) *Pharmacovigilance*. 2nd ed.: John Wiley & Sons, pp 183–194.
Bates, D.W., Cullen, D.J., Laird, N., Petersen, L.A., Small, S.D., Servi, D., Laffel, G., Sweitzer, B.J., Shea, B.F., Hallisey, R. and Vander Vliet, M. (1995). Incidence of adverse drug events and potential adverse drug events: implications for prevention. *Journal of American Medical Association*, 274(1), pp.29–34.
Bénard-Laribière, A., Miremont-Salamé, G., Pérault-Pochat, M.C., Noize, P., Haramburu, F. and EMIR Study Group on behalf of the French network of pharmacovigilance centres. (2015). Incidence of hospital admissions due to adverse drug reactions in France: the EMIR study. *Fundamental & Clinical Pharmacology*, 29(1), pp.106–111.
Biswas, P. (2013). Pharmacovigilance in Asia. *Journal of Pharmacology & Pharmacotherapeutics*, 4, S7.
Black, A. and K. Somers, Drug-related illness resulting in hospital admission. *Journal of the Royal College of Physicians of London*, 1984. 18(1): p. 40.
Caduff-Janosa, P. (2017). Lost in regulation. *Pharmacovigilance*. Springer, pp 9–19.
Classen, D.C., Pestotnik, S.L., Evans, R.S., Lloyd, J.F. and Burke, J.P. (1997). Adverse drug events in hospitalized patients: excess length of stay, extra costs, and attributable mortality. *Journal of American Medical Association*, 1997. 277(4): p. 301–306.
DRAP. (2019). Pakistan National Pharmacovigilance Guidelines (Draft). 1 ed. Islamabad, PK: Drug Regulatory Authority of Pakistan. Available: https://dra.gov.pk/docs/Draft%20Pakistan%20National%20Pharmacovigigilance%20guidlines%204-9-2019.pdf [Accessed February 22 2020].
Edwards, I. R. & Biriell, C. (1994). Harmonisation in pharmacovigilance. *Drug Safety*, 10, 93–102.
Edwards, I. R. & Aronson, J. K. (2000). Adverse drug reactions: definitions, diagnosis, and management. *The Lancet*, 356, 1255–1259.
EMA. (2003). Post-approval safety data management: definitions and standards for expedited reporting E2D. Published in the Federal Register, 2003. 68(178): p. 53983–53984.

EMA. (2005). ICH Topic E 2 E Pharmacovigilance Planning (Pvp). London, UK: European Medicines Agency.

Faich, G. A. (1996). US adverse drug reaction surveillance 1989–(1994). *Pharmacoepidemiology and Drug Safety*, 5, 393–398.

FDA. (2005). Good Pharmacovigilance Practices and Pharmacoepidemiologic Assessment. *In:* RESEARCH, C. F. D. E. A. R. C. F. B. E. A. (ed.). USA: Food and Drug Administration.

FDA. (2018). *FDA Adverse Event Reporting System (FAERS): Latest Quarterly Data Files* [Online]. USA: Food and Drug Administration. Available: https://www.fda.gov/drugs/questions-and-answers-fdas-adverse-event-reporting-system-faers/fda-adverse-event-reporting-system-faers-latest-quarterly-data-files [Accessed September 15 2019].

FDA. (2019a). *MedWatch: The FDA Safety Information and Adverse Event Reporting Program* [Online]. USA: U.S. Food and Drug Administration. Available: https://www.fda.gov/Safety/MedWatch/default.html [Accessed August 15 2019].

FDA. (2019b). *MedWatch: The FDA Safety Information and Adverse Event Reporting Program* [Online]. USA: Food and Drug Administration. Available: https://www.fda.gov/safety/medwatch-fda-safety-information-and-adverse-event-reporting-program [Accessed September 15 2019].

Gibson, B. R., Suh, R. & Tilson, H. (2008). The US drug safety system: role of the pharmaceutical industry. *Pharmacoepidemiology and Drug Safety*, 17, 110–114.

Gottlieb, S. (2005). Opening Pandora's pillbox: using modern information tools to improve drug safety. *Health Affairs*, 24(4), 938–948.

Government of Canada. (2018). Canada Vigilance Program. 2018 [Online]. Available: https://www.canada.ca/en/health-canada/services/drugs-health-products/medeffect-canada/canada-vigilance-program.html [Accessed September 15 2019].

Government of Pakistan. (2007). *Health Systems Profile-Pakistan* [Online]. World Health Organization. Available: http://apps.who.int/medicinedocs/documents/s17305e/s17305e.pdf [Accessed August 30 2019].

Government of Pakistan. (2012). Batch J093: The Pathology of Negligence (Report of the Judicial Inquiry Tribunal to Determine the Causes of Deaths of Patients of the Punjab Institute of Cardiology, Lahore in (2011)–2012. Punjab, PK.

Government of Pakistan. (2016). National Vision 2016–2025 for Coordinated Priority Actions to Address Challenges of Reproductive, Maternal, Newborn, Child, Adolescent Health and Nutrition. 2016: Islamabad, PK. p. 32.

Granas, A. G., Buajordet, M., Stenberg-Nilsen, H., Harg, P. & Horn, A. M. 2007. Pharmacists' attitudes towards the reporting of suspected adverse drug reactions in Norway. *Pharmacoepidemiology and Drug Safety*, 16, 429–434.
Green, C. F., Mottram, D. R., Rowe, P. H. & Pirmohamed, M. (2001). Attitudes and knowledge of hospital pharmacists to adverse drug reaction reporting. *British Journal Of Clinical Pharmacology, 51*, 81–86.
Green, J. A. & Norris, P. (2015). Quantitative Methods in Pharmacy Practice Research. *Pharmacy Practice Research Methods*. Springer.
Greene, J. C., Caracelli, V. J. & Graham, W. F. (1989). Toward a conceptual framework for mixed-method evaluation designs. *Educational Evaluation and Policy Analysis*, 11, 255–274.
Griffin, J. and J. Weber, Voluntary systems of adverse reaction reporting, in Medicines: Regulation, Research and Risk, G. JP, Editor. 1992, The Queen's University: Belfast.
Hadi, M. A., Neoh, C. F., Zin, R. M., Elrggal, M. E. & Cheema, E. (2017). Pharmacovigilance: pharmacists' perspective on spontaneous adverse drug reaction reporting. *Integrated Pharmacy Research & Practice*, 6, 91.
Hartmann, K., Koller Doser, A. & Kuhn, M. (1999). Postmarketing safety information: how useful are spontaneous reports? *Pharmacoepidemiology and Drug Safety*, 8, S65-S71.
Heeley, E., Waller, P. & Moseley, J. (2005). Testing and implementing signal impact analysis in a regulatory setting. *Drug Safety*, 28, 901–906.
Houghton, J., Pinto, L. P., Woods, F., Richens, A. & Routledge, P. (1996). The Welsh Adverse Drug Reactions Scheme: experience of a UK regional monitoring centre. *Adverse Drug Reactions and Toxicological Reviews*, 15, 93–107.
Hussain, R., et al., (2018). A qualitative exploration of knowledge, attitudes and practices of hospital pharmacists towards adverse drug reaction reporting system in Lahore, Pakistan. *Journal of pharmaceutical policy and practice*, 11(1): p. 16.
Hussain, R., M.A. Hassali, and S.M. Rana, (2019). Evaluation of an educational intervention on physicians' knowledge about adverse drug reaction reporting system. *Journal of Public Health*, p. 1–4.
Inman, W. (1986). Editor's introduction and commentary. *In:* WH, I. (ed.) *Monitoring for Drug Safety*. Boston: MTP Press Limited.
Inman, W. (1996). Attitudes to adverse drug reaction reporting. *British Journal of Clinical Pharmacology*, 41.
Kunac, D.L., M. Harrison-Woolrych, and M.V. Tatley, Pharmacovigilance in New Zealand: the role of the New Zealand Pharmacovigilance Centre in

facilitating safer medicines use. *The New Zealand Medical Journal* (Online), 2008. 121(1283).

Lazarou, J., Pomeranz, B.H. and Corey, P.N. (1998). Incidence of adverse drug reactions in hospitalized patients: a meta-analysis of prospective studies. *Journal of the American Medical Association*, 279(15), pp.1200–1205.

Lexchin, J. (2006). Is there still a role for spontaneous reporting of adverse drug reactions? *Canadian Medical Association Journal*, 174, 191–192.

Li, Q., Zhang, S.-M., Chen, H.-T., Fang, S.-P., Yu, X., Liu, D., Shi, L.-Y. & Zeng, F.-D. (2004). Awareness and attitudes of healthcare professionals in Wuhan, China to the reporting of adverse drug reactions. *Chinese Medical Journal*, 117, 856–861.

Light, K. P., Lovell, A. T., Butt, H., Fauvel, N. J. & Holdcroft, A. (2006). Adverse effects of neuromuscular blocking agents based on yellow card reporting in the UK: are there differences between males and females? *Pharmacoepidemiology and Drug Safety*, 15, 151–160.

Linger, M. & Martin, J. (2018). Pharmacovigilance and expedited drug approvals. *Australian Prescriber*, 41, 50.

Mcdowell, S. E., Coleman, J. J. & Ferner, R. (2006). Systematic review and meta-analysis of ethnic differences in risks of adverse reactions to drugs used in cardiovascular medicine. *British Medical Journal*, 332, 1177–1181.

Mclernon, D. J., Bond, C. M., Hannaford, P. C., Watson, M. C., Lee, A. J., Hazell, L., Avery, A. & Collaboration, Y. C. (2010). Adverse drug reaction reporting in the UK. *Drug Safety*, 33, 775–788.

MHRA. (2019). Yellow Card. [Online]. United Kingdom: Medicines and Healthcare products Regulatory Agency. Available: https://yellowcard.mhra.gov.uk/monitoringsafety/ [Accessed February 22 2020].

Montastruc, J.-L., Sommet, A., Lacroix, I., Olivier, P., Durrieu, G., Damase-Michel, C., Lapeyre-Mestre, M. & Bagheri, H. (2006). Pharmacovigilance for evaluating adverse drug reactions: value, organization, and methods. *Joint Bone Spine*, 73, 629-632.

Nkeng, L., Cloutier, A.-M., Craig, C., Lelorier, J. & Moride, Y. (2012). Impact of regulatory guidances and drug regulation on risk minimization interventions in drug safety. *Drug Safety*, 35, 535–546.

NZPVC. (2019). *CARM* [Online]. New Zealand Pharmacovigilance Centre. Available: https://nzphvc.otago.ac.nz/carm [Accessed August 15 2019].

Osborne, C.A., 2010. Adverse drug reactions: investigating to reporting. *Journal of the Canadian Academy of Child and Adolescent Psychiatry*, 19(1), p.46.

Oshikoya, K. A. & Awobusuyi, J. O. (2009). Perceptions of doctors to adverse drug reaction reporting in a teaching hospital in Lagos, Nigeria. *BMC Clinical Pharmacology*, 9, 14.

Palaian, S. (2018). Pharmacovigilance Practices and Activities: Issues, Challenges, and Future Direction. *Social and Administrative Aspects of Pharmacy in Low- and Middle-Income Countries*. Elsevier.

Pinkston, V. & Swain, E. (1998). Management of adverse drug reactions and adverse event data through collection, storage, and retrieval. *Detection of New Adverse Drug Reactions*, 4, 282.

Pirmohamed, M., James, S., Meakin, S., Green, C., Scott, A.K., Walley, T.J., Farrar, K., Park, B.K. and Breckenridge, A.M. (2004). Adverse drug reactions as cause of admission to hospital: prospective analysis of 18 820 patients. *British Medical Journal*, 329(7456), pp.15–19.

Praus, M., Schindel, F., Fescharek, R. and Schwarz, S., 1993. Alert systems for post-marketing surveillance of adverse drug reactions. *Statistics in Medicine*, 12(24), pp.2383–2393.

Psaty, B.M., Furberg, C.D., Ray, W.A. and Weiss, N.S., 2004. Potential for conflict of interest in the evaluation of suspected adverse drug reactions: use of cerivastatin and risk of rhabdomyolysis. *Journal of American Medical Association*, 292(21), pp.2622–2631.

Ramesh, M., J. Pandit, and G. Parthasarathi. (2003) Adverse drug reactions in a south Indian hospital—their severity and cost involved. *Pharmacoepidemiology and Drug Safety*, 12(8): p. 687–692.

Rolfe, G. (2006). Validity, trustworthiness and rigour: quality and the idea of qualitative research. *Journal of Advanced Nursing*, 53, 304–310.

Rolfes, L., et al., (2014). Important information regarding reporting of adverse drug reactions: a qualitative study. *International Journal of Pharmacy Practice*, 22(3): p. 231–233.

Schneeweiss, S., Hasford, J., Göttler, M., Hoffmann, A., Riethling, A.K. and Avorn, J. (2002). Admissions caused by adverse drug events to internal medicine and emergency departments in hospitals: a longitudinal population-based study. *European Journal of Clinical Pharmacology*, 58(4), pp.285–291.

Shamim, S., Sharib, S. M., Malhi, S. M., Muntaha, S.-U., Raza, H., Ata, S., Farooq, A. S. & Hussain, M. (2016). Adverse drug reactions (ADRS) reporting: awareness and reasons of under-reporting among health care professionals, a challenge for pharmacists. *Springer Plus*, 5, 1778.

Ståhl, M., Lindquist, M., Edwards, I. & Brown, E. (2004). Introducing triage logic as a new strategy for the detection of signals in the WHO Drug Monitoring Database. *Pharmacoepidemiology and Drug Safety*, 13, 355–363.

Stephens, T. & Brynner, R. (2009). *Dark remedy: the impact of thalidomide and its revival as a vital medicine*, Basic Books.

Strom, B. L. (2019). What is pharmacoepidemiology? In: Strom, B. L. (Ed.), *Pharmacoepidemiology*. 6th ed. New York: John Wiley & Sons, pp 1–26.

Su, C., Ji, H. & Su, Y. (2010). Hospital pharmacists' knowledge and opinions regarding adverse drug reaction reporting in Northern China. *Pharmacoepidemiology and Drug Safety*, 19, 217–222.

Sultana, J., Cutroneo, P. & Trifirò, G. (2013). Clinical and economic burden of adverse drug reactions. *Journal of Pharmacology & Pharmacotherapeutics*, 4, S73.

TGA. (2015). Medicines and vaccines post-market vigilance - statistics for (2015). Australia: Therapeutic Goods Administration.

TGA. (2017). *Reporting problems* [Online]. Australia: Therapeutic Goods Administration. Available: https://www.tga.gov.au/reporting-problems [Accessed September 15 2019].

Toklu, H. Z. & Uysal, M. K. (2008). The knowledge and attitude of the Turkish community pharmacists toward pharmacovigilance in the Kadikoy district of Istanbul. *Pharmacy World & Science*, 30, 556–562.

UMC. (2017a). What happens to reports of problems with medicines? Uppsala Monitoring Centre. Available from: https://www.who-umc.org/safer-use-of-medicines/safer-use-of-medicines-the-basics/what-happens-to-reports [Accessed December 12 2019].

UMC. (2017b). Vigiflow. [Online]. Uppsala Monitoring Centre. [Avaialble]: https://www.who-umc.org/globalpharmacovigilance/vigiflow/. [Accessed December 25 2019].

UMC. (2018a). The story of UMC and the WHO Program [Online]. Uppsala Monitoring Centre. Available: https://www.whoumc.org/global-pharmaco-vigilance/who-program/the-story-of-umc-and-thewho-program/ [Accessed September 15 2019].

UMC. (2018b). Communication in pharmacovigilance [Online]. Uppsala Monitoring Centre. Available: https://www.whoumc.org/globalpharmaco-vigilance/communicationinpharmacovigilance/patient-centered-communications [Accessed December 15 2019].

UMC. (2019a). Members of the WHO Program for International Drug Monitoring [Online]. Geneva: Uppsala Monitoring Centre. Available: https://www.who-umc.org/global-pharmacovigilance/members/whoprogram-members/ [Accessed January 15 2020].

UMC. (2019b). Detecting signals [Online]. Uppsala Monitoring Centre. Available: https://www.who-umc.org/research-scientificdevelopment/signal-detection/ [Accessed January 12 2020].

USAID (2017). National Guideline on the Pharmacovigilance System in Bangladesh. Arlington, VA.

van Grootheest, K., Olsson, S., Couper, M. & De Jong-Van Den Berg, L. (2004). Pharmacists' role in reporting adverse drug reactions in an international perspective. *Pharmacoepidemiology and Drug Safety*, 13, 457–464.

Waller, P. C., Coulson, R. A. & Wood, S. M. (1996). Regulatory pharmacovigilance in the United Kingdom: current principles and practice. *Pharmacoepidemiology And Drug Safety*, 5, 363–375.

Waller, P. C. & Lee, E. H. (1999). Responding to drug safety issues. *Pharmacoepidemiology and Drug Safety*, 8, 535–552.

Waller, P., Heeley, E. & Moseley, J. (2005). Impact analysis of signals detected from spontaneous adverse drug reaction reporting data. *Drug Safety*, 28, 843–850.

Waller, P. C. (2006). Making the most of spontaneous adverse drug reaction reporting. *Basic & Clinical Pharmacology & Toxicology*, 98, 320–323.

Waller, P. & Harrison-Woolrych, M. (2010). *An introduction to pharmacovigilance*, Wiley Online Library.

Wazir, H. (2017). DRAP to introduce regulations for post-marketing surveillance of drugs. Pakistan Today. Available: https://www.pakistantoday.com.pk/2017/08/20/drap-to-introduce-regulations-for-post-marketing-surveillance-of-drugs/ [Accessed February 21 2020].

White, T. J., Arakelian, A. & RHO, J. P. (1999). Counting the costs of drug-related adverse events. *Pharmacoeconomics*, 15, 445–458.

WWiktorowicz, M., Lexchin, J., Moscou, K., Silversides, A. and Eggertson, L., 2010. *Keeping an eye on prescription drugs, keeping Canadians safe*. Toronto: Health Council of Canada.

WHO. (2002). The Importance of Pharmacovigilance – Safety Monitoring of Medicinal Products [Online]. United Kingdom: World Health Organization. Available: http://apps.who.int/medicinedocs/en/d/Js4893e/ [Accessed February 22 2020].

WHO. (2013). *Deadly medicines contamination in Pakistan* [Online]. World Health Organization. Available: http://www.who.int/features/(2013)/pakistan_medicine_safety/en/ [Accessed August 12 2019].

WHO. (2014). Pharmacovigilance: ensuring the safe use of medicines. Geneva. Avaialble: https://apps.who.int/medicinedocs/pdf/s6164e/s6164e.pdf [Accessed February 22 2020].

WHO. (2015). Essential medicines and health products [Online]. Switzerland: World Health Organization. Available: https://www.who.int/medicines/areas/quality_safety/safety_efficacy/PV_fast_facts/en/ [Accessed January 30 2020].

WHO. (2019a). Annual Meeting of Representatives of National Pharmacovigilance Centres participating in the WHO Program for International Drug Monitoring [Online]. Geneva: World Health Organization. Available: https://www.who.int/medicines/regulation/medicines-safety/npvcmeeting/en/ [Accessed February 12 2020].

WHO. (2019b). Essential medicines and health products: Adverse drug reactions monitoring [Online]. World Health Organization. Available: https://www.who.int/medicines/areas/quality_safety/safety_efficacy/advdrugreactions/en/ [Accessed December 12 2019].

Wu, T.Y., Jen, M.H., Bottle, A., Molokhia, M., Aylin, P., Bell, D. and Majeed, A., 2010. Ten-year trends in hospital admissions for adverse drug reactions in England 1999–2009. *Journal of the Royal Society of Medicine*, 103(6), pp.239–250.

Zhou, L., Harrison-Woolrych, M. and Coulter, D.M., 2003. Use of the New Zealand Intensive Medicines Monitoring Programme to study the levonorgestrel-releasing intrauterine device (Mirena). *Pharmacoepidemiology and drug safety*, 12(5), pp.371–377.

2

Managing the Pharmaceutical Supply Chain—To Sustainability and Beyond

Liz Breen, Marina Papalexi, and Ying Xie

Introduction

One might question why we need to focus on the pharmaceutical supply chain (PSC). This entity is such an important part of medicines access and provision, yet in past decades this activity has been very much under-estimated, undervalued and under-nurtured, leading to deficiencies in its strategic management. The PSC is a global system responsible for

L. Breen (✉)
School of Pharmacy and Medical Sciences, University of Bradford, Bradford, UK
e-mail: l.breen@bradford.ac.uk

M. Papalexi
Faculty of Business and Law, Manchester Metropolitan University, Manchester, UK
e-mail: M.Papalexi@mmu.ac.uk

Y. Xie
Faculty of Business and Law, Anglia Ruskin University, Chelmsford, UK
e-mail: ying.xie@anglia.ac.uk

Z. Babar (ed.), *Global Pharmaceutical Policy*,
https://doi.org/10.1007/978-981-15-2724-1_2

sustainably sourcing and delivering medicines and medical products from manufacturers to healthcare providers via logistic service providers (LSPs), to improve patient health and wellbeing. It is a very clear and simple agenda, but in reality it is a very complex system involving hundreds of stakeholders and governed by multiple regulatory and advisory bodies.

By its very nature sustainability has a number of definitions; at a basic level these include *the quality of being able to continue over a period of time* and *the quality of causing little or no damage to the environment and therefore able to continue for a long time* (Cambridge Dictionary 2019). The 1987 Brundtland Commission Report of the United Nations Economic Development Commission developed guidance principles for sustainability and defined it as *meeting the needs of the present without compromising the ability of future generations to achieve their own goals* (United Nations 1987). Other definitions are aligned with what is known as the Triple Bottom Line of sustainability (Elkington 1998). This helps organizations evaluate their performance aligned with three key areas to become more sustainable (activities should consider and deliver to social, environmental and economic aspects) and that they should include people's skills, abilities and values (Sarkis et al. 2010; Pagell and Gobeli 2009; Gualandris et al. 2015).

Sustainability of our world, our healthcare system and our PSC is a goal that we endeavour to successfully deliver to. In achieving this we use the resources we need *without* depleting all the resources that we have. This is particularly pertinent to healthcare and the sourcing and availability of active pharmaceutical ingredients and medicines.

In 2016, the United Nations introduced the Sustainable Development Goals (SDGs), a set of worldwide objectives designed to end poverty, protect the planet and guarantee that all individuals have peace and prosperity by 2030. The 17 goals replace the 8 Millennium Development Goals from 2000 with integrated and indivisible SDGs across the three sustainability pillars of economic growth, social inclusion and environmental protection (Halisçelik and Soytas 2019). Healthcare and medicines feature prominently in this agenda.

Challenges to a sustainable future can be seen throughout the PSC, beginning upstream with sourcing raw materials to downstream closer to primary care and the patient. This discussion will focus on various dimensions that we consider problematic and destructive to the effective functioning of this supply chain and the healthcare system it services. It will begin with describing the current landscape of the pharmaceutical sector and the stakeholders within this. It will then consider key threats to sustainability before considering the most important aspect, the patient at the heart of this supply chain.

Medicines Supply—The Current Landscape

In order to examine medicines supply chain issues, it is pertinent to firstly be cognisant of the nature and fabric of this supply chain; to do this we use the UK as a case example. The medicines supply chain within the UK follows a traditional model adopted by many countries globally. This is typically the sourcing of products from manufacturer to pharmacy (hospital and community) via wholesaler (also known as logistics service provider) or direct. The dynamics within this supply chain are constantly changing with formation of key alliances, e.g. companies such as Pfizer (2007) and AstraZeneca (2019) choosing to form partnerships with key pharmaceutical wholesalers (Alliance Healthcare and AAH, respectively) to offer an exclusive direct-to-pharmacy service (Chemist and Druggist 2009; PSNC 2019; Alliance Healthcare 2017). According to the Healthcare Distribution Association (HDA), changes within this supply chain have encouraged suppliers to develop into "integrated health care service providers" (HDA 2016). *The distribution industry must change, with wholesalers taking more of a role in central dispensing, informatics and big data, as well as reacting to continued consolidation, online pharmacies and new picking and delivery mechanisms* (HDA 2016:1).

Figure 2.1 summarizes the supply chain stakeholder influence within England (UK) and the role of pharmacy within this (Breen et al. 2018). Breen et al. (2018:58) demonstrate the relationships between these stakeholders by the type of influence as shown by line type and depth; e.g. the General Pharmaceutical Council (GPhC) has a regulatory influence over

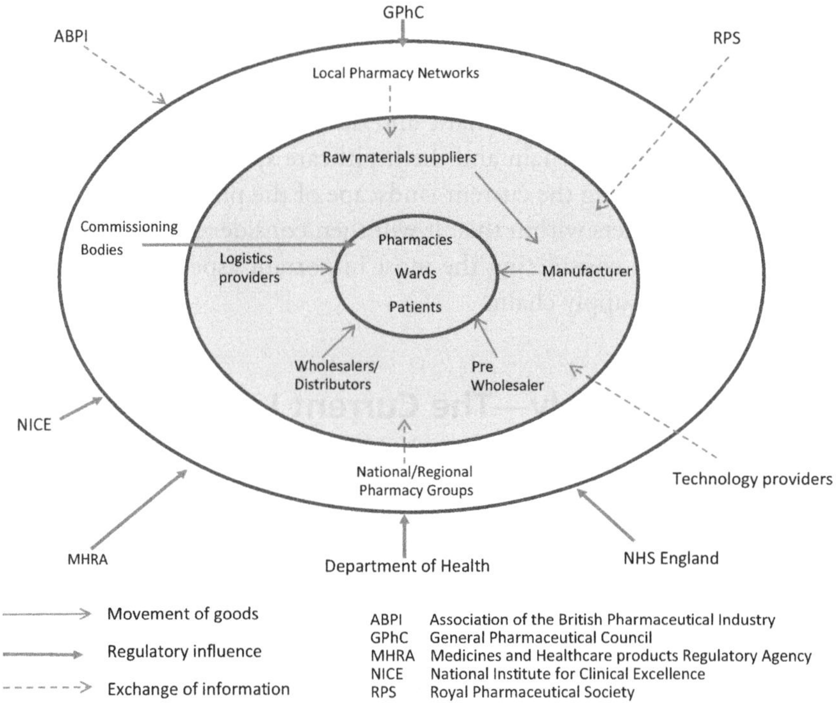

Fig. 2.1 Influence of stakeholders within the PSC (Breen et al. 2018)

three tiers of the supply chain, whereas the Royal Pharmaceutical Society (RPS) has advisory influence over the inner two tiers of the supply chain.

Putting the Patient at the Centre of the PSC

Service processes are characterized by the fact that the customer provides significant input into the production process (Grönroos and Ojasalo 2004). That input can be of three general types: the customer himself/herself, goods from the customer and/or information from the customer (Sampson 1999). Customers do not only provide input (they themselves, information, requests, complaints), but they also take part in the service process, influencing both the process performance, i.e. efficiency, and the perception of quality of the service produced (Grönroos and Ojasalo 2004). Customers are more than mere consumers of output; they are co-producers of the process (Grönroos and Ojasalo 2004); patients can be considered likewise. Co-design of services and the role of patients within this has risen in popularity in previous years (The Point of Care Foundation 2019; Goodrich 2018; Soni and Freeman 2018) and is now considered a "must-have" input into service design, research funding bids and healthcare operations business cases, to ensure appropriateness and accuracy and to support shared decision-making (as opposed to the previously existing patriarchal systems where the patient had no voice and input into their healthcare).

According to Richards et al. (2015:1), *we must harness the energy, insight and expertise of patients, carers, and the communities that support them to help drive change...patient centred care is central to the mission of healthcare.* The patient therefore has the perfect front-row seat of both the products manufactured and moved within the PSC and the service that they experience. They are therefore both the best critic and advocate of this service. There is a constant invitation for patients to feedback their views to the NHS and healthcare systems, but does this mean that all medicines and services designed to improve patients' health are designed with them in mind?

An example of where the patient's role is imperative in the PSC is the return of unused medicines to pharmacy. The driver for this system is reduction of risk within the domestic environment, but the burden of effort is placed on the patient and not on the system, and designing a return-friendly system would increase patient engagement with the returns process (Xie and Breen 2012) but what would this look like? The returns process will only happen if the patient or a patient representative facilitates this. This issue has risen in currency due to concerns of patients hoarding medicines and hence increasing the risk of non-adherence, accidental ingestion, etc. (RPS 2019a, RPS 2019b). Research undertaken by Breen (2016) proposed enhancements to this system to reduce the burden placed on patients. This would involve collecting medicines from domestic properties (as per American practice) or having the capacity to drop them at a collection point within their community (as per battery recycling). Both returns channels can be designed and executed to ensure optimal medicines are returned to community pharmacies.

Medicines Availability

A basic supply interpretation of the pharmaceutical supply chain is that it is linear (as shown in the figure below); however, this is not always the case. Within this supply chain, there are various levels of complexity, compounded by institutional competitiveness and complexity, gaming, lack of visibility, bureaucracy and political influence (Fig. 2.2).

In the PSC most improvement initiatives have concentrated more on reducing the pharmaceutical inventory (PI) and consequently the supply chain costs (SCC). However, Hendricks and Singhal (2005) believe that supply chain strategies (SCS) that focus on cost reduction are ineffective because they have ignored the risks from supply chain disruptions. In addition to this, they identify several consequences of a failure to manage risks effectively, which include financial losses, negative impact on product quality and an organization's reputation and conflict amongst the organization's stakeholders. Moreover, economic, political and social developments increase the risk of supply chain disruptions, as supply chains are gradually becoming longer and more complex (Khan and Burnes 2007).

With the increasing complexity of the supply chain and the growing number of new companies in the pharmaceutical sector, e.g. generics, coupled with increasing demands for medicines (more patients, patients living longer but with more conditions leading to polypharmacy), the potential risk of disconnect and fragility has increased. Breen, in 2008, identified key risks within the PSC (as reported from an experienced body of pharmaceutical stakeholders), the fragmentation of the supply chain being the risk most highly ranked; see Table 2.1 (Breen 2008). In second place was the lack of visibility of stock leading to stock-outs and short supplies; this is still very much a live issue today (Morris 2019).

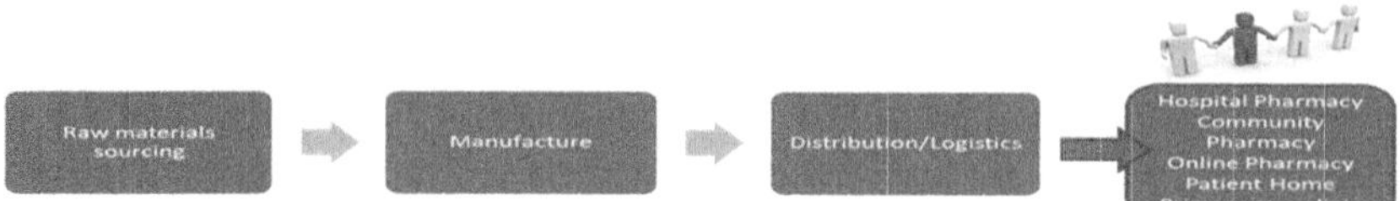

Fig. 2.2 A basic linear pharmaceutical supply chain

Table 2.1 Risks identified in the pharmaceutical supply chain in 2005

Risk	Rating
Fragmentation of SC—No single source, multiple channels, no communication, unilateral decisions	10
Lack of visibility of stock	9
Unexpected increase in demand	8.5
Demand versus capacity	8.5
Information flow or lack of information	8.5
Lack of forecasting—Customer side	8.5
Availability of raw material—True and commercially induced. Regulatory issues—Manufacturing licensing/change of standards/drug recalls	8
Demand/economics—Not able to respond to demand	8
Inadequate buffer stock—JIT/lean	8
Contracting treated as a commodity—Big contract equals big risk. Drives competitors out of market	8
Transportation—Unavailability of fuel, congestion, weather, illness	7.5
Manufacturer defence tactics	7.5
Diversion of manufacturing capacity	7.5
External influences—Disaster recovery	7.5
Stock holding—More concentrated	7
Exploitation	6.5
Dispensing/picking error—Medication/packaging, prescription management	6.5
Decrease in capacity linked to profit	6.5
Too much information	6.5
Short-term SC planning	6.5
Operational in–/efficiencies, e.g. systems operating properly	6
Nonstandard practice—Customized policies per hospital. Lack of common codes, etc.	6
Counterfeiting	6
Increase in demand due to NICE approval, patient involvement, press	6
Rationalization of range	5.5
Cash flow/cash management—Threat associated with small companies and hospitals	5.5
Storage/cold chain	5.5
Reimbursement policies not consistent	5.5
Response of industry to shortages—Communication?	5.5
Loss of expertise—Unsophisticated supply chain purchasing/practice?	5
Risk of litigation—Influence on market?	5
Hubs—Introduce more complexity	4.5
Lack of knowledge regarding manufacturing process or source of supply	4.5
Theft	4.5
Prioritization—Conflict between patients and profits	4

Medicines availability has continued to be a threat to patient care over the years (Awad et al. 2016; Lyengar et al. 2016) and is still a major thorn in the side of healthcare strategists. Within the UK this has received even more attention with the onset of Brexit, the political removal of the UK from the European Union; there has been an immense fear of products not being available via normal distribution channels (O'Carroll 2019; Andalo 2018; Breen and Vann Yaroson 2018). Patients, as might be expected, have been very concerned as to the ramification of supply disruptions on their medications, especially those reliant on these for long-term conditions, but even basic products such as naproxen experienced stock-outs (The Week 2019). Measures have been put in place by the government to address access to European stock and distribution routes, but what other measures could be considered within the UK? An example of good practice in medicines sourcing by patients is that employed in the Spanish PSC. Using commercial platforms, patients can now source medication available within a specific geographic area and "hold" stock in that location to be collected. This is highly convenient for the patient as it saves time and reduces emotional frustration in trying to find medicines (Lázaro and Acosta Gómez 2019).

Innovation in the Pharmaceutical Supply Chain

Several scholars have investigated the PSC and to what extent innovation could optimize it. These, once explored, can be translated into tangible operational practices. Innovation implemented within the PSC has been divided into two main categories: (a) theoretical innovations (Burgess and Radnor 2013; Baker 2014) and (b) technological innovations (Wamba et al. 2013; Cranfield et al. 2015).

Theoretical Innovations

Regarding the theoretical innovations, the application of a reverse logistics approach to manage and improve the reverse components in order to minimize pharmaceuticals waste has been reported (Cardoso et al. 2013;

Xie and Breen 2014). Reverse logistics has been described as *the process of planning, implementing and controlling the efficient, cost-effective flow of raw materials, in process inventory, finished goods and related information from the point of consumption to the point of origin for the purpose of recapturing or creating value or for proper disposal* (Rogers and Tibben-Lembke 1999:2).

A representative example of reverse logistics application is that of Aurora Health Care Pharmacy, which keeps returns at less than 2% of its total inventory despite stringent regulations related to expiration dates, manufacturer recalls and proper disposal of drugs (Morton 2006). In addition, Xie and Breen (2012), in their research, designed a green community PSC that reduces preventable pharmaceutical waste and effectively disposes of inevitable pharmaceutical waste, using a cross-boundary green PSC approach that requires every actor in the PSC to participate in environmentally friendly practices (Fig. 2.3).

Kumar et al. (2009) analysed the PSC using the define, measure, analyse, improve and control (DMAIC) process for improvement of reverse logistics. They found that specific information on the PSC was limited because much of the reverse logistics for pharmaceuticals is handled through third-party providers.

The application of lean tools and techniques could be used to help pharmacies manage their inventory, eliminate waste and reduce costs. Although lean thinking, which is a method that increases efficiency through the removal of non-value-adding activities (Brandao de Souza 2009; Young and McClean 2009), was derived from the automobile manufacturing industry, over the last decade it has been adopted by other industries, such as public sector services and healthcare (Zhang et al. 2012; Bamford et al. 2015; Cheng et al. 2015). Papalexi et al. (2015) focused on the implementation of the Kanban system (a lean and just-in-time (JIT) technique, which was created to control inventory levels and the production and supply of components) on the supply chain for a group of cooperative pharmacists proposing that the organization can store 56.8% fewer products and spend 71.8% less money, by adopting the Kanban system. There are also documented reports highlighting the implementation of just-in-time (JIT) approaches (lean tools that supply materials to each stage of production only when required) (Ndubisi et al.

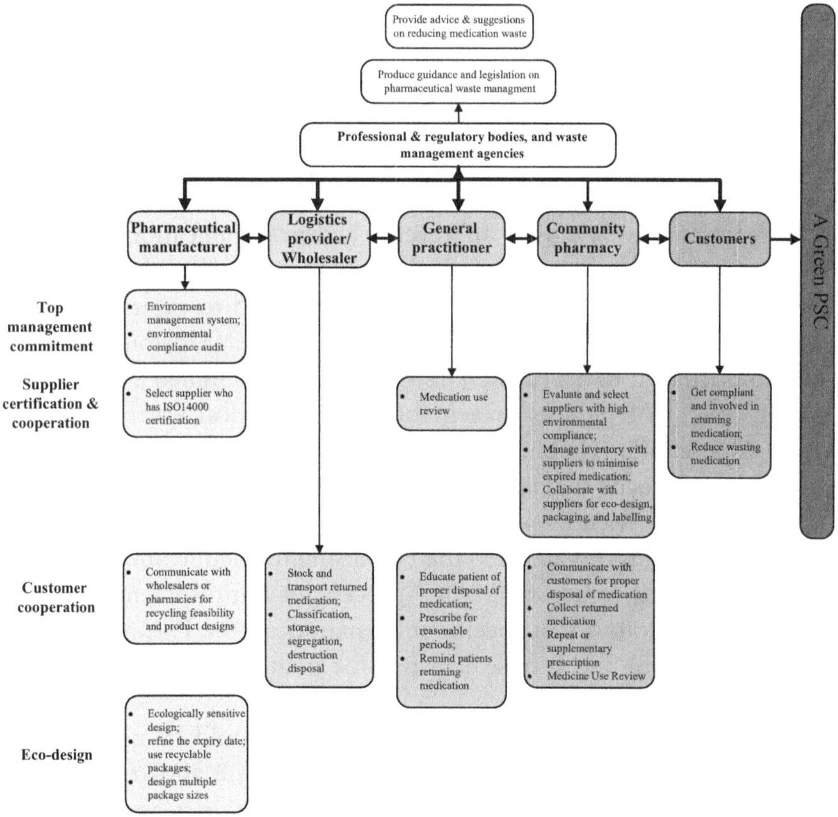

Fig. 2.3 The cross-boundary green PSC (XGPSC) approach (Xie and Breen 2012)

2005; Braga et al. 2015) and inventory control systems such as vendor-managed inventory (VMI) (Mustaffa and Potter 2009; Bhakoo et al. 2012). Bhakoo et al. (2012:219) defined VMI as *a system whereby the supplier takes responsibility for monitoring the retailer's inventory levels and makes periodic replenishment decisions regarding order quantities, delivery mode and timing of replenishments*. Kim (2005) stated that improved information reliability, fewer errors and a 30% reduction in the inventory were some of the benefits recorded by applying VMI. Mustaffa and Potter (2009) reported several significant benefits are derived from the VMI application: increased service quality, decreased stock-outs and elimination of the bullwhip effect.

Simulation modelling and outsourcing of noncritical medical supplies were examined by scholars such as Nicholson et al. (2004), Samuel et al. (2010) and Battini et al. (2013). Similarly, those approaches were aimed at reducing inventory costs without influencing the quality of services. In a Canadian hospital, a "stockless system" was implemented (Rivard-Royer et al. 2002). This system used a hospital's central store for distributing the low-volume products, whilst the high-volume products were delivered directly to the point of each patient care unit. Daly et al. (2015) and Lücker and Seifert (2017) proposed that the pharmaceutical sector should adopt approaches that enable late-stage customization and manage multiple co-existing agile supply chains to be able to deal with future trends, sustaining a broader range of more specialized products at lower volumes (Voura et al. 2011) and satisfying current market and volume demands (Daly et al. 2015).

Technological Innovations

Besides the theoretical innovations discussed, there have been several reported initiatives focusing on developing technological innovations. Although healthcare organizations generate large amounts of data which used to be stored in hard copy form, the current trend is to digitalize them, a fact that might enable healthcare organizations to be more productive (Raghupathi and Raghupathi 2014). These large amounts of data provide significant information and support the healthcare functions such as population health management (Burghard 2012; Fernandes et al. 2012). Health data sets are considered as large and complex, mainly due to their diversity and importance, that makes them difficult to manage without integrated software and/or hardware (Frost and Sullivan 2013). According to Raghupathi and Raghupathi (2014), there is a potential to improve care, save lives and lower costs through identifying associations and understanding patterns and trends within healthcare data. Information technology (IT) systems can create and develop platforms in order for the large volumes of data and information to be captured, stored and manipulated effectively (Feldman et al. 2012). Real-time data are crucial within the healthcare sector because they allow the right treatments to be applied as early as possible and sometimes they can mean the difference between life and death (Raghupathi and Raghupathi 2014).

eHealth, which is a system that uses big data to provide digital services in healthcare, has been introduced in most of the developed countries. Walter and Lazic-Peric (2017:67) stated that *digital platforms link pharmacies and patients and enable them to jointly manage the patient's health* via *such services as appointment and prescription refill reminders, medication intake reminders, health tracking tools* (e.g. *weight loss, smoking cessation), immunization tracking, health measurement and progress tools* (e.g. *diabetes) and live chat tools to facilitate communication between patients and pharmacists.* The application of radiofrequency identification (RFID) technology, which is an automatic identification and data capture technology, has been suggested to enhance inventory management, warehouse management and transportation management (Papert et al. 2016; Yang et al. 2018; Breen 2006). Although some applications of RFID in the healthcare sector (FossoWamba et al. 2013) already show the potential of this system, Çakıcı et al. (2011) stated that RFID cannot be as effective without operational redesign to suit the technology. There are also other potential problems with RFID, such as privacy, data security and trust issues as well as very high costs for implementation (Kuo and Chen 2008). However, despite this, with a need to push for sustainability, RFID is a good way of reducing costs longer term and improving efficiency. More recent research has focused on the need to enhance visibility within the supply chain (as per the current good distribution practice (GDP) guideline) through the use of automatic identification (auto-ID) technology solutions such as securPharm with passive radiofrequency identification tags, transport containers with sensor nodes and a supply chain visibility dashboard (Papert et al. 2016).

Workforce Development

According to Health Education England (HEE 2019:6), *a growing concern is the availability of a workforce with the right skills to deliver the service now, while developing talent to deliver future service requirements.* In order to meet the needs of the NHS Long Term Plan (NHS England

2019), strategic changes need to take place within the pharmacy workforce.

In previous years there have been concerns as to the predominance of pharmacists available to deliver services globally (Almaghaslah et al. 2018; Rutter et al. 2018; Bates et al. 2018; Ekpenyong et al. 2018), and this issue continues to cause concerns with changes in NHS funding and also external factors such as Brexit. Within the UK recent policies and strategic documents have outlined the role and strategic direction of pharmacy in future years (NHS England's Next Steps on the Five Year Forward View (2017) and Five Year Forward View (2014), Royal Pharmaceutical Society's Now or Never: Shaping Pharmacy for the Future (2013), Department of Health's Improving the Use of Medicines for Better Outcomes and Reduced Waste: An Action Plan (2012)). All of these promote the critical nature of this profession and service within the UK healthcare system. They all also propose new roles and extended service provision across the NHS (in both hospitals/secondary care and in the community/primary care, Marques et al. 2018; Edwards et al. 2019) for pharmacists and pharmacy. In response we have seen the introduction of emergency department pharmacists (Greenwood et al. 2019), primary care pharmacists in general practice (Mann et al. 2018), care home pharmacists (Pharmaceutical Journal 2018) and veterinary pharmacists (Pharmaceutical Journal 2015).

Such changes have also encouraged the development of more appropriate and innovative service models, which deliver optimal care and shift care closer to the patients (whilst also reducing the burden on acute/hospital care). This has required the development of the workforce to become more agile and flexible in designing optimal care and moving between modes of care and service models. Workforce development is a priority as evidenced by the World Health Organization (WHO 2017) and more locally within the UK by the Nuffield Trust (2019) reporting concerns of healthcare workforce capability over the next ten years. The RPS (2019a, 2019b:1) has responded to this stating that *the forthcoming Workforce Implementation Plan will need to enable healthcare professionals to deliver the NHS Long Term Plan, to reduce pressure on the NHS and improve the way we deliver patient care. This must include support for pharmacists, with a focus on education, health and wellbeing and their continuing professional development if we are to see the biggest positive impact of these changes.*

Pharmacists as healthcare providers, therefore, can build on their professional clinical capabilities in adopting new roles. In order to do so they will have to adapt and develop new skills such as management/operational skills. The foundation for this development was laid over 20 years ago by the creation of the "seven-star pharmacist", by the World Health Organization (1997), which set the minimum international standards and expectations for all current and future pharmacists' roles. The seven-star pharmacist consisted of core roles: manager, leader, care-giver, decision-maker, communicator, lifelong learner and teacher (Thamby and Subramani 2015). The manager domain encompassed effective resources management (human, physical and financial) and information governance (WHO 1997). The seven-star concept has now been updated to include two additional roles, that of researcher and entrepreneur to deliver the new nine-star pharmacist (Thamby and Subramani 2015).

Conclusions

Healthcare organizations have one of the most crucial roles in the society as they are responsible for providing high-quality healthcare services. Investments and constant improvement are required for the healthcare system to enhance its performance and improve the individual patient care experience in terms of quality, access and reliability (Papalexi 2017; Chassin 2013). However, globally, healthcare expenditure is growing rapidly, governmental cost-cutting measures put extensive pressure on healthcare organizations to reduce their expenses without sacrificing service quality (Ferreira et al. 2018; Narayanamurthy et al. 2018). Bhakoo et al. (2012:217) stated that *supply-related costs constitute approximately 30 per cent of hospital expenditure;* the perceived high cost and high level of wastage associated with pharmaceuticals increase the overall healthcare expenditure. Therefore, healthcare organizations aim to optimize the pharmaceutical supply chain to achieve cost saving, waste elimination and still deliver high-quality services. Healthcare literature suggests that the adoption of innovative interventions could enhance healthcare supply chains and assist healthcare organizations to manage economic challenges (Pohjosenperä et al. 2018).

Within the healthcare environment, numerous forces are influencing the redesign of the PSC as the current model is unsustainable (Price Waterhouse Coopers 2019). *By 2020, health care will shift in focus from treatment to prevention; pharmaceutical companies will provide total health care packages; the current linear phase research and development process will give way to in-life testing and live licensing, in collaboration with regulators and health care providers; the traditional blockbuster sales model will disappear; the supply chain function will become revenue generating as it becomes integral to the health care package and enables access to new channels and more sophisticated direct-to-consumer distribution channels will diminish the role of wholesalers* (Price Waterhouse Coopers, 2019:1). Other developments which are pushing boundaries within this sector and this supply are key collaborations at critical stages in the supply chain. One example is that of Verily, Google's healthcare spin-off company, and the Novartis, Otsuka, Pfizer and Sanofi collaboration to revolutionize clinical trials (PM Live, 2019) which are traditionally *outdated, cumbersome and inefficient systems not built around patient needs* (Business Wire 2019).

So how does the PSC become sustainable as an enterprise now and beyond? Achieving universal health coverage by 2030, as part of the Sustainable Development Goals (SDGs), depends on access to quality essential health services and safe and effective use of drugs and vaccines (WHO 2017); it also relies heavily on access to accurate and timely data to inform strategic decisions in all matters pertaining to essential resources. Sustainability has a triple agenda: to respond to society, to have a positive economic impact and to be environmentally conscious. There is evidence of all three elements within the PSC globally but there is also evidence that there is more to be done in each one of these. The development of innovative and smart strategies, service models and an agile workforce is critical to delivering a sustainable PSC, fit for purpose now and beyond.

References

Alliance Healthcare (2017) Alliance Healthcare UK wins new distribution contract with Pfizer. Available at: http://www.alliance-healthcare.co.uk/latest-news/-/asset_publisher/jL0I/content/alliance-healthcare-uk-wins-new-distribution-contract-with-pfizer?redirect=http%3A%2F%2Fwww.alliance-healthcare.co.uk%2Flatest-news%3Fp_p_id%3D101_INSTANCE_jL0I%26p_p_lifecycle%3D0%26p_p_state%3Dnormal%26p_p_mode%3Dview%26p_p_col_id%3Dcolumn-1%26p_p_col_count%3D1%26_101_INSTANCE_jL0I_advancedSearch%3Dfalse%26_101_INSTANCE_jL0I_keywords%3D%26_101_INSTANCE_jL0I_delta%3D10%26_101_INSTANCE_jL0I_cur%3D8%26_101_INSTANCE_jL0I_andOperator%3Dtrue Accessed: 15 June 2019.

Almaghaslah, D., Alsayari, A., Asiri, R. and Albugami, N. (2018). Pharmacy workforce in Saudi Arabia: Challenges and opportunities: A cross-sectional study. The International Journal of Health Planning and Management, 34(1), pp. 583–593.

Andalo, D (2018). Don't stockpile drugs for Brexit, government tells community pharmacists. Accessed: 23/8/18. Available at: https://www.pharmaceutical-journal.com//news-and-analysis/news/dont-stockpile-drugs-for-brexit-government-tells-community-pharmacist/20205360.fullarticle?firstPass=false#cxrecs_

Awad, H., Al-Zu'bi, Z. and Abdallah, A. (2016). A Quantitative Analysis of the Causes of Drug Shortages in Jordan: A Supply Chain Perspective. International Business Research, 9(6), p. 53.

Baker, G. (2014). Improving Healthcare Using Lean Processes. Healthcare quality, 17(2), pp. 18–19.

Bamford, D., Forrester, P., Dehe, B. and Leese, R. (2015). Partial and iterative Lean implementation: Two case studies. International Journal of Operations and Production Management. 35(5), pp. 702–727.

Bates, Bates I., John, C., Meilianti, S., Bader, L. (2018) Pharmacy Workforce Intelligence: Global Trends Report, International Pharmaceutical Federation.

Battini, D., Faccio, M., Persona, A. and Sgarbossa, F. (2013). Modelling the Growing Process of Integrated Healthcare Supply Networks. International Journal Of System Dynamics Applications, 2(1), pp. 1–13.

Bhakoo, V., Singh, P. and Sohal, A. (2012). Collaborative management of inventory in Australian hospital supply chains: practices and issues. Supply Chain Management: An International Journal, 17(2), pp. 217–230.

Braga, M., Tyler, M., Rhoads, J., Cacchio, M., Auerbach, M., Nishisaki, A. and Larson, R. (2015). Effect of just-in-time simulation training on provider performance and patient outcomes for clinical procedures: a systematic review. BMJ Simulation And Technology Enhanced Learning, bmjstel-2015-000058.

Brandao de Souza, L. (2009). Trends and Approaches in Lean Healthcare. Leadership in Health Services 22 (2), pp. 121–139.

Breen L. and Vann Yaroson, E. (2018) Medicines Shortages are already a reality but a no deal Brexit could make it worse. The Conversation. Available at: https://theconversation.com/medicine-shortages-are-already-a-reality-but-a-no-deal-brexit-could-make-it-worse-102218 Accessed: 12 February 2019.

Breen, L., Urban, R. and Zaman, H. (2018) The Health Supply Chain in the United Kingdom. Pharmacists in the Supply Chain Technical Report, International Federation of Pharmacists (FIP). https://fip.org/files/fip/publications/Pharmacists_in_the_supply_chain_The_role_of_the_medicines_expert_in_ensuring_quality_and_availability.pdf Accessed: 11 May 2019.

Breen, L. (2016) Medicines Optimisation – extracting the last vestiges of value from your medicines, Journal of Medicines Optimisation, 2 (3), pp 46–49.

Breen, L (2008) A Preliminary examination of risk in the Pharmaceutical Supply Chain (PSC) in the National Health Service (NHS) (UK), Journal of Service Science and Management, 1 pp 193–199.

Breen L, (2006) Give me back my empties or else! – A Preliminary analysis of customer compliance in reverse logistics practices (UK), Management Research News, 29 (9) pp 532–551.

Burgess, N., and Radnor, Z. (2013). Evaluating Lean in healthcare. International Journal Of Health Care Quality Assurance, 26(3), pp. 220–235.

Burghard, C. (2012). Big Data and Analytics Key to Accountable Care Success. IDC Health Insights.

Business Wire (2019) Ochsner Health System and Pfizer Partner to Develop Innovative Models for Clinical Trials. Available at: https://www.businesswire.com/news/home/20190219005624/en/Ochsner-Health-System-Pfizer-Partner-Develop-Innovative Accessed: 15 June 2019.

Çakıcı ÖE, Groenevelt H and Seidmann A (2011) Using RFID for the management of pharmaceutical inventory—system optimization and shrinkage control. Decision Support Systems. 51(3), pp. 627–637

Cambridge Dictionary (2019) Definition of sustainability. Available at: https://dictionary.cambridge.org/dictionary/english/sustainable. Accessed: 15 June 2019.

Cardoso, S., Barbosa-Póvoa, A. and Relvas, S. (2013). Design and planning of supply chains with integration of reverse logistics activities under demand uncertainty. European Journal Of Operational Research, 226(3), pp. 436–451.

Chassin, M. (2013). Improving The Quality Of Health Care: What's Taking So Long?. Health Affairs, 32(10), pp. 1761–1765.

Chemist and Druggist (2009) Pfizer renews its DTP deal with Alliance Healthcare. Available at: https://www.chemistanddruggist.co.uk/news/pfizer-renews-its-dtp-deal-alliance-healthcare Accessed 14 June 2019.

Cheng, S., D. Bamford, M. Papalexi and B. Dehe. (2015). Improving Access to Health Services – Challenges in Lean Application. International Journal of Public Sector Management, 28 (2), pp. 121–135.

Cranfield, S., Hendy, J., Reeves, B., Hutchings, A., Collin, S., and Fulop, N. (2015). Investigating healthcare IT innovations: a "conceptual blending" approach. Journal Of Health Organization And Management, 29(7), pp. 1131–1148.

Daly, R., Harrington, T.S., Martin, G.D. and Hutchings, I.M. (2015). Inkjet printing for pharmaceutics – a review of research and manufacturing. International Journal of Pharmaceutics. Article first published online: 12th March.

Doyle, C., Howe, C., Woodcock, T., Myron, R., Phekoo, K. and McNicholas, C. et al. (2013). Making change last: applying the NHS institute for innovation and improvement sustainability model to healthcare improvement. Implementation Science, 8(1), pp. 127.

Edwards, Z., Bennett, MI., Blenkinsopp, A. (2019). A community pharmacist medicines optimisation service for patients with advanced cancer pain: a proof of concept study. International Journal of Clinical Pharmacy. 41(3), pp. 700–710.

Ekpenyong, A., Udoh, A., Kpokiri, E. and Bates, I. (2018). An analysis of pharmacy workforce capacity in Nigeria. Journal of Pharmaceutical Policy and Practice, 11(1).

Elkington, J. (1998), "Accounting for the Triple Bottom Line", Measuring Business Excellence, 2(3), pp. 18–22. https://doi.org/10.1108/eb025539.

Feldman, B., Martin, E.M. and Skotnes, T. (2012). Big Data in Healthcare Hype and Hope. Dr. Bonnie 360, Retrieved from: http://www.west-info.eu/files/big-data-inhealthcare.pdf.

Fernandes, L., O'Connor, M. and Weaver, V. (2012). Big data, bigger outcomes. Journal American Health Information Management Association, pp. 38–42.

Ferreira, D., Marques, R., and Nunes, A. (2018). Economies of scope in the health sector: The case of Portuguese hospitals. European Journal of Operational Research, 266 (2), pp. 716–735.
FossoWamba, S., Anand, A. and Carter, L. (2013). A literature review of RFID-enabled healthcare applications and issues. International Journal of Information Management, 33(5), pp. 875–891.
Frost & Sullivan. (2013). Drowning in Big Data? Reducing Information Technology Complexities and Costs for Healthcare Organizations. Retrieved from: http://www.emc.com/collateral/analyst-reports/frost-sullivan-reducing-informationtechnologycomplexities-ar.pdf.
Goodrich, J. (2018) Why experience-based co-design improves the patient experience. The Journal of Health Design. Available at: https://www.journalofhealthdesign.com/JHD/article/view/45 Accessed: 22 June 2019.
Greenwood, D., Tully, M.P., Martin, S. and Steinke, D. (2019). The description and definition of Emergency Department Pharmacist Practitioners in United Kingdom (the ENDPAPER study). International Journal of Clinical Pharmacy, 41, pp. 434–444.
Grönroos, C. and Ojasalo, K., (2004), Service Productivity: Towards a conceptualisation of the transformation or inputs into economic results in services, Journal of Business Research, Vol. 57, pp. 414–423.
Gualandris, J., Klassen, R., Vachon, S. and Kalchschmidt, M. (2015). Sustainable evaluation and verification in supply chains: Aligning and leveraging accountability to stakeholders. Journal of Operations Management, 38(1), pp. 1–13.
Halisçelik, E. and Soytas, M. (2019). Sustainable development from millennium 2015 to Sustainable Development Goals 2030. Sustainable Development
Healthcare Distribution Association (2016) About us. Available at: http://www.hdauk.co.uk/ Accessed: 15 June 2019
Health Education England (2019) Advancing Pharmacy Education and Training: A Review. https://www.hee.nhs.uk/sites/default/files/documents/Advancing%20Pharmacy%20Education%20and%20Training%20Review.pdf. Accessed: 14 June 2019.
Hendricks, K.B. and Singhal, V.R. (2005) An empirical analysis of the effects of supply chain disruption on long-run stock price performance and equity risk of the firm. Production and Operations Management. 14(1), pp. 35–52.
Khan, O. and Burnes, B. (2007). Risk and supply chain management: creating a research agenda. The International Journal of Logistics Management. 18(2), pp. 197–216.

Kim, D. (2005) An integrated supply chain management system: a case study in healthcare sector. Lecture Notes in Computer Science. 3590, pp. 218–27.

Kumar S., Dieveney E. and Dieveney A. (2009) Reverse logistic process control measures for the pharmaceutical industry supply chain. International Journal of Productivity and Performance Management, 58(2), pp. 188–204

Kuo, C.H. and Chen, H.G. (2008) The Critical Issues about Deploying RFID in Healthcare Industry by Service Perspective. Proceedings of the 41st Annual Hawaii International Conference on System Sciences (HICSS 2008). Hawaii, IEEE Computer Society Washington, DC, USA

Lücker F. and Seifert, R. W. (2017). Building up Resilience in a Pharmaceutical Supply Chain through Inventory, Dual Sourcing and Agility Capacity. Omega. 73, pp. 114–124.

Lyengar S., Hedman, L., Forte G. and Hill S. (2016) Medicine shortages: a commentary on causes and mitigation strategies. BMC Medicine (2016) 14, pp. 124.

Maher, L., Plsek, P. and Bevan, H. (2008) Making a bigger difference: a guide for NHS front-line staff and leaders on assessing and stimulating service innovation. NHS Institute for Innovation and Improvement.

Mann, D., Anderson, C., Avery, A.J., Waring, J. and Boyd, M.J. (2018). Clinical Pharmacists in General Practice: Pilot Scheme. Available at: https://www.nottingham.ac.uk/pharmacy/documents/generalpracticeyearfwdrev/clinical-pharmacists-in-general-practice-pilot-scheme-full-report.pdf/ Accessed 12 May 2019.

Martín Lázaro, R., Acosta Gómez JA (2019) Tecnología, desabastecimiento y rentabilidad de un nuevo servicio para las farmacias. Infarma, European Congress of Pharmacy Office and Salon of Medicines and Parapharmacy, Barcelona 2019.

Marques, I et al (2018). Pharmacist joint-working with general practices: evaluating the Sheffield Primary Care Pharmacy Programme. A mixed-methods study. British Journal of General Practice. Available at: https://doi.org/10.3399/bjgpopen18X101611. Accessed: 12 April 2019.

Morris, P. (2019) Responding to disruptions in the pharmaceutical supply chain. Clinical Pharmacist, 2(2), pp. 54–63.

Morton, R. (2006) Reverse spells "headache relief". Logistics Today. 47(9), pp. 35–6.

Mustaffa, N.H. and Potter, A., (2009). Healthcare supply chain management in Malaysia: a case study. Supply Chain Management: An International Journal. 14 (3), pp. 234–243.

Narayanamurthy, G., Gurumurthy, A., Subramanian, N., and Moser, R. (2018). Assessing the readiness to implement lean in healthcare institutions – A case study. International Journal Of Production Economics, 197, pp. 123–142.

Ndubisi, N.O., Jantan, M., Hing, L.C. and Ayub, M.S. (2005) Supplier selection and management strategies and manufacturing flexibility. Journal of Enterprise Information Management. 18(3), pp. 330–49.

NHS England (2019) NHS Long Term Plan. https://www.england.nhs.uk/long-term-plan/. Accessed: 14 May 2019.

NHS England (2017) Next Steps on the NHS Five Year Forward View. Available at: https://www.england.nhs.uk/wp-content/uploads/2017/03/NEXT-STEPS-ON-THE-NHS-FIVE-YEAR-FORWARD-VIEW.pdf Accessed: 22 June 2019.

NHS England (2014) Five Year Forward View. Available at: http://www.england.nhs.uk/wp-content/uploads/2014/10/5yfv-web.pdf Accessed: 11 May 2019.

Nicholson, L., Vakharia, A.J. and Erenguc, S.S. (2004). Outsourcing inventory management decisions in healthcare: models and application. European Journal of Operational Research, 154(1), pp. 271–90.

O'Carroll L. (2019) Brexit "already causing medicine shortages" at pharmacies in England. The Guardian. Available at: https://www.theguardian.com/politics/2019/apr/09/brexit-medicine-shortages-pharmacies-england Accessed: 22 June 2019.

Pagell, M. and Gobeli, D. (2009). How Plant Managers' Experiences and Attitudes Toward Sustainability Relate to Operational Performance. Production and Operations Management, 18(3), pp. 278–299.

Papalexi, M., Bamford, D. and Dehe, B. (2015). A case study of Kanban implementation within the Pharmaceutical Supply Chain. International Journal of Logistics Research and Applications. 1–17, ISSN 1367-5567.

Papalexi, M. (2017). An investigation into the aspects of innovation within the downstream domain of the pharmaceutical supply chain. Doctoral thesis. The University of Huddersfield.

Papert, M., Rimpler, P. and Pflaum, A. (2016). Enhancing supply chain visibility in a pharmaceutical supply chain: Solutions based on automatic identification technology, International Journal of Physical Distribution & Logistics Management, 46 (9), pp. 859–88.

Pharmaceutical Services Negotiating Committee (2019) AstraZeneca announce changes to their distribution arrangements. Available at: https://psnc.org.uk/our-news/astrazeneca-announce-changes-to-their-distribution-arrangements/ Accessed: 15 June 2019.

PM Live (2019) Verily unveils next-gen trials alliance with Novartis, Pfizer. Available at: https://www.pmlive.com/pharma_news/verily_unveils_next-gen_trials_alliance_with_novartis,_pfizer_1288930 Accessed: 15 June 2019

Pohjosenperä, T., Kekkonen, P., Pekkarinen, S., and Juga, J. (2018). Service modularity in managing healthcare logistics. The International Journal Of Logistics Management. 30(1), pp. 174–194

Price Waterhouse Coopers (2019) Pharma 2020: The vision. Available at: https://www.pwc.com/gx/en/industries/pharmaceuticals-life-sciences/publications/pharma-2020/pharma-2020-vision-path.html Accessed: 22 June 2019.

Raghupathi, W., and Raghupathi, V. (2014). Big data analytics in healthcare: promise and potential. Health Information Science and Systems, 2(1), 3.

Richards, T., Coulter, A. and Wicks, P. (2015) Time to deliver patient centred care, BMJ, pp. 350.

Rivard-Royer, H., Landry, S. and Beaulieu, M. (2002). Hybrid stockless: a case study: lessons for health-care supply chain integration. International Journal of Operations & Production Management. 22(4), pp. 412–24.

Rogers, D.S. and Tibben-Lembke, R.S. (1999), Going Backwards: Reverse Logistics Trends and Practices, Reverse Logistics Executive Council Press, Pittsburgh, PA.

Royal Pharmaceutical Society (2013) Now or Never: Shaping Pharmacy for the Future. Available at: http://www.rpharms.com/promoting-pharmacy-pdfs/moc-report-full.pdf Accessed: 11th May 2019

Royal Pharmaceutical Society (2019a) Building up the pharmacy workforce. Available at: https://www.rpharms.com/about-us/news/details/Building-up-the-pharmacy-workforce Accessed: 22 June 2019.

Royal Pharmaceutical Society (2019b) Unused medicines and expiry dates, Available at: https://www.rpharms.com/about-us/news/details/Unused-medicines-and-expiry-dates- Accessed: 22 June 2019.

Rutter, V., Chan, A., Tuck, C., Bader, L., Babar, Z. and Bates, I. (2018). Weaving the health and pharmaceutical care agenda through the themes of the commonwealth heads of government meeting (CHOGM), London 2018. Journal of Pharmaceutical Policy and Practice, 11(1).

Sampson, S.E., (1999), Understanding service businesses, Brigham Young University.

Samuel, C., Gonapa, K., Chaudhary, P. and Mishra, A. (2010). Supply chain dynamics in healthcare services. International Journal Of Health Care Quality Assurance, 23(7), pp. 631–642.

Sarkis, J., Gonzalez-Torre, P. and Adenso-Diaz, B. (2010). Stakeholder pressure and the adoption of environmental practices: The mediating effect of training. Journal of Operations Management, 28(2), pp. 163–176.

Soni, A. and Freeman, E. (2018.) G14(P) Understanding young people with diabetes: using experience based co-design to provide a patient-centred diabetes transition service Archives of Disease in Childhood. 2018;103:A6.

Thamby, S. and Subramani, P. (2015). The Nine-star pharmacies: an overview. Journal of Young Pharmacist, 7(4), pp. 281–284.

The Nuffield Trust (2019) Closing the gap: Key areas for action on the health and care workforce. Available at: https://www.nuffieldtrust.org.uk/research/closing-the-gap-key-areas-for-action-on-the-health-and-care-workforce Accessed: 22 June 2019.

The Pharmaceutical Journal (2018) Government announces extra role for pharmacists in care homes as part of £3.5bn funding package. https://www.pharmaceutical-journal.com/news-and-analysis/news/government-announces-extra-role-for-pharmacists-in-care-homes-as-part-of-35bn-funding-package/20205790.article?firstPass=false Accessed: 30 May 2019.

The Pharmaceutical Journal (2015) Why I chose veterinary pharmacy instead of community or hospital. https://www.pharmaceutical-journal.com/careers-and-jobs/careers-and-jobs/career-qa/why-i-chose-veterinary-pharmacy-instead-of-community-or-hospital/20200126.article Accessed: 15 April 2019.

The Point of Care Foundation (2019) EBCD: Experience-based co-design toolkit. Available at: https://www.pointofcarefoundation.org.uk/resource/experience-based-co-design-ebcd-toolkit/ Accessed: 22 June 2019.

The Week (2019) NHS medicine shortage: what medicines are affected? Available at: https://www.theweek.co.uk/brexit/99058/pharmacists-warn-of-shortages-of-commonly-prescribed-drugs Accessed: 22 May 2019.

United Nations (1987) Report of the World Commission on Environment and Development: Our Common Future. Available at: http://www.un-documents.net/our-common-future.pdf Accessed 21 May 2019.

Voura, C., Schroedl, N., Gruber, M.M., Strohmeier, D., Eitzinger, B., Bauer, W., Brenn, G., Khinast, J.G. and Zimmer, A., (2011). Printable medicines: a microdosing device for producing personalised medicines. Pharm. Technol. Eur. 23, pp. 32–36.

Walter, E. and Lazic-Peric, A. (2017). Distribution profile and efficiency of the European pharmaceutical full-line wholesaling sector. Institute for

Pharmaeconomic Research. Available at: http://girp.eu/files/GIRP-IPF%20 Study%202016.pdf Accessed: 17 May 2019.
Wamba, S., Anand, A. and Carter, L. (2013). RFID Applications, Issues, Methods and Theory: A Review of the AIS Basket of TOP journals. Procedia Technology, 9, pp. 421–430.
World Health Organization, (2004) WHO review of NICE in the United Kingdom. WHO Drug Information. 17(4).
World Health Organization. (1997). The role of the pharmacist in the health care system: preparing the future pharmacist: curricular development: report of a third WHO Consultative Group on the Role of the Pharmacist, Vancouver, Canada, 27–29. Available at: http://www.who.int/iris/handle/10665/63817/ Accessed 12 May 2019.
World Health Organization (2017) International Bank for Reconstruction and Development/The World Bank. Tracking universal health coverage: 2017 global monitoring report. Geneva: WHO; Available at: http://www.who.int/healthinfo/universal_health_coverage/report/2017/en/, Accessed 26 July 2018.
Xie, Y. and Breen, L. (2012) Greening community pharmaceutical supply chain in UK: a cross boundary approach. Supply Chain Management: An International Journal. 7(1), pp. 40–53.
Xie, Y. and Breen, L. (2014). Who cares wins? A comparative analysis of household waste medicines and batteries reverse logistics systems. Supply Chain Management: An International Journal. 19(4), pp. 455–474.
Yang, K., Botero, U., Shen, H., Forte D. and Tehranipoor M. (2018). A Split Manufacturing Approach for Unclonable Chipless RFIDs for Pharmaceutical Supply Chain Security. IEEE.
Young, T., and S. McClean. (2009). Some Challenges Facing Lean Thinking in Healthcare. International Journal of Quality in Health Care. 21, pp. 309–310.
Zhang, Z., D. Bamford, C. Moxham, and B. Dehe. (2012). Strategy Deployment Systems within the UK Healthcare Sector: A Case Study. International Journal of Productivity and Performance Management 61 (8), pp. 863–880.

3

Generic Medicines and Biosimilars: Impact on Global Pharmaceutical Policy

Mohamed Izham Mohamed Ibrahim
and Ahmed Awaisu

Background

The generally high healthcare expenditure in most countries of the world poses challenges for the government in terms of healthcare financing. Pharmaceuticals account for a large proportion of this expenditure, representing 1.5% of GDP in Organisation for Economic Co-operation and Development (OECD) countries, on average (Gothe et al. 2015; Theodorou et al. 2009).

Biosimilar and interchangeable products, such as generic medicines, can offer additional treatment options and may reduce healthcare costs. Generic drugs and biosimilars are versions of brand-name drugs and may offer more affordable treatment choices to patients. Third-party payers, especially governments, increasingly promote the utilization of generic medicines to decrease the escalating healthcare expenditure and medicine expenditure (Choudhry et al. 2016; Hassali et al. 2014a; King and

---

M. I. Mohamed Ibrahim (✉) • A. Awaisu
College of Pharmacy, Qatar University, Doha, Qatar
e-mail: mohamedizham@qu.edu.qa

Z. Babar (ed.), *Global Pharmaceutical Policy*,
https://doi.org/10.1007/978-981-15-2724-1_3

Kanavos 2002). A generic medicine is defined as "a medication created to be the same as an existing approved brand-name drug in dosage form, safety, strength, route of administration, quality, and performance characteristics" (US FDA). According to the US FDA, it is "a pharmaceutical product, usually intended to be interchangeable with an innovator product that is manufactured without a license from the innovator company and marketed after the expiry date of the patent or other exclusive rights". A generic medicine is identical or bioequivalent to a brand-name medicine, i.e. the originator, in terms of dosage formulation, route of administration, safety profile, strength, quality, performance characteristics and intended use (Birkett 2003; Razmaria 2016).

Generic medicines are considered to be clinically interchangeable and have quality, efficacy and safety profiles similar to those of innovator branded medicines. However, they have lower acquisition costs than the originator branded medicines (Liberman and Roebuck 2010; Shafie and Hassali 2008). Therefore, generic medicines offer therapeutic outcomes similarly to branded medicines and lead to significant healthcare savings (Choudhry et al. 2016; Hassali et al. 2014a; King and Kanavos 2002). Therefore, the use of generic medicines is promoted in many developed and developing countries (King and Kanavos 2002), and generic medicines play a vital role in the efficient allocation and utilization of financial health resources for pharmaceuticals. Policies have been implemented to promote the utilization of generic medicines in many countries, including the US, European countries, and the UK. Previous reviews have reported on policy measures that address the supply chain and demand aspects and analysed how these measures impact the uptake of generic medicines in both low- and high-income countries (Dylst and Simoens 2010; Kaplan et al. 2012; King and Kanavos 2002).

A biosimilar is a generic version of a biological product or medicine (Kramer 2011). It is a biotechnologically manufactured product. Biological medicines offer treatment options for patients with chronic and often disabling disorders, such as cancers, diabetes and autoimmune disease. They comprise large and generally complex molecules that are produced from living organisms and prudently scrutinized to guarantee consistent quality. According to the FDA, "the biologic product is highly similar to the reference product notwithstanding minor differences in clinically inactive components and that there are no clinically meaningful differences between the biologic product and the reference product in terms of safety, purity, and potency of the product" (US FDA n.d.; EMA n.d.). A biosimilar is highly similar to a reference product that has been licensed for use (NHS England 2019). After expiry of the patent product, the biosimilar is submitted to regulatory agencies for marketing authorization, and the FDA reviews the molecular structure and bioactivity. Usually, studies are carried out to demonstrate that biosimilars are similar in terms of safety, potency and purity. Such studies look at the clinical aspects, immunogenicity, pharmacokinetics and pharmacodynamics of the biosimilar (US FDA n.d.). According to Knuts, the knowledge concerning immunogenicity, interchangeability and substitution is constantly evolving (Knuts 2016; EMA yr). The FDA ensures that biosimilars undergo a stringent process of evaluation to meet its higher standards. They must be manufactured in approved facilities, and they undergo post-marketing surveillance to ensure continued safety (US FDA n.d.). Biosimilar medicines are not considered generic equivalents to the originator biological medicine because the two products are similar but not identical, i.e. biosimilars are not exact versions of the originator (NHS England 2019).

Clinical, Economic and Social Aspects

In most jurisdictions, generic medicines have to be proven to be bioequivalent to their branded innovator counterparts. While bioequivalent generic medications exist for many original drug products, whether they are clinically equivalent remains a subject of controversy (Gothe et al. 2015). Although brand substitution with generic medications is a common cost-containment strategy in the healthcare system globally, the impact of this practice on clinical, economic and patient-reported outcomes needs to be extensively and carefully explored (Choudhry et al. 2016; Gothe et al. 2015; Straka et al. 2017). Studies have investigated the clinical and economic impact of switching from brand-name to generic medicines in several therapeutic areas, and recent reviews have summarized them (Choudhry et al. 2016; Gothe et al. 2015; Straka et al. 2017). Commonly studied therapeutic classes in terms of clinical and economic outcomes include antiepileptics, antipsychotics, antiarrhythmics, anticoagulants, antihypertensives, antihypercholesterolemics and immunosuppressants.

In general, studies analysing the overall clinical and economic consequences of generic substitution are scarce. A 2015 review by Gothe and colleagues assessed whether generic substitution was associated with positive clinical and economic outcomes in ten therapeutic areas (Gothe et al. 2015). The clinical outcomes included, but were not limited to, medication adherence, adverse drug events, dosage adjustment and concomitant therapy. On the other hand, economic outcomes included drug acquisition costs, healthcare utilization (i.e. outpatient and inpatient service costs) and copayments. The investigators found that in 67% of the 97 reported clinical outcome comparisons, the clinical effects were not significantly different between generic drugs and their off-patent branded counterparts. Conversely, in 64% of 22 reported economic comparisons, generic substitution practice was associated with higher costs of care. Therefore, in the absence of well-designed studies comparing one generic product to another, generic substitution cannot guarantee cost savings.

Although generic medications may represent appropriate alternatives to branded medications, this is not always the case. For instance, the safety of substituting generics for branded drugs with narrow therapeutic indices, such as digoxin, antiepileptics, anticoagulants, antiarrhythmic drugs and thyroid medications, has been a much-debated and controversial issue. This suggests the need for an evidence base to demonstrate the impact of generic substitution on clinical and economic outcomes. In a more recent review, Straka et al. found that generic substitution may negatively impact medication adherence and may be associated with poorer clinical outcomes and more adverse events (Straka et al. 2017). Furthermore, generic switching may sometimes result in an increased total cost of care due to increased incidence of physician office visits or hospitalizations.

A meta-analysis by Kesselheim et al. summarized the clinical evidence of safety and effectiveness between generic and brand-name medications for cardiovascular diseases (Kesselheim et al. 2008). The study included 47 studies (38 RCTs) covering nine classes of cardiovascular medications (diuretics, β-blockers, statins, calcium channel blockers, antiplatelet agents, angiotensin-converting enzyme inhibitors, anticoagulants, α-blockers and antiarrhythmic drugs). The authors found clinical equivalence in most of the RCTs included in the review. The aggregate effect size indicated no evidence of superiority of brand-name medications over generic medications. Therefore, the evidence base does not support the notion that branded medications are superior to generic drugs used in cardiovascular disease management. Despite this, more than half (53%) of 43 editorials noted negative views about generic medicines or generic substitution. In fact, most editorials advocate against the interchangeability of branded vs. generic drugs.

Furthermore, Kesselheim et al. conducted a systematic review and meta-analysis to determine whether brand-name antiepileptic drugs were superior to generics in maintaining seizure control (Kesselheim et al. 2010). The review included 15 studies (9 RCTs and 6 observational studies). In the meta-analysis of seven RCTs, the authors found no difference in the odds of uncontrolled seizure for patients receiving generic medications when compared with those receiving brand-name medications (aggregate odds ratio, 1.1; 95% CI, 0.9–1.2). On the other hand, the observational studies included in the review showed some trends in terms of health resource utilization and adverse events. In an earlier systematic review of 70 studies, Crawford and associates explored the potential problems with generic switching of antiepileptic drugs and found potential therapeutic failure associated with increased risk of seizure frequency and potential for adverse drug events as well as variation in response to the generic antiepileptic drugs (Crawford et al. 2006).

Previous observational studies, mainly questionnaire-based surveys among healthcare professionals and patients, have reported varying results (i.e. both positive and negative findings). For instance, some studies have reported a negative impact of generic substitution on adherence to drug therapy and noted negative perceptions of patients and healthcare professionals towards generic medicines. Some concerns raised are related to the safety and efficacy of the generic medicines and the confusion experienced by some patients. One systematic review of 52 observational studies investigated the perceptions about generic medicines among patients and the lay public, physicians and pharmacists (Colgan et al. 2015). A large proportion of physicians, pharmacists and laypeople held negative perceptions of generic medicines. In this review, laypeople were significantly more likely to view generic medications as less effective than branded medications compared to doctors and pharmacists. Surprisingly, pharmacists were significantly more likely to view generics as of inferior quality compared to branded medications than doctors and laypeople. Furthermore, pharmacists and physicians had significantly greater safety concerns about generic medicines than did the general public. Overall, a greater proportion of laypeople held negative views about generic substitution policy or practice compared to the professional groups. However, these findings from aggregated observational data should be interpreted with caution, given that the included studies are very heterogeneous, the sampling techniques are very diverse and the tools used to evaluate perceptions are highly varied. Toverud et al. (2015) conducted a systematic review of physicians' and pharmacists' perspectives on the use of generic medicines globally (Toverud et al. 2015). Generally, physicians and pharmacists indicated awareness of the cost-saving advantages of generic medications and their important role in improving access to medicines. However, the 24 studies presented clear differences between developed and developing countries regarding physicians' and pharmacists' perceptions of generic drugs, where the professionals in developed healthcare systems trusted the quality of the generic medicines and offered them to patients regardless of their socioeconomic status. Moreover, pharmacists appeared to have better knowledge of the concept of bioequivalence and other aspects of generic medicines than physicians. These findings are also in concert with those of Hassali et al., who documented the perspectives of physicians towards generic medicines in low- and middle-income countries (LMICs) compared with high-income countries (Hassali et al. 2014b). The reviewers noted the main difference that physicians from high-income countries generally demonstrated positive views and attitudes regarding generic medicines, while those from LMICs had mixed views (Hassali et al. 2014b).

Biosimilars have great potential to treat all kinds of diseases, including cancer (Reno 2018). Biosimilars that go through a lengthy review by the FDA provide the same benefits for patients as the original drug. A clinician in consultation with the patient may decide to prescribe a biological medicine for an individual patient, whether an originator or biosimilar medicine. When dispensing, the pharmacist should not automatically substitute a biosimilar medicine for the originator (NHS England 2019). Choy and Jacobs (2014) emphasized that biosimilars must be approximately identical to their reference biologics in terms of efficacy, side effect risk profile and immunogenicity. Furthermore, immunogenicity is a main element throughout the stepwise biosimilar development process (Choy and Jacobs 2014). Reinisch and Smolen (2015) stressed that safety concerns, including hypersensitivity reactions, immunogenicity and an increased risk for other adverse effects, are vital aspects of the development of biosimilars. A systematic review was carried out by Feagan and co-workers (2019) to evaluate the evidence assessing the efficacy and safe of switching between biosimilar and reference infliximab in patients with various disorders. The findings have not indicated significant risks related to a single switch between biosimilar and reference infliximab. The authors also suggested for more data due to the lack of experimental studies to generate high level of evidence. Another systematic review conducted showed that the results provide reassurance that the risk of immunogenicity-related safety concerns or diminished efficacy is unchanged after switching from a reference biologic to a biosimilar medicine (Cohen et al. 2018). They also reported that most of the publications did not report differences in immunogenicity, safety or efficacy. It is challenging to develop a biosimilar with a safety profile similar to that of the reference product due to the complex molecular structure and manufacturing procedure involved. Furthermore, the molecular structure of biologic products is sensitive to changes in formulation, packaging and storage. An immune response may lead to altered efficacy (i.e. modified or loss of effect, cross-reaction with endogenous protein, altered pharmacokinetics) or compromised safety (i.e. anaphylaxis, hypersensitivity reactions and infusion reactions) (Schellekens 2002; Purcell and Lockey 2008).

A biosimilar must undergo additional testing to be considered interchangeable. According to the US FDA (n.d.), a biosimilar must have clinical efficacy equivalent to that of its reference product, and there must be no changes in safety or efficacy when switching between the biosimilar and its reference product. Small changes in the production and purification process of the biological can have major implications for its safety and effectiveness profile. The purpose of ensuring that a biosimilar is substitutable is to allow switching without referring to the physician. As mentioned by Yoo (2014), the main concerns raised regarding biosimilars are immunogenicity, efficacy, adverse effects when switching from a biologic to a biosimilar and possible long-term effects.

The interchangeability of biologics and biosimilars requires further study. The case of switching from a biosimilar to a biologic if the biosimilar does not produce significant clinical improvement should also be explored, especially in view of the number of biologic-naïve patients who may start with a biosimilar rather than with biologic therapy (Yoo 2014). One concern with switching is the inadequate data concerning disease-specific pharmacokinetics and dynamics (van Bodegraven and Boone 2018); more information is needed regarding switching between biosimilars and originator biologic agents (Feagan 2017). To ensure that a biosimilar reaches its potential in ordinary clinical use, an intensive post-licensing monitoring system must be established. This is the only way to establish the true similarity between the original biologic and its biosimilar (Pineda et al. 2015).

Another challenge with biosimilars is the nocebo effect, which is "a negative effect of a pharmacological or non-pharmacological medical treatment that is induced by patients' expectations, and that is unrelated to the physiological action of the treatment" (Pouillon et al. 2018). This type of negative placebo effect and presumably psychogenic aspect may compromise the benefits of biosimilars. It may be observed as an unexplained, unfavourable therapeutic effect that arises after switching and that disappears after reinitiating the originator and regaining the beneficial effects. Nocebo effects are independent of a (biological) compound and may be explained by study design, therapeutic effectiveness, and patients' and physicians' knowledge and expectations (van Bodegraven and Boone 2018).

The high cost of biologics has become a central issue in the effort to control healthcare costs (Blackstone and Joseph 2013). The high costs of biologics often limit their sustainable accessibility to patients, even though they have proven to be effective in treating or managing many diseases (Kaida-Yip et al. 2018). Biologic drugs have become a burden on pharmacy budgets in most countries, especially LMICs (Feagan 2017). As mentioned above, biosimilars are not generic drugs—they are highly similar to the originator biologic agents but are less expensive (Feagan 2017; EMA n.d.). Biosimilars go through fewer clinical trials than do their reference biologics, although the manufacturing process still involves production within living cells. This eventually decreases the production cost and the biosimilar drug cost compared to the reference biologic (Kaida-Yip et al. 2018). Biosimilars are less costly than originator biologic agents primarily because they do not have to undergo the intensive clinical development process associated with the approval of an originator. Furthermore, biosimilars do not incur high costs for marketing, market access and post-marketing research and development. These differences yield an opportunity for savings, which can potentially be passed onto consumers and payers (Feagan 2017).

A biosimilar that is produced at a lower cost than its originator can, by reducing costs, ensure accessibility to patients without compromising effectiveness, quality and safety (Camila do Reis et al. 2016). Liu et al. (2019) conducted a systematic review to study the economic impact of non-medical switching from biologic originators to their biosimilars. Cost estimation/simulation studies demonstrated the cost reduction associated with non-medical switching. It is reported that the economic impacts of biosimilar non-medical switching separately from drug costs are emerging. Those that reported such results found increased healthcare resource utilization in patients with biosimilar non-medical switching.

According to Crespi-Lofton and Skelton (2017), although the potential benefits of biosimilars are clear, certain factors may limit their uptake. These barriers include prescriber-pharmacist communication, legislation and regulations, technology, limited patient and healthcare practitioner knowledge and perceptions of biological products and scientific advancement or lack of long-term data. Smeeding et al. (2019) listed several key considerations for assessing biosimilar uptake, i.e. clinical efficacy, toxicity and immunogenicity, supplier manufacturing ability, cost savings to payer and supplier reliability. Generally, patient acceptance of biosimilars will depend on the ease of the physicians in prescribing biosimilars and educating patients about them. Physicians' confidence in biosimilars will depend on additional clinical trials and the amount of available data. Improving insurance coverage of new biosimilars will also increase patient access to biosimilars (Kaida-Yip et al. 2018). Physician awareness of the similarities and differences between original biopharmaceuticals and biosimilars, as well as their impact on efficacy and safety, is crucial. Stringent pharmacovigilance procedures and strategies (i.e. safety specifications, pharmacovigilance plans, evaluation of the need for risk minimization activities and risk minimization plans) are required to detect potential differences in safety signals between biosimilars and their reference products. Such activities permit national authorities to determine a drug's performance in the marketplace (Calvo and Zuniga 2011; Casadevall et al. 2013).

Policies in Relation to Generic Medicines and Biosimilars

To promote the uptake and quality use of generic medicines, relevant regulations and policy recommendations have to be in place. Some commonly reported policies for promoting the uptake and use of generic medicines globally include the following: bioequivalence testing, marketing application prior to patent expiry of the innovator product, reference pricing, financial incentives for pharmacists, physician budgets, new information technology systems for prescribing, generic substitution and prescribing policy and patient copayments (Dylst et al. 2013; Kaplan et al. 2012; King and Kanavos 2002). Typically, countries and healthcare systems use a combination of these policies to promote the use of generics and achieve better health outcomes and optimal cost savings (Choudhry et al. 2016, Dylst et al. 2013). Policy measures for the promotion and greater use of generic medicines can be broadly categorized into supply-side measures and demand-side measures (Dylst and Simoens 2010; Dylst et al. 2013; King and Kanavos 2002). Key policy measures related to supply include generic drug marketing regulation, reference pricing, pricing of branded originator products and monitoring the degree of price competition in pharmaceutical markets (King and Kanavos 2002). On the other hand, policy measures related to demand include policies influencing prescribing and dispensing practices and copayment regulations that account for the difference in price between branded and generic medicines (Dylst et al. 2013; King and Kanavos 2002). Nevertheless, it is challenging to quantify the monetary savings for the healthcare system attributable to these broad categories.

Regulatory approvals of market generic medicines are reported to have a direct impact on competition in the pharmaceutical market (King and Kanavos 2002). The competition is driven by the timing of the application for generic approval and the time needed to process the application. In North America and some European countries, the activities required to secure the regulatory authorization to market generic medicines include bioequivalence studies, and the application for approval should be submitted prior to the expiration of exclusivity rights. This timing enables the manufacturers of generic medicines to compete in the post-patent market in an expedited manner, resulting in price competition and lowering the prices of the medication in question. In the US, drug application approval times are also significantly reduced through the FDA Abbreviated New Drug Application (ANDA). In this approval process, generic manufacturers are not required to include preclinical and clinical data for safety and effectiveness (US FDA).

Furthermore, some countries with well-established pharmaceutical markets may impose regulations on pharmaceutical prices, including the prices of generic medicines. Such countries may also establish a reference price system for patent-expired substances. Many European countries, including the UK, have various regulatory mechanisms in place to control the prices of new medicines and generics (King and Kanavos 2002). In addition to promoting cost savings, such measures related to price controls on generic medicines may counteract the potential adverse demand and supply problems. Some healthcare systems also regulate the reimbursement of pharmaceuticals to promote the use of generic medicines. One approach is through reference pricing, in which similar products are grouped together, and a relative price to be reimbursed by health insurance schemes is determined.

Demand-side policies for generic medicines may be implemented to elicit a response from physicians, pharmacists and patients (Dylst et al. 2013). Financial incentives target physicians and, increasingly, pharmacists. On the other hand, one of the approaches to persuade patients is through cost payment that favours generic medicines. In particular, pharmacists may receive discounts and rebates from wholesalers and/or manufacturers as an incentive to dispense one drug over another. Another important measure is generic substitution policy, which allows a pharmacist to dispense a generic version of a brand-name medicine, even when a physician has prescribed the brand-name drug (Posner and Griffin 2011; Royal Dutch Pharmacists Association 2012). Pharmacists may be accorded wide or limited/restricted authority concerning generic substitution, which differs across countries. Studies have shown that patients respond positively to generic substitution, particularly when a copayment is required for a more expensive branded product (Dylst et al. 2013, Young 1994).

Policies to promote the use of generic medicines and their enforcement are somewhat variable between developed and developing economies. King and Kanavos (2002) reviewed the generic medicine policies implemented in countries with a high rate of generic drug use with consideration of market structures that facilitate strong competition. Significant savings are achieved in these countries as a result of the significant price differences between brand-name and generic medicines. Hassali et al. (2014a) reviewed the role of generic medicine policies in the healthcare systems in eight countries (Australia, Finland, Japan, Malaysia, Sweden, Thailand, the UK and the US) (Hassali et al. 2014a). They documented the different key policies adopted to promote generic medicines, such as generic substitution in the US, generic prescription in the UK and mandatory generic substitution in Finland and Sweden (Hassali et al. 2014a). They also identified barriers to and facilitators of the implementation of generic medicine policies and generic medicine use globally. Despite the existence of numerous policies promoting the use of generic medicines globally, a few policy evaluation studies seek to determine their impact on generic medicine utilization. A review undertaken to determine the impact of pro-generic policies on generic medicine utilization in LMICs found only a few relevant studies (Kaplan et al. 2012).

The increasing healthcare expenditure and the discrepancy between spending and achieved outcomes globally have made it necessary to use less costly but equally effective generic medicines instead of their innovator branded counterparts. Supply-side and demand-side generic medicine policies are complementary and should be used in combination for synergy. Policies to increase the financial responsibility of healthcare systems and facilitate the prescription of generic medicines should be advocated and adopted globally.

The development of a biosimilar follows a scientifically rigorous step-wise process. In addition, a biosimilar follows a totality-of-the-evidence approach that emphasizes biologic, physicochemical and preclinical studies to establish biosimilarity, with clinical development focused on confirming and resolving any uncertainties regarding biosimilarity (US FDA 2012, 2014). To meet the FDA requirements, clinical development of the biosimilar begins with studies to show comparable pharmacokinetics and pharmacodynamics with the reference product in a relevant population (US FDA 2014). Once pharmacokinetic, pharmacodynamic and immunogenicity similarity to the reference product has been demonstrated, at least one phase 3 clinical comparability trial is conducted to confirm similar efficacy and safety in a sensitive population (Berghout 2011). Alten and Cronstein (2015) mentioned that the key considerations in evaluating phase 3 clinical studies of biosimilars are safety, efficacy, patient population, dose, comparability, power/sample size, endpoints, study duration and statistical analysis. The expiration of patents for biologics removes a barrier to the development and commercialization of biosimilars. The barriers to biosimilar entry into the marketplace are much more difficult to overcome than those faced by generic manufacturers (Blackstone and Joseph 2013). Biologics are produced from living organisms; thus, the related manufacturing issues are more important than those in the chemical drug market. In the US and Europe, biosimilar drugs must undergo structural analyses, functional assays, animal studies and clinical studies. Throughout each step of the abbreviated approval process, the biosimilar drug is compared to its reference biologic and assessed for similarity (Kaida-Yip et al. 2018). Smeeding et al. (2019) highlighted significant concerns in addition to cost that payers should consider when evaluating biosimilars. These considerations are safety, analytical/functional similarity, and efficacy, the potential added value beyond cost and manufacturing considerations, including the reliability of logistics and supply.

Conclusions

In summary, biosimilars, such as lower-cost biologics and generic medicines, have the potential to improve patient access to high-level drug therapies and alleviate the financial strain chronic illnesses represent for healthcare systems worldwide. Numerous aspects, such as safety, pricing, manufacturing, entry barriers, physician acceptance and marketing, make the biosimilar market develop differently from the generic market. The high cost to enter the market and the size of the biologic drug market make entry attractive but risky. Another limitation of biosimilars and generic medicines is physician and patient recognition and approval, with many patients favouring to stay on biologics and physicians desiring to prescribe biologics. There is a need to create trust among physicians. For supporting a sustainable biosimilar and generic medicines market, gain sharing can be used as an incentive to prescribe, dispense or use these products.

Patient access to cost-effective and safe treatment is a main aim for the healthcare system. With the growing availability and use of biosimilars and generic medicines, including those determined to be interchangeable, the possibility to reduce costs and improve patient access to treatment grows. Nevertheless, the size of such growth is, in part, dependent on various stakeholders' decisions to provide, pay for and use these products in a safe and considerate manner. Continuing stakeholder cooperation, educational activities and review of current government and payer policies are essential to optimize the uptake of generic medicines and biosimilars.

Important Links and Websites

Below are a few important links for further reading:

US Food & Drug Administration. Generic Drugs.https://www.fda.gov/drugs/buying-using-medicine-safely/generic-drugs

US Food & Drug Administration. Generic Drugs: Questions & Answers. https://www.fda.gov/drugs/questions-answers/generic-drugs-questions-answers

The Association for Accessible Medicines. Generic Medicines. https://accessiblemeds.org/generic-medicines

Generics and Biosimilars Initiative Journal: http://gabi-journal.net/

Guidelines for Substitution of Generics in the Netherlands http://www.gabionline.net/layout/set/print/Guidelines/Guidelines-for-substitution-of-generics-in-The-Netherlands

Davit et al. Comparing generic and innovator drugs: a review of 12 years of bioequivalence data from the United States Food and Drug Administration. Ann Pharmacother. 2009;43(10):1583–97. Available at: https://doi.org/10.1345/aph.1M141

IQVIA Institute for Human Data Science: Reports. Available from: https://www.iqvia.com/institute/reports/reports-archive

The Center for Biosimilars. Available at: https://www.centerforbiosimilars.com/news/nhs-publishes-update-on-the-use-of-biosimilars

United States Food & Drug Administration. Available at: https://www.fda.gov/drugs/therapeutic-biologics-applications-bla/biosimilars

Dove Medical Press. Available at: https://www.dovepress.com/biosimilars-archive113

The Pharmaceutical Journal. Available at: https://www.pharmaceutical-journal.com/104319.subject?firstPass=false

References

Birkett, D. J. 2003. Generics – equal or not? *Australian Prescriber* 26, 85–87.

Choudhry, N. K., Denberg, T. D. & Qaseem, A. 2016. Improving Adherence to Therapy and Clinical Outcomes While Containing Costs: Opportunities From the Greater Use of Generic Medications: Best Practice Advice From the Clinical Guidelines Committee of the American College of Physicians. *Ann Intern Med,* 164, 41–9.

Colgan, S., Faasse, K., Martin, L. R., Stephens, M. H., Grey, A. & Petrie, K. J. 2015. Perceptions of generic medication in the general population, doctors and pharmacists: a systematic review. *BMJ Open,* 5, e008915.

Crawford, P., Feely, M., Guberman, A. & Kramer, G. 2006. Are there potential problems with generic substitution of antiepileptic drugs? A review of issues. *Seizure,* 15, 165–76.

Dylst, P. & Simoens, S. 2010. Generic Medicine Pricing Policies in Europe: Current Status and Impact. *Pharmaceuticals (Basel, Switzerland)*, 3, 471–481.

Dylst, P., Vulto, A. & Simoens, S. 2013. Demand-side policies to encourage the use of generic medicines: an overview. *Expert Rev Pharmacoecon Outcomes Res*, 13, 59–72.

Gothe, H., Schall, I., Saverno, K., Mitrovic, M., Luzak, A., Brixner, D. & Siebert, U. 2015. The Impact of Generic Substitution on Health and Economic Outcomes: A Systematic Review. *Appl Health Econ Health Policy*, 13 Suppl 1, S21–33.

Hassali, M. A., Alrasheedy, A. A., Mclachlan, A., Nguyen, T. A., Al-Tamimi, S. K., Ibrahim, M. I. & Aljadhey, H. 2014a. The experiences of implementing generic medicine policy in eight countries: A review and recommendations for a successful promotion of generic medicine use. *Saudi Pharm J*, 22, 491–503.

Hassali, M. A., Wong, Z. Y., Alrasheedy, A. A., Saleem, F., Mohamad Yahaya, A. H. & Aljadhey, H. 2014b. Perspectives of physicians practicing in low and middle income countries towards generic medicines: a narrative review. *Health Policy*, 117, 297–310.

Kaplan, W. A., Ritz, L. S., Vitello, M. & Wirtz, V. J. 2012. Policies to promote use of generic medicines in low and middle income countries: a review of published literature, 2000–2010. *Health Policy*, 106, 211–24.

Kesselheim, A. S., Misono, A. S., Lee, J. L., Stedman, M. R., Brookhart, M. A., Choudhry, N. K. & Shrank, W. H. 2008. Clinical equivalence of generic and brand-name drugs used in cardiovascular disease: a systematic review and meta-analysis. *Jama*, 300, 2514–26.

Kesselheim, A. S., Stedman, M. R., Bubrick, E. J., Gagne, J. J., Misono, A. S., Lee, J. L., Brookhart, M. A., Avorn, J. & Shrank, W. H. 2010. Seizure outcomes following the use of generic versus brand-name antiepileptic drugs: a systematic review and meta-analysis. *Drugs*, 70, 605–21.

King, D. R. & Kanavos, P. 2002. Encouraging the use of generic medicines: implications for transition economies. *Croat Med J*, 43, 462–9.

Liberman, J. N. & Roebuck, M. C. 2010. Prescription drug costs and the generic dispensing ratio. *J Manag Care Pharm*, 16, 502–6.

Posner, J. & Griffin, J. P. 2011. Generic substitution. *British journal of clinical pharmacology*, 72, 731–732.

Razmaria, A. A. 2016. Generic Drugs Generic Drugs JAMA Patient Page. *JAMA*, 315, 2746–2746.

Royal Dutch Pharmacists Association 2012. Guideline for generic substitution. The Hague, The Netherlands.

Shafie, A. A. & Hassali, M. A. 2008. Price Comparison between Innovator and Generic Medicines Sold by Community Pharmacies in the State of Penang, Malaysia. *Journal of Generic Medicines,* 6**,** 35–42.

Straka, R. J., Keohane, D. J. & Liu, L. Z. 2017. Potential Clinical and Economic Impact of Switching Branded Medications to Generics. *Am J Ther,* 24**,** e278–e289.

Theodorou, M., Tsiantou, V., Pavlakis, A., Maniadakis, N., Fragoulakis, V., Pavi, E. & Kyriopoulos, J. 2009. Factors influencing prescribing behaviour of physicians in Greece and Cyprus: results from a questionnaire based survey. *BMC Health Serv Res,* 9**,** 150.

Toverud, E. L., Hartmann, K. & Hakonsen, H. 2015. A Systematic Review of Physicians' and Pharmacists' Perspectives on Generic Drug Use: What are the Global Challenges? *Appl Health Econ Health Policy,* 13 Suppl 1**,** S35–45.

Us Food & Drug Administration. *What standards must generic medicines meet to receive FDA approval?* [Online]. Available: https://www.fda.gov/drugs/questions-answers/generic-drugs-questions-answers [Accessed].

Young, J. D. 1994. Prescribing generic drugs. *The British journal of general practice: the journal of the Royal College of General Practitioners,* 44**,** 139–140.

Alten, R, Cronstein, BN. Clinical trial development for biosimilars. Seminars in Arthritis and Rheumatism 2015; 44:S2–S8. doi:https://doi.org/10.1016/j.semarthrit.2015.04.002.

Berghout, A. Clinical programs in the development of similar biotherapeutic products: Rationale and general principles. Biologicals. 2011 Sep;39(5):293–6. doi:https://doi.org/10.1016/j.biologicals.2011.06.024

Blackstone, EA, Joseph, PF. The economics of biosimilars. Am Health Drug Benefits. 2013 Sep;6(8):469–78. https://www.ncbi.nlm.nih.gov/pubmed/24991376

Calvo, B, Zuniga, L. InTech. Risk management plan and pharmacovigilance system- biopharmaceuticals: biosimilars, http://www.intechopen.com/books/risk-management-trends/risk-managementplan-and-pharmacovigilance-system-biopharmaceuticals-biosimilars; 2011

Casadevall, N, Edwards, IR, Felix, T, Graze, PR, Litten, JB, Strober, BE, Warnock, DG. Pharmacovigilance and biosimilars: considerations, needs and challenges. Expert Opin Biol Ther. 2013 Jul;13(7):1039–47. doi: https://doi.org/10.1517/14712598.2013.783560.

Choy, E, Jacobs, IA. Biosimilar safety considerations in clinical practice. Safety issues – Semin Oncol. 2014 Feb;41 Suppl 1:S3–14. doi: https://doi.org/10.1053/j.seminoncol.2013.12.001.

Cohen, HP, Blauvelt A, Rifkin RM, Danese S, Gokhale SB, Woollett G. Switching Reference Medicines to Biosimilars: A Systematic Literature Review of Clinical Outcomes. Drugs. 2018 Mar;78(4):463–478. doi: https://doi.org/10.1007/s40265-018-0881-y.

Crespi-Lofton, J, Skelton, JB. The growing role of biologics and biosimilars in the United States: Perspectives from the APhA Biologics and Biosimilars Stakeholder. J Am Pharm Assoc (2003). 2017 Sep – Oct;57(5):e15–e27. doi: https://doi.org/10.1016/j.japh.2017.05.014.

do REIS, C, Ricardo, T, Fernando, M, Rui Santos, C. Biosimilar medicines – Review. International Journal of Risk and Safety in Medicine, 2016 vol. 28, no. 1, pp. 45–60, 2016. DOI: https://doi.org/10.3233/JRS-160672

European Medicines Agency (EMA). Biological medicine. https://www.ema.europa.eu/en/glossary/biological-medicine

European Medicines Agency (EMA). Improving understanding of biosimilars in the EU. 13/09/2018. https://www.ema.europa.eu/en/news/improving-understanding-biosimilars-eu

European Medicines Agency (EMA). Biosimilar medicines: Overview. https://www.ema.europa.eu/en/human-regulatory/overview/biosimilar-medicines-overview (n.d.)

Feagan, B. Benefits, concerns, and future directions of biosimilars in inflammatory bowel disease. Gastroenterol Hepatol (N Y). 2017;13(12):745–747. https://www.ncbi.nlm.nih.gov/pmc/articles/PMC5763561/

Feagan, BG, Lam, G, Ma, C, Lichtenstein, GR. Systematic review: efficacy and safety of switching patients between reference and biosimilar infliximab. Aliment Pharmacol Ther. 2019 Jan;49(1):31–40. doi: https://doi.org/10.1111/apt.14997

Kaida-Yip, F, Deshpande, K, Saran, T, Vyas, D. Biosimilars: Review of current applications, obstacles, and their future in medicine. World J Clin Cases. 2018;6(8):161–166. doi:https://doi.org/10.12998/wjcc.v6.i8.161. https://www.ncbi.nlm.nih.gov/pmc/articles/PMC6107532/

Knuts, B. Biosimilars, no generic biologicals! J Pharm Belg. 2016 Dec;(4):24–29;

Kramer, I. Biosimilars. Ther Umsch. 2011 Nov;68(11):659–66. doi: https://doi.org/10.1024/0040-5930/a000227.

Liu, Y, Yang, M, Garg, V, Wu, EQ, Wang, J, Skup, M. Economic impact of non-medical switching from originator biologics to biosimilars: a systematic literature review. Advances in Therapy August 2019, Volume 36, Issue 8, pp 1851–1877

NHS England. What is a Biosimilar Medicine? Medicines and Diagnostics Policy Unit, Specialised Commissioning, NHS England and NHS Improvement. 30 May 2019. https://www.england.nhs.uk/wp-content/uploads/2015/09/biosimilar-guide.pdf.

Pineda, C, Caballero-Uribe, CV, de oliveira, MG, Lipszyc, PS, Lopez, JJ, Moreira, MMM, Azevedo, VF. Recommendations on how to ensure the safety and effectiveness of biosimilars in Latin America: a point of view. Clin Rheumatol (2015) 34:635–640. DOI https://doi.org/10.1007/s10067-015-2887-0

Pouillon, L, Socha, M, Demore, B, Thilly, N, Abitbol, V, Danese, S & Peyrin-Biroulet, L. The nocebo effect: a clinical challenge in the era of biosimilars. Expert Review of Clinical Immunology 2018;14:739–49. DOI: https://doi.org/10.1080/1744666X.2018.1512406

Purcell, RT, Lockey, RF. Immunologic responses to therapeutic biologic agents. J Investig Allergol Clin Immunol 2008;18:335–42.

Reinisch, W, Smolen, J. Biosimilar safety factors in clinical practice. Seminars in Arthritis and Rheumatism 2015; 44: S9–S15.

Reno, J. Biosimilar drugs could save money and lives. So why don't we use them? July 27, 2018. https://www.healthline.com/health-news/biosimilar-drugs-save-money-and-lives-why-dont-we-use-them#1

Schellekens, H. Bioequivalence and the immunogenicity of biopharmaceuticals. Nature Reviews Drug Discovery 2002; 1:457–462.

Smeeding, J, Malone, DC, Ramchandani, M, Stolshek, B, Green, L, Schneider, P. Biosimilars: Considerations for Payers. P T. 2019;44(2):54–63.

United States Food and Drug Administration (US FDA). Scientific Considerations in Demonstrating Biosimilarity to a Reference Product. http://www.fda.gov/downloads/Drugs/GuidanceComplianceRegulatoryInformation/Guidances/UCM291128.pdf

United States Food and Drug Administration (US FDA). What is biosimilar. https://www.fda.gov/media/108905/download

United States Food and Drug Administration (US FDA). Biological Product Definitions. Available from: https://www.fda.gov/downloads/Drugs/DevelopmentApprovalProcess/HowDrugsareDevelopedandApproved/ApprovalApplications/TherapeuticBiologicApplications/Biosimilars/UCM581282.pdf

United States Food and Drug Administration (US FDA). Guidance for industry. Clinical pharmacology data to support a demonstration of biosimilarity to a reference product. 2014. http://www.fda.gov/downloads/drugs/guidancecomplianceregulatoryinformation/guidances/ucm397017.pdf.

United States Food and Drug Administration (US FDA). Guidance for industry. Scientific considerations in demonstrating biosimilarity to a reference product. 2012. http://www.fda.gov/downloads/Drugs/GuidanceComplianceRegulatoryInformation/Guidances/UCM291128.pdf.

van Bodegraven, A. A., Boone, N.W. Editorial: nocebo effect and switching to biosimilars. Alimentary Pharmacology & Therapeutics 2018;47:850–51. https://onlinelibrary.wiley.com/doi/full/10.1111/apt.14509.

Yoo, DH. The rise of biosimilars: potential benefits and drawbacks in rheumatoid arthritis. Expert Rev. Clin Immunol. 2014;10:981–983. https://www.ncbi.nlm.nih.gov/pmc/articles/PMC6107532/#B20

4

Global Access to Cancer Medicines

Hye-Young Kwon and Yujeong Kim

Introduction

Prevalence of Cancer

According to the WHO, cancer was the second leading cause of death in 2015 (World Health Organization 2018a), with the global cancer burden increasing to 18.1 million cases and 9.6 million cancer deaths worldwide (Bray et al. 2018). Nearly one in six deaths worldwide is due to cancer, and approximately 70% of these deaths occur in low- and middle-income

H.-Y. Kwon (✉)
School of Pharmacy, Seoul National University, Seoul, South Korea

Strathclyde Institute of Pharmacy and Biomedical Science, University of Strathclyde, Glasgow, UK

Y. Kim
School of Pharmacy, Ewha Woman's University, Seoul, South Korea

Health Insurance Review and Assessment Agency (HIRA), Wonju, South Korea

Z. Babar (ed.), *Global Pharmaceutical Policy*,
https://doi.org/10.1007/978-981-15-2724-1_4

countries (LMICs). The most commonly diagnosed cancer in the world was lung cancer (11.6% of the total cases), and it caused the highest proportion of deaths (18.4% of total cancer deaths) in 2014. The incidence of breast cancer was 11.6%, followed by colorectal (10.2%), prostate (7.1%), stomach (5.7%) and liver cancer (4.7%). Lung cancer had the highest mortality rate (18.4%), followed by colorectal (9.2%), stomach (8.2%), liver (8.2%) and breast cancers (6.6%) (World Health Organization. New Global Cancer Country Profiles [Internet] n.d.).

Globally, the cancer incidence rate and mortality rate varied across countries; within countries, these were related to the extent of economic development and social and lifestyle factors (Bray et al. 2018).

Regardless of the income level of countries, cancer mortality was generally high. In most cancer types, the incidence of cancer is two or three times higher in the high/very high Human Development Index (HDI)[1] countries compared to the low/medium HDI countries, but the difference in mortality between the two groups is less, because of the higher incidence of fatality in the low HDI countries (Bray et al. 2018).

Cancer incidence was 21.0% in America, 23.4% in Europe and 1.4% in Oceania; cancer mortality was 14.4% in America, 20.3% in Europe and 0.7% in Oceania. On the other hand, the incidence of cancer was 5.8% in Africa and 48.4% in Asia, and its mortality was 7.3% in Africa and 57.3% in Asia. Thus, the Global North[2] had a similar cancer incidence of cancer but a relatively low mortality rate compared to the Global South[3] (World Health Organization. New Global Cancer Country Profiles [Internet] n.d.). Cancer mortality rates of wealthy countries have been declining slightly due to screening, early detection, and

---

[1] HDI (Human Development Index): It is created by the United Nations Development Programme to highlight the importance of national policy decisions beyond economic growth in assessing development outcomes (United Nations Development Programme 2016). HDI can help identify cancer transitions and four-tier HDI was used to further assess the cancer burden according to a binary proxy of development (low and medium HDI vs. high and very high HDI).

[2] The Global North indicates high-income countries including the USA, Canada, Europe, developed parts of Asia (Japan, the Four Asian Tigers, Hong Kong, Singapore, South Korea and Taiwan), Australia and New Zealand.

[3] The Global South indicates low- and middle-income countries including Africa, Latin America, developing Asia and Middle East (Torre et al. 2016; Hoen 2014; Introduction: Concepts of the Global South (GSSC) n.d.; North And South, the (Global) [Internet] n.d.).

development and availability of treatment therapy, while they have been increasing in LMICs due to smoking, excess body weight and physical inactivity (Torre et al. 2016).

Currently, 14 million people are diagnosed with cancer annually, with expected increases to 19 million by 2025, 22 million by 2030 and 24 million by 2035. More than 60% of the world's cancer cases are from Africa, Asia and Latin America (Hoen 2014). Nonetheless, cancer treatments are not widely available in LMICs. According to the WHO (2002), only about 5% of the global resources for cancer are consumed in developing countries (Economist Intelligence Unit 2009), yet these countries accounted for 80% of the disability-adjusted years of life lost to cancer globally (World Health Organization. Metrics: Disability-Adjusted Life Year (DALY) [Internet] n.d.).

Cancer Therapy

Previously, chemotherapy was the mainstay of cancer treatment. However, recently, high-cost biological pharmaceuticals (e.g. monoclonal antibody) have been developed, resulting in cancer treatment becoming more expensive (e.g. annual course of the breast-cancer trastuzumab is up to $50,000 in the US) (Richardson 2013). In particular, the recent anticancer paradigm has become more expensive with the paradigm shift due to the development of personalized medicine through immuno-oncology and gene therapy (Quintiles IMS Institute 2017; Annadurai and Danasekaran 2016).

Between 2011 and 2016, a total of 68 new therapies for cancer treatment were approved for 22 indications worldwide, including immuno-oncology agents that revolutionized the therapeutic paradigm in many types of cancers and more than 600 molecules in late-stage development (Quintiles IMS Institute 2017). In particular, the immuno-oncology PD-1 (programmed cell death protein 1) and PD-L1 (programmed cell death-ligand 1) inhibitors have shown a rapid uptake based on the remarkable clinical profile and their success with multiple cancers (Quintiles IMS Institute 2017; Alsaab et al. 2017).

The availability of anticancer drugs varies greatly from region to region, with the majority of new cancer drugs being available in the US and Germany. It was observed that the listing of new cancer drugs varied from 61% to 100% in each country (Quintiles IMS Institute 2017). Spending on anticancer drugs and supportive oncology care has increased since 2011, and therapies launched over the last five years were estimated to account for more than 20% of global anticancer drug sales in 2016 (Quintiles IMS Institute 2017).

The global cost of anticancer therapeutics and supportive care drugs increased from $91 billion in 2012 to $113 billion in 2016; 46% of the total global oncology cost is borne by the US. The increase in costs in the US was mainly attributed to the availability of new drugs. The longer duration of treatment with new drugs, the use of combination therapy with high-cost new drugs and the potential for patients receiving multiple lines of treatment may have contributed to the additional costs. The use of newer drugs and the increase in the use of older branded medicines are factors contributing to the cost increase in other areas (Quintiles IMS Institute 2017).

The anticancer drug market is expected to grow by 6% to 9% annually by 2021; when global oncology costs exceed $147 billion, patent expiry and competition due to the entry of biosimilars will lower the cost (Quintiles IMS Institute 2017).

Characteristics of Cancer Drugs

Uncertainty in Effectiveness

In recent years, many anticancer drugs have been approved on the basis of uncontrolled study designs or surrogate endpoints that cannot guarantee a significant improvement in patients (Sacca n.d.; Prasad et al. 2015); some have been marketed on a fast track through conditional marketing authorization, which is yet to prove its efficacy for overall survival or quality of life through post-marketing studies. However, no substantive evidence has been found to indicate that any of these medicines prolonged or improved life after four years of market entry (Cohen 2017; FDA n.d.). Thus, there is clinical uncertainty about the long-term effect (e.g. overall survival) of several of these anticancer agents in real-world settings (Cohen 2017).

Davis et al. (2018) analysed 48 oncology drugs approved for 68 indications by the European Medicines Agency (EMA) from 2009 to 2013. Furthermore, they ascertained that there was no evidence for improvement in the quality of life or quality of life extension for 57% or 39 of these drugs over available alternatives (Madersbacher and Kramer 2018). Only anticancer drugs for 24 indications (35%) showed a significantly prolonged survival, with an average of 2.7 months (median) and a range of 1.0 to 5.8 months in overall survival. Fifty-seven percent of the indications were approved through a fast track, with efficacy presented through their surrogate variables (tumour size reduction or progression-free survival (PFS)) that replaced overall survival (OS) or quality-of-life indicators. However, whether their high prices are well-deserved is questionable since no clinical effects were seen.

A study on the cost-effectiveness of anticancer drugs conducted by Salas-Vega et al. (2017) found that new anticancer drugs did not always provide superior clinical benefit and safety over existing drugs (Salas-Vega et al. 2017). The study which analysed the overall survival and quality of life of 62 anticancer drugs approved by the US FDA and EMA between 2003 and 2013 revealed that the overall survival increased by 3.5 months on average. Among the drugs, 23 drugs extended survival for more than three months or longer and 6 for less than three months (Salas-Vega et al. 2017). There was no clear evidence of prolonging survival for approximately 30% of these anticancer drugs compared to the incumbent medicines. In particular, 16 of them did not demonstrate improvement of OS compared to existing alternatives (Salas-Vega et al. 2017).

High Prices

As mentioned above, the recently developed anticancer drugs do not have clear clinical effectiveness, but their prices are relatively high. In recent decades, cancer treatment costs, often reaching tens of thousands of US dollars per patient per year, have exceeded the costs of medicines used for treating other diseases (World Health Organization 2018b). The price of cancer drugs, for example, is growing at a higher rate than the public and private expenditure for healthcare, which is a challenge for healthcare systems and individuals even in high-income countries. The cost of anticancer drugs recently range from $5000 to $10,000 per month in the US (Fojo and Grady 2009). The unsustainability of the high prices of new medicines has become a global issue that hampers access to these medicines in LMICs as well as high-income countries (Hoen 2014). The biggest issue for accessibility to anticancer drugs is drug prices (Siddiqui and Rajkumar 2012). Pharmaceutical companies have claimed legitimacy for higher prices, citing the rationale for compensating for their investments for R&D of new products (Hoen 2014; Institute for New Economic Thinking 2017). However, the claim of pharmaceutical companies of higher prices for new medicines is not convincing, and there is a lack of transparency in the R&D costs of manufacturers (Hoen 2014). To address the high price problem, delinking R&D costs from the price of medicines and international collaboration for sharing costs for innovation have been proposed (Hoen 2014).

In most high-income countries, the government conducts the health technology assessment (HTA) on high-cost cancer drugs within the national health service or social health insurance to list financially affordable drugs (WHO Regional Office for Africa 2016). In terms of access to medicines, HTA agencies in each country address the issues pertaining to the uncertainty of clinical effectiveness and high cost that consequently attribute the financial uncertainty to the insurer or government (World Health Organization 2018b; Lopes et al. 2017).

Recently, the American Society of Clinical Oncology (ASCO) and the European Society for Medical Oncology (ESMO) have published the ASCO Value Framework and ESMO Magnitude of Clinical Benefit Scale, respectively, by defining the value of cancer drugs in systematic consideration of their clinical benefits, side effects and improvement in patient symptoms or quality of life in the context of cost in order to support the decision-making of clinical doctors and patients (Lin et al. 2018).

Uncertainty in Affordability

Even if the clinical benefits of some new anticancer drugs are doubtful, they will pose a financial risk due to their high prices, resulting in the risk of side effects for patients and waste of important social resources (Gammie et al. 2015). It is difficult to list the recent influx of high cost and clinically uncertain anticancer drugs based on the incremental cost-effective ratio (ICER) threshold when performing HTA, and the financial burden of these medicines is solely charged to the patients, which consequently results in a problem of access to cancer medicines. In order to facilitate access to these new cancer drugs, some countries have a separate programme (e.g. Cancer Drugs Fund (CDF) in the UK, Life Saving Drugs Program (LSDP) in Australia, a 5% independent Agenzia Italiana del Farmaco (AIFA) fund in Italy) or a special arrangement, such as managed entry agreements (MEAs) for sharing the risks embedded in new cancer drugs with the pharmaceutical companies.

Access to Cancer Medicines

Access to Medicines: Definition and Indicators

The WHO claims that access to medicines is a universal and basic right for people to attain a high standard of health. This is perceived as a part of the rights to health by international law since 1946 (World Health Organization n.d.). For access to medicines, the WHO specifies at a minimum the availability of high-quality and essential medicines (WHO. Essential Medicines [Internet] n.d.).

Availability, acceptability, accessibility and quality are elements that must be addressed when considering access to medicines (Perehudoff et al. 2016). Availability refers to the development, distribution and use of medicines and is directly related to factors such as the R&D of pharmaceuticals, marketing approval in domestics and supply shortage. Acceptability refers to the possibility of domestic acceptance, considering appropriate dosage, dose and cultural factors. Accessibility is a concept that includes physical accessibility, economic affordability and information accessibility that affect the use of medicines. Finally, quality is the assurance that the medicines are of high quality and will contribute to people's health and welfare (Bigdeli et al. 2013; Swiss Agency for Development and Cooperation (SDC) 2004).

Vogler and colleagues (2018) (World Health Organization/European Observatory 2018) defined access to medicines as ensuring that patients have timely and affordable access to the medicines that are safe and effective and highlighted the access to medicines in terms of pricing, reimbursement and procurement policies in the lifecycle of medicines (World Health Organization/European Observatory 2018). In particular, they further explored the policies related to access to medicines, including external reference pricing, MEAs, HTAs, horizon scanning, specific funds, amortization and tendering.

Ensuring timely and affordable access to safe and effective medicines is considered one of the three common objectives of the healthcare system, along with stimulating innovation that provides incentives for research that will lead to innovative medicines that effectively target real therapeutic needs and safeguard sustainability, which involves developing the mechanisms to purchase these medicines at affordable prices in order to protect the sustainability of pharmaceutical budgets (World Health Organization/European Observatory 2018).

Babar et al. (2019) considered the outcomes that affect access to medicines, which encompass both the availability and access to medicines as well those that enable an individual (financially and physically) to obtain and receive relevant care involving the respective medicine. In particular, they have classified the pharmaceutical policy that can affect the accessibility of medicines into three broad categories: the national health system, pricing and reimbursement. The following nine subcategories were then reviewed: national health policy, pharmacy system, marketing authorization and regulation, prescription non-prescription medicine switch, orphan drug policies, generic drug substitution, national pharmaceutical schedule and HTA, patient copayment and MEAs.

Current Status of Access to Cancer Medicines

Recently, access to high-cost anticancer drugs has become a major challenge in many countries, because of the lack of insurance coverage and the resulting financially unaffordable cost to patients. These medicines are often unavailable because the NHI system does not allow them to be listed based on the HTA (Blauvelt et al. 2018). This is more challenging in low-income countries. Consequently, access to anticancer drugs is a common issue for both the Global South and North where the high cost of these medicines is burdensome for all countries (Hoen 2014). Regarding access to cancer drugs, two factors, namely, affordability and availability, were reviewed by contrasting the difference in both the North and South to simplify the current aspect. These two terms were defined by the WHO (2018b):

- *Availability: Presence of medicines in national formulary available to patients for free or for a fixed fee*
- *Affordability: For the health system—Proportion of spending on cancer medicines compared to existing expenditure on medicines or other health products and services. For individual patients—The number of days' wages needed to pay for the cost of treatment*

Availability of Cancer Drugs

According to the report by IQVIA (2017) analysing 42 anticancer drugs launched between 2011 and 2015, the availability of these drugs varied geographically. The highest number of available products was 37 in the US and 35 in Germany and was significantly less in other developed countries (Quintiles IMS Institute 2017). Of 42 new cancer drugs, more than half have been launched across eight countries, indicating that access to novel oncology therapies is a continuing problem even in developed countries. The situation was even worse in emerging economies[4]

[4] The markets include China, Brazil, India, Russia, Mexico, Turkey, Poland, Saudi Arabia, Indonesia, Egypt, Philippines, Pakistan, Vietnam, Bangladesh, Argentina, Algeria, Colombia, South Africa, Chile, Nigeria and Kazakhstan, which were defined as pharmerging markets characterized by less

(Rickwood 2017). Only four of the new cancer drugs launched between 2011 and 2015 were available in India, Indonesia and China in 2016 (Quintiles IMS Institute 2017).

The most comprehensive assessment on the international availability of anticancer drugs was conducted in 49 European countries in 2014 (Cherny et al. 2016) and in 63 non-European countries in 2016 (Cherny et al. 2017), with an online survey of the availability of anticancer drugs in the national drug list. Two studies have shown that countries with low income, as indicated by gross domestic product (GDP) per capita, had lower availability of medicines, or availability only with higher patient out-of-pocket costs. In the high-income and upper middle-income countries, most of the medicines incorporated in the EML were listed and available to patients free-of-charge or on a subsidized basis. In particular, this tendency was significant for higher-cost medicines including medicines that require genetic profiling (e.g. trastuzumab and erlotinib) (Cherny et al. 2016; Cherny et al. 2017). LMICs have shown less accessibility, and even a generic version of anticancer drugs incorporated in the EML available in many countries must be paid for in full by the patients. According to the findings, 32% of cancer medicines listed in the EML were available in the lower middle-income countries, and 57.7% were available in low-income countries only when the patients bore all the costs. The two most frequently cited obstacles to listing on the national formulary to provide better access to medicines were the lack of reliable suppliers and budgetary restraints (Cherny et al. 2017). In addition, the price of anticancer drugs that the suppliers are willing to supply is higher than the price that can be paid in the healthcare system.

In conclusion, cancer patients in LMICs only have access to some of the cancer drugs listed on the EML and at full cost as an out-of-pocket expense, and the accessibility is limited by an unreliable supply. Moreover, in countries other than highly developed countries, recently approved medicines targeting metastatic cancers are often unavailable or available only when patients are charged more. This leads to profound inequity in access to cancer medicines.

---

than $30 k GDP per capita and greater than $1bn absolute prescription medicines market growth potential between 2014 and 2019 (World Health Organization 2018b).

Affordability of Anticancer Drugs

The expenditures of anticancer drugs are escalating faster than the increasing rate of cancer patients (World Health Organization 2018b). Globally, the upsurge of spending on cancer drugs has surpassed that of total health expenditures, especially in several low-income countries. The increase in spending on cancer drugs is attributed to the increase in drug prices. The prices and related costs of cancer medicines will not be affordable in the long term for healthcare systems worldwide.

When the cost of cancer medicines becomes unaffordable and unsustainable, health systems may be forced to restrict health expenditure by limiting demand and containing spending. In particular, the demand for pharmaceuticals in low-income countries is sensitive to changing prices. Thus, the increased price of cancer drugs may compel governments in low-income countries to reduce the procurement and supply of these medicines resulting in compromising the timely access to these medicines (FDA n.d.; England NHS2014). If these medicines are not covered by health insurance, the unaffordable prices will prevent these medicines from being used for a substantial portion of cancer patients. For example, the monthly costs of biological cancer medicines in Pakistan were higher than 20% of the monthly household income after spending on food (Saqib et al. 2018). Only 58.1% of non-biological cancer medicines were affordable (Saqib et al. 2018).

The per person budget for cancer drugs can be estimated by dividing the expenditure threshold of cancer drugs by the number of new cancer patients, assuming that the expenditure threshold could range from 1% to 5% of the total health expenditure. Accordingly, the per person budget for cancer drugs was estimated to range from $800 to $3800 in low-income countries, $1600 to $8000 in lower middle-income countries, $3100 to $15,600 in upper middle-income countries and $8100 to $40,600 in high-income countries (World Health Organization 2018b).

Upon calculating the estimated annual cost of standard treatment regimens for selected cancers based on the recommended dosage in the clinical guidelines and on the prices of the anticancer drugs, the estimated cost of treatment often exceeds annual budgets per patient despite the generous assumption that anticancer drugs alone consume 1% to 5% of total healthcare finances; the estimated cost of treatment often exceeds annual budgets per estimated patient (see Table 4.1) (World Health Organization 2018b).

Table 4.1 Estimated annual budget for, and costs of, cancer medicines per patient by country income level

Economic status	Standard regimen[a]	Low	Lower middle	Upper high	High
Selected countries		**India**	**South Africa**	**Australia**	**US**
Per patient budget		\$800–\$3800	\$1600–\$8000	\$3100–\$15,600	\$8100–\$40,600
Estimated annual costs of cancer medicines[b]					
Breast cancer Early stage HER2 positive	Doxorubicin, cyclophosphamide, docetaxel, trastuzumab [adjuvant AC-TH]	\$18,500	\$33,900	\$41,800	\$71,700
Colon cancer Stage III	Capecitabine, oxaliplatin [adjuvant CAPOX or XELOX]	\$2200	\$1300	\$1200	\$7300
Liver cancer Advanced	Sorafenib	\$700	\$12,700	\$28,700	\$90,800
Prostate cancer	Goserelin, bicalutamide	\$3600	\$3300	\$4100	\$7100
Castration-sensitive metastatic	Docetaxel [ADT plus DOCE]				
Lung cancer	Vinorelbine, cisplatin	\$1800	\$800	\$1200	\$500
Metastatic non-small cell	Erlotinib for EGFR positive	\$1700	\$27,300	\$13,400	\$76,700
Lymphoma Non-Hodgkin-diffuse large B-cell	Rituximab, cyclophosphamide, doxorubicin, vincristine, prednisolone [R-CHOP21]	\$6700	\$20,000	\$17,800	\$48,100
Leukaemia	Imatinib	\$800	\$13,300	\$23,200	\$96,700
Chronic myeloid	Dasatinib	\$800	\$20,000	\$40,200	\$109,400

Note: [a]Please refer to the WHO Essential Medicines List and clinical guidance for specific details of the treatment regimens. [b]Costs were estimated for a full-course or 12- month treatment. Cost calculations were based on body surface area of 1.8m^2 or body weight of 75 kg where necessary. Please note that the cost estimates are indicative only. Numbers represent US$ in 2016

Source: WHO (2018a), recomposed by authors

In fact, the nominal cost for the treatment was lower in low-income countries, while the cost of treatment adjusted with purchasing power parity (PPP) exceeded the estimated cost in high-income countries. This means that anticancer drugs are relatively more expensive in low-income countries when purchasing power is taken into account. Even when supported by an insurance scheme, patients often suffer from financial distress due to the high cost of anticancer drugs, especially for new drugs, so-called targeted cancer therapy. Consequently, the number of people who survive cancer is expected to increase over the next several decades, but if the current price trend persists, the unaffordability of anticancer drugs will worsen. Given the diverse evidence suggesting the unaffordability of anticancer drugs, governments and stakeholders should consider implementing policies that modify current high prices internationally (Huntington et al. 2015).

Efforts to Improve Access to Medicines

High-Income Countries

In order to solve the issues pertaining to the access to high-cost cancer medicines, high-income countries have adopted MEAs or a separate fund applicable to the medicines that are of a high cost or lack sufficient evidence on clinical efficacy due to the limited number of patients.

Managed Entry Agreements (MEAs)

MEAs (i.e. risk sharing agreements) can be defined as "an arrangement between a manufacturer and payer/provider that enables access to (coverage/reimbursement of) a health technology subject to specified conditions" (World Health Organization 2018b; World Health Organization/European Observatory 2018). These arrangements can use a variety of mechanisms to address uncertainty about the performance of technologies (e.g. clinical efficacy, efficacy and cost-effectiveness) and to manage the adoption of technologies in order to maximize their effective use or limit their budget impact (World Health Organization 2018b). MEAs facilitate access to high-cost medicines, particularly cancer drugs or orphan drugs. Two types of MEAs are available: financial-based and performance-based. The financial-based form typically specifies conditions that are directly related to drug prices, volume used or both. For example, Italian authorities have implemented "value-based pricing" as well as "price-volume agreements" to manage the prices of expensive, innovative drugs that involve large patient populations. This form is commonly applied for anticancer drugs in other European countries. MEAs generally impose confidential terms but entail discounts, rebates, free stock and capping of utilization to a threshold volume or number of patients.

On the other hand, the performance-based type requires payments to be contingent when achieving certain pre-agreed health outcomes or other milestones when implemented. For example, health authorities do not pay or provide discounts for patients who do not respond to treatment under performance-based MEAs. Data collected by setting up a registry or a phase IV clinical trial provides evidence for this. For example, the UK's National Institute for Health and Care Excellence (NICE) contracted with the manufacturer of bortezomib on the condition that the manufacturer would refund to the insurers, retrospectively, the costs of bortezomib for non-responders, while patients responding to medicines can be insured as usual.

According to Pauwels and colleagues' study (2017), among 164 cases of MEAs applied to cancer drugs in Europe, discounts (34%) were the most popular incentive followed by a money-back guarantee (22%), a free/discounted treatment initiation (19%), a patient utilization cap (4%), a combination of these mentioned factors (3%) or an outcome guarantee (1%). The remaining 18% of the cases were unknown owing to reasons of confidentiality (Pauwels et al. 2017).

The application of MEAs, especially performance-based MEAs to be robustly enforced, requires excellent governance. In order to avoid the unequal distribution of limited resources for complex monitoring and contract management, conditions need to be manageable from the implementation side. Thus, when implementing a performance-based approach, strong background support is required from the information infrastructure, including the use of electronic health records to monitor patient health performance (World Health Organization 2018b).

There are also challenges surrounding the MEAs, including achieving acceptable risk distribution to both manufacturers and regulators (e.g. certainty of future payoffs), linking research outcomes in a specific clinical context to pricing arrangements, minimizing potentially high transaction and administrative costs, discouraging pharmaceutical companies from seeking higher prices in expectation of the MEAs and implementing clinically and politically acceptable contracts for patients and physicians when abolishing the MEAs due to the failure to achieve a pre-agreed milestone (KCE 2018).

This agreement facilitates access to high-cost cancer drugs by helping patients receive insurance benefits and sharing the financial and clinical uncertainties embedded in the medicines between both manufacturers and insurers. However, this is also criticized for being a compromise wherein the insurer has adopted the high pricing strategy of pharmaceutical companies as a compliant.

Independent Funds

Apart from the national health benefit programme, the independent fund can be used for high-cost drugs. For example, the Cancer Drugs Fund (CDF) in the UK was established in 2010 to improve the accessibility to drugs (including anticancer drugs) that have not been evaluated, have been evaluated by the NICE but not recommended or are under evaluation (Aggarwal et al. 2017). This programme aims to improve the accessibility of cancer drugs within the NHS, reduce delays and provide funding for orphan indications or rare conditions that the NICE does not generally assess (Davies et al. 2012). Since 2010, the CDF has made treatments accessible to more than 55,000 patients. The CDF began with an initial budget of £50 million per annum in 2014. However, the cost of maintaining funds has risen sharply to £200 million in 2013/2014, £280 million in 2014/2015 and £340 million in 2015/2016. At the time of unification with NICE, the total budget of the CDF was £1.27 billion, which was equivalent to the one-year total spent on all cancer drugs in the NHS (2014).

There is a similar form of an independent fund in other countries for drugs that are not necessarily cancer drugs: the Life Saving Drugs Program (LSDP) in Australia (Australian Department of Health n.d.), the Special Drug Program (SDP) in Canada (Government of Canada n.d.), the 5% AIFA fund in Italy (AIFA 2019), the Contestable Fund for Medicines for Rare Disorders in New Zealand (PHARMAC n.d.), and the New Medicines Fund in Scotland (Scotland launches medicines fund for rare conditions [Internet] n.d.). These independent funds aim to improve patient access by funding high-cost medicines that are not suitable to the standard pharmaceutical benefit schemes within the national health service or insurance (Cherny et al. 2016; Cherny et al. 2017; Saqib et al. 2018; Huntington et al. 2015; Pauwels et al. 2017).

Low and Middle Income Countries (LMICs)

Low and Middle Income Countries (LMICs) have not systematically developed their healthcare system; often, no insurance benefits for medicines can be found. In addition, the manufacturing technology of pharmaceuticals, mainly concentrated in developed countries, is poor or even absent in LMICs. The supply and procurement of medicines are not performed sufficiently; thus, the availability of anticancer drugs is low (World Health Organizationt 2018b). The WHO's EML complementary contains only 9 (18%) of the 51 cancer drugs newly approved by the US FDA since 1995, including antineoplastics and immunosuppressives (World Health Organization 2017), implying a lack of available cancer drugs in these countries. Since it is difficult for LMICs to purchase new high-priced cancer drugs compared to high-income countries for economic reasons, traditional complementary, alternative medicines (TCAM) are mainly used (54.5%) for lower middle- and low-income countries; however, it is not easy to use even these medicines (Hill et al. 2019). Consequently, the supply of medicines is highly dependent on the official development assistance (ODA), but some countries have made efforts for the self-sufficiency of medicines, such as through compulsory licensing.

Compulsory Licensing

In some countries, the compulsory licensing of anticancer drugs has provided access to the drug at low prices to the public. However, this is allowed not in many countries. India and Thailand are the only countries that have granted compulsory licensing for pharmaceuticals (Hoen 2014).

In January 2013, India's Ministry of Health recommended compulsory licensing of three anticancer drugs to the Department of Industrial Policy and Promotion (DIPP): dasatinib, trastuzumab and ixabepilone (DIPP n.d.). The only case, however, where compulsory licensing was granted for pharmaceuticals in India was the case of sorafenib tosylate, a hepatocarcinogen, under Section 84 of the Indian Patents Act, at the request of the generic company Natco Ltd. in March 2012 (Official Journal of the Patent Office 2011).

According to the law, the Indian Patent Controller can file a counterclaim against patenting. Since 2006, generic companies and civic groups have successfully prevented the use of pre- and post-grant oppositions to grant anticancer patents. There were cases for imatinib (Glivec) and sunitinib (Sutent®) (Complete list of oppositions [Internet] n.d.). This resistant action towards patenting imatinib (Glivec®) fomented a fierce opposition from the US pharmaceutical industry and policymakers (170 Members of Congress Send Letter to Obama n.d.), and accordingly, the Alliance for Fair Trade with India was established focusing on India's intellectual property (IP) policy (US Businesses Launch Coalition For Fair Trade With India [Internet] n.d.).

In Thailand, from 2006 to 2008, seven drugs were granted compulsory licensing, four of which were anticancer drugs, namely, letrozole (early breast cancer), docetaxel (breast cancer), erlotinib (small-cell lung cancer) and imatinib (chronic myeloid leukaemia). Prior to compulsory licensing, a series of drug price negotiations were conducted with patent holders, but the proposed drug price cuts were not considered sufficient, or the added conditions were disallowed. However, the implementation of the government license for imatinib was subsequently deferred based on the condition that the originator Glivec® would be provided free-of-charge to low-income patients under the government health insurance scheme and the Novartis Glivec International Patient Assistance Program (GIPAP).

Compulsory licensing in Thailand was a "government use" version. Thai law (Section 51 of the Thai Patent Act BE 2522) has allowed the government to exercise authority over patents for the benefit of the general public. This is in accordance with the full international law, such as the TRIPS agreement (Quintiles IMS Institute 2017).

The reason for compulsory licensing in Thailand is part of a set of cost-containment measures to provide universal health coverage. The Thai Universal Health Coverage Plan is intended to extend healthcare to low-income households and to provide medicines under the plan for access to medicines that are included on the National List of Essential Medicines. The compulsory licensing of anticancer drugs in Thailand has played an important role in improving the accessibility of those drugs and lowering the cost of patented drugs; no adverse effect on the economy was observed in the short term (Braun n.d.).

Free Donation Through Patient Support Programmes

Some of these programmes also provide access through the free supply of anticancer drugs due to the participation of pharmaceutical companies. For example, Novartis has provided patients with Glivec free-of-charge or for subsidized support through the Glivec International Patient Assistance Program (GIPAP) and Glivec US Patient Assistance. Initiated in 2002, GIPAP was implemented in more than 75 LMICs, and in India, more than 75,000 were provided (Glivec International Patient Assistance Program (GIPAP) [Internet] n.d.). Roche also assisted patients who pay out-of-pocket costs through patient assistance programmes. Bayer's patient assistance programme aided the cost of 27 days of the month for sorafenib as each of the first three days was borne by the patient ($493). However, the cost of sorafenib for the patient in Bayer's assistant programme was still 4.5 times higher than its generic drugs ($110) (Hoen 2014).

Differential Pricing Strategies

Pharmaceutical companies also provide drugs with lowered prices in low-income countries (e.g. countries in Africa) based on price differentiation strategies. For example, Roche was engaged in developing differential pricing programmes in LMICs, including for anticancer drugs. Herceptin® was tested with a tiered pricing scheme in connection with the patient's ability to pay (Hoen 2014). To do so, Roche called for international cooperation against the external referencing and the parallel importation from countries outside of the same economic development level. Another approach to minimize the impact of external referencing or parallel imports is to use "second brands". For example, Roche provides the same drug as Herceptin under the new name Herclon® through an agreement with Emcure in India (Hoen 2014). By doing so, the price of Herceptin is not affected by the price differentiation between countries.

Discussion

In order to address the issue of accessibility to these anticancer drugs, collaborations at national and international levels, including between the Global North and South, the pharmaceutical industry, local national health authorities, the WHO and other non-profit and patient-oriented organizations, are needed. A strong commitment by national policymakers is required as well.

Recently, the Dutch and Belgian Ministries of Health announced international cooperation for HTA and pharmaceutical pricing in June 2018. Since then, a coalition, including Belgium, the Netherlands, Luxembourg, Austria and Ireland, has jointly launched an agreement to conduct HTA and drug price negotiations for Biogen's Spinraza®. Such cross-national coordination is required in the field of horizon scanning, information sharing and policy exchange, HTA and pricing and reimbursement (A landmark for international collaboration on HTA n.d.). In addition, the Italian government proposed to the WHO in February 2019 a call for international actions to set international standards for drug-pricing transparency, which would allow pharmaceutical companies to disclose drug prices, R&D costs and production costs in order to expand access to pharmaceuticals (Italy proposes the WHO n.d.).

The universal healthcare system assures access to cancer medicines; however, its sustainability is challenged due to the high cost of recently developed cancer drugs. This is an aspect affecting access to medicines, even in high-income countries. Accordingly, procurement policies, such as pricing and reimbursement, are important factors that can improve the affordable accessibility of high-cost cancer drugs. Since the high price of anticancer drugs is a barrier to the treatment and prevention of cancer in all countries, it is necessary to regulate the price of medicines at an affordable level by guaranteeing reasonable profits through regional and global cooperation.

References

World Health Organization. Global Health Observatory. Geneva: [Internet]. [cited 2018a Jan 21]. http://who.int/gho/database/en

Bray F, Ferlay J, Soerjomataram I, Siegel RL, Torre LA, Jemal A. Global cancer statistics 2018: GLOBOCAN estimates of incidence and mortality worldwide for 36 cancers in 185 countries. CA Cancer J Clin [Internet]. 2018;68(6):394–424. http://www.ncbi.nlm.nih.gov/pubmed/30207593

World Health Organization. New Global Cancer Country Profiles [Internet]. https://www.who.int/cancer/country-profiles/en

Torre LA, Siegel RL, Ward EM, Jemal A. Global cancer incidence and mortality rates and trends - An update. Cancer Epidemiol Biomarkers Prev. 2016;25(1):16–27.

Hoen E, Access to cancer treatment: A study of medicine pricing issues with recommendations for improving access to cancer medication, Oxfam. 2014. https://www.ciaonet.org/attachments/27387/uploads

Economist Intelligence Unit. Breakaway: The global burden of cancer—challenges and opportunities. Econ. 2009;1–73.

World Health Organization. Metrics: Disability-Adjusted Life Year (DALY) [Internet]. http://www.who.int/healthinfo/global_burden_disease/metrics_daly/en/

Richardson E. Health Policy Brief: Biosimilars. Heal Policy Br. 2013
Quintiles IMS Institute. Global Oncology Trends 2017: Advances, complexity & cost. 2017 May;1–47
Annadurai K, Danasekaran R, Mani G Personalized medicine: A paradigm shift towards promising health care. J Pharm Bioallied Sci. 2016;8(1):77–8.
Alsaab HO, Sau S, Alzhrani R, Tatiparti K. PD-1 and PD-L1 Checkpoint Signaling Inhibition for Cancer Immunotherapy: Mechanism, Combinations, and Clinical Outcome. Frontiers in Pharmacology 2017;8(August):1–15.
Sacca L. The uncontrolled clinical trial: scientific, ethical, and practical reasons for being. Intern Emerg Med. 5(3):201–4.
Prasad V, Kim C, Burotto M, Vandross A. The Strength of Association Between Surrogate End Points and Survival in Oncology. JAMA Intern Med. 2015;175(8):1389–98.
Cohen D. Cancer drugs: High price, uncertain value. BMJ [Internet]. 2017;359(October):1–4. https://doi.org/10.1136/bmj.j454315.
FDA increasingly approves drugs without conclusive proof they work [Internet]. https://www.pbs.org/newshour/health/fda-increasingly-approves-drugs-without-conclusive-proof-they-work
Madersbacher S, Kramer G. Re: Availability of Evidence of Benefits on Overall Survival and Quality of Life of Cancer Drugs Approved by European Medicines Agency: Retrospective Cohort Study of Drug Approvals 2009–2013. Eur Urol. 2018;73(4):635–6.
Salas-Vega S, Iliopoulos O, Mossialos E. Assessment of overall survival, quality of life, and safety benefits associated with new cancer medicines. JAMA Oncol. 2017;3(3):382–90.
World Health Organization. Technical report: pricing of cancer medicines and its impacts: a comprehensive technical report for the World Health Assembly [Internet]. 2018b. 112 p. Available from: https://apps.who.int/iris/handle/10665/277190
Fojo T, Grady C. How much is life worth: Cetuximab, non-small cell lung cancer, and the $440 billion question. J Natl Cancer Inst. 2009;101(15):1044–8.
Siddiqui M, Rajkumar SV. The High Cost of Cancer Drugs and What We Can Do About It. Mayo Clin Proc. 2012;87(10):935–43.
Institute for New Economic Thinking. Working Paper No.60: US Pharma's Financialized Business Model. 2017(July 13);649186(60).
WHO Regional Office for Africa. Assessment of Medicine Pricing and Reimbursement Systems in Health Insurance Schemes in Selected African Countries. July 2016 https://apps.who.int/iris/bitstream/handle/10665/246416/9789290233145-eng.pdf?sequence=1

Lopes G, Vulto A, Wilking N, van Harten W, Meier K, Simoens S. Potential Solutions for Sustaining the Costs of Cancer Drugs. Eur Oncol Haematol [Internet]. 2017;13(02):102. http://www.touchoncology.com/articles/potential-solutions-sustaining-costs-cancer-drugs

Lin D, Lee SY, Makarov D V., Levy BP, Grossbard ML, Becker DJ. Exploration of the ASCO and ESMO value frameworks for cancer drugs. J Clin Oncol. 2018;34(15_suppl):6512–6512.

Gammie T, Lu CY, Ud-Din Babar Z. Access to orphan drugs: A comprehensive review of legislations, regulations and policies in 35 countries. PLoS One. 2015;10(10):1–24.

World Health Organization. Access to essential medicines as part of the right to health [Internet]. https://www.who.int/medicines/areas/human_rights/en/

WHO. Essential Medicines [Internet]. https://www.who.int/medicines/services/essmedicines_def/en/

Perehudoff SK, Toebes B, Hogerzeil H. Essential medicines in national constitutions: Progress since 2008. Health Hum Rights. 2016;18(1):141–56.

Bigdeli M, Jacobs B, Tomson G, Laing R, Ghaffar A, vDujardin B, et al. Access to medicines from a health system perspective. Health Policy Plan. 2013;28(7):692–704.

Swiss Agency for Development and Cooperation (SDC). ACCESS TO MEDICINES: Medicines supply: Lessons learnt in Tanzania and Mozambique: A capitalisation report established in the frame of the SDC Backstopping Mandate 2004 of the Social Development Division's Health Desk. 2004: 1–16

World Health Organization/European Observatory on Health Systems and Policies (2018).POLICY BRIEF 30: Ensuring access to medicines: How to redesign pricing, reimbursement and procurement? 2018: 1–36. http://www.euro.who.int/en/about-us/partners/

Zaheer Babar, Gammie T, Seyfoddin A, Hasan SS, Curley LE. Patient access to medicines in two countries with similar health systems and differing medicines policies: Implications from a comprehensive literature review. Res Soc Adm Pharm. 2019;15(3):231–43.

Blauvelt B, Jazieh AR, McClung M, Eniu A, Zafar Y, Carlson R, et al. Facing the Global Challenges of Access to Cancer Medication. J Glob Oncol. 2018;(4):1–7.

Rickwood S. Prescription medicines trends: an overview and perspective on two therapy areas. 2017; Available from: https://www.who.int/phi/2-Sarah-Rickwood.pdf

Cherny NI, Sullivan R, Torode J, Saar M, Eniu A. ESMO European Consortium Study on the availability, out-of-pocket costs and accessibility of antineoplastic medicines in Europe. Ann Oncol. 2016;27(8):1423–43.

Cherny NI, Sullivan R, Torode J, Saar M, Eniu A. ESMO International Consortium Study on the availability, out-of-pocket costs and accessibility of antineoplastic medicines in countries outside of Europe. Ann Oncol. 2017;28(11):2633–47.

Saqib A, Iftikhar S, Sarwar MR. Availability and affordability of biologic versus non-biologic anticancer medicines: A cross-sectional study in Punjab, Pakistan. BMJ Open. 2018;8(6).

Huntington SF, Weiss BM, Vogl DT, Cohen AD, Garfall AL, Mangan PA, et al. Financial toxicity in insured patients with multiple myeloma: A cross-sectional pilot study. Lancet Haematol. 2015;2(10):e408–16.

Pauwels K, Huys I, Vogler S, Casteels M, Simoens S. Managed entry agreements for oncology drugs: Lessons from the European experience to inform the future. Front Pharmacol. 2017;8(APR):1–8.

KCE. How to improve the Belgian process for managed entry agreements? An analysis of the Belgian and international experience. 2018;75 https://kce.fgov.be/sites/default/files/atoms/files/KCE_288_Improve_Belgian_process_managed_entry_agreements_Report.pdf

Aggarwal A, Fojo T, Chamberlain C, Davis C, Sullivan R. Do patient access schemes for high-cost cancer drugs deliver value to society ?— lessons from the NHS Cancer Drugs Fund. Ann Oncol. 2017;(Aug);28(8):1738–1750. doi: https://doi.org/10.1093/annonc/mdx110

Davies JE, Neidle S, Taylor DG. Developing and paying for medicines for orphan indications in oncology : utilitarian regulation vs equitable care ? Br J Cancer [Internet]. 2012;106(1):14–7. Available from: https://doi.org/10.1038/bjc.2011.544

England NHS. NHS England consultation : Proposals for a sustainable Cancer Drug Fund. 2014

Australian Department of Health. Life Saving Drugs Program Criteria and Conditions. [Internet]. https://www.health.gov.au/internet/main/publishing.nsf/Content/lsdp-criteria

Government of Canada. Special Access Programme - Drugs [Internet].https://www.canada.ca/en/health-canada/services/drugs-health-products/special-access/drugs/special-access-programme-drugs-1.html

AIFA. The independent research on drugs. 2019 [Internet] http://www.aifa.gov.it/en/content/independent-research-drugs

PHARMAC. Contestable fund for medicines for rare disordershttps://www.pharmac.govt.nz/news/consultation-2014-07-08-rare-disorders/

Scotland launches medicines fund for rare conditions [Internet]. https://www.pharmaceutical-journal.com/news-and-analysis/scotland-launches-medicines-fund-for-rare-conditions-updated/11115004.article

World Health Organization. WHO Model List of Essential Medicines: 20th list, March 2017;(March):1–62. http://www.who.int/medicines/publications/essentialmedicines/en/

Hill J, Mills C, Li Q, Smith JS. Prevalence of traditional, complementary, and alternative medicine use by cancer patients in low income and lower-middle income countries. Glob Public Health. 2019;14(3):418–30.

DIPP to issue CLs for Herceptin, Dasatini & Ixabepiloone – End of the line for Big Pharma's patents in the Indian market? [Internet]. https://spicyip.com/2013/01/dipp-to-issue-cls-for-herceptin.html

Official Journal of the Patent Office. Issue 32/2011, 12/08/2011;13337–13363. Publication of the Patent Office. https://docs.google.com/viewer?a=v&pid=sites&srcid=ZGVmYXVsdGRvbWFpbnxzcGljeWlwZmlsZXN8Z3g6NDFlNjAxZDIyOTY0MjMyMg

Complete list of oppositions [Internet]. www.patentoppositions.org

170 Members of Congress Send Letter to Obama Criticizing India on Interllectual Property. https://www.keionline.org/22245

US Businesses Launch Coalition For Fair Trade With India [Internet]. https://www.ip-watch.org/2013/06/18/us-businesses-launch-coalition-for-fair-trade-with-india/

Braun JV. Use of Compulsory Licenses Selected National Experiences. http://unctad.org/Sections/dite_totip/docs/tot_ip_0018_en.pdf

Glivec International Patient Assistance Program (GIPAP) [Internet]. https://accessaccelerated.org/initiative/glivec-international-patient-assistance-program-gipap/

A landmark for international collaboration on HTA and pharmaceutical pricing. https://www.linkedin.com/pulse/landmark-international-collaboration-hta-pricing-neil-grubert

Italy proposes the WHO set international standards for drug-pricing transparency [Internet]. https://www.statnews.com/pharmalot/2019/02/14/italy-who-drug-prices-transparency/

United Nations Development Programme. Human Development Report 2016: Human Development for Everyone. 2016. http://hdr.undp.org/en/content/human-development-report-2016-human-development-everyone

Introduction: Concepts of the Global South (GSSC) https://web.archive.org/web/20160904205139/http://gssc.uni-koeln.de/node/451

North And South, the (Global) [Internet]. https://www.encyclopedia.com/social-sciences/applied-and-social-sciences-magazines/north-and-south-global#D

World Health Organization, National cancer control programmes: policies and managerial guidelines (2nd edition), Geneva. 2002.

Davis C, Naci H, Gurpinar E et al., Availability of Evidence of Benefits on Overall Survival and Quality of Life of Cancer Drugs Approved by European Medicines Agency: Retrospective Cohort Study of Drug Approvals 2009–2013. Eur Urol. 2018;73(4):635–6.

Vogler S, Paris V, Panteli D. Ensuring access to medicines: How to redesign pricing, reimbursement and procurement? Addressing Policy Failures In Pharmaceuticals Series Editor: Elias Mossialos. 2018; Available from: http://www.euro.who.int/en/about-us/partners/

5

Medicines Pricing: Limitations of Existing Policies and New Models

Sabine Vogler

Abbreviations

AIDS	Acquired immune deficiency syndrome
DNDi	Drugs for Neglected Diseases initiative
EPR	External price referencing
EU	European Union
EUnetHTA	European network for health technology assessment
GAVI	Global Alliance for Vaccines and Immunisation
GCC	Gulf Cooperation Council
HAI	Health Action International
HIV	Human immunodeficiency virus
HTA	Health technology assessment
ICER	Incremental cost-effectiveness ratio

S. Vogler (✉)
WHO Collaborating Centre for Pharmaceutical Pricing and Reimbursement Policies, Pharmacoeconomics Department, Gesundheit Österreich GmbH (GÖG/Austrian National Public Health Institute), Vienna, Austria
e-mail: sabine.vogler@goeg.at

Z. Babar (ed.), *Global Pharmaceutical Policy*,
https://doi.org/10.1007/978-981-15-2724-1_5

JPA	Joint Procurement Agreement
LMIC	Low- and middle-income countries
MCDA	Multiple-criteria decision analysis
MEA	Managed entry agreement(s)
MWPP	Manufacturer (price), wholesale (price), pharmacy (retail price net) and pharmacy (retail price gross); alternatively manufacturer, wholesaler, pharmacy and patient
NHS	National health service
OECS	Pharmaceutical Procurement Service of the Organization of Eastern Caribbean States
PAHO	Pan-American Health Organization
PPRI	Pharmaceutical pricing and reimbursement information
R+D	Research and development
RCT	Randomized controlled trial(s)
RWD	Real-world data
RWE	Real-world evidence
SADC	Southern African Development Community
UHC	Universal health coverage
UN	United Nations
UNFPA	United Nations Population Fund
UNICEF	United Nations International Children's Emergency Fund
USD	United States dollar
VBP	Value-based pricing
WHA	World Health Assembly
WHO	World Health Organization
WTP	Willingness-to-pay

Introduction

Medicine pricing policies are defined as 'regulations and processes used by government authorities to set the price of a medicine as part of exercising price control' (WHO Collaborating Centre for Pharmaceutical Pricing and Reimbursement Policies 2018). Why is there a need to regulate prices of medicines by governments? Why not leave it to market mechanisms? How effective are these pricing policies? The introductory section presents key concepts and facts around medicine prices and provides a rationale for governments' interventions to ensure affordable access to medicines.

Who Pays the Price?

Economic theory teaches that sellers and buyers meet in a marketplace and exchange goods and services, with or without payment. Health care is, however, **not a common consumer market**. There are more parties involved as the example of medicines shows:

- Relating to the seller: The pharmaceutical company and its intermediaries including the pharmacy or a retailer
- Relating to the consumer: The patient who may, or may not, pay for the medication and whose choice is—in case of prescribed medicines—determined by the doctor
- Relating to the payer: The medicine is paid either by the patient or a third-party payer (e.g. a public payer such as a social health insurance or a national health service or a private health insurance) or both (cost-sharing)

There are different parties that pay (or co-pay) a medicine price and different parties that receive money in return for producing, trading, selling/dispensing and handling the medicine and providing related services with medicine dispensation (e.g. counselling). As a result, there are also price types that relate to the different stages in the supply chain (see Fig. 5.1).

Are Medicines Affordable?

According to the WHO, so-called **essential medicines** (i.e. those that satisfy the priority health-care needs of the population) should be available within the context of functioning health systems at all times in

Paying the price		Receiving money from medicine's sale/dispensing	Price components (price types)
Patient and his/her carer Third-party payer, e.g. social health insurance, national health service, private health insurance, health maintenance organization	→	Community pharmacy, hospital pharmacy Retailer, drugstore Wholesaler, distributor, importer Pharmaceutical company State (Ministry of Finance), via taxes	*Pharmacy retail price gross/net (incl./excl. taxes)* *Wholesale price (pharmacy purchasing price)* *Ex-factory price (manufacturer price)* *Cost, insurance and freight* *Landing price* *Hospital price* *Reimbursement price*

Fig. 5.1 Parties involved in paying for and obtaining parts of the medicine and implications on the price components. Note: Major taxonomies to describe price components are the one of the World Health Organization/Health Action International (WHO/HAI) methodology to measure medicine prices, availability, affordability and price components (WHO, HAI 2008) which defines five stages (manufacturer's selling price, 'landed price', wholesale selling price or central medical stores price, retail price (in the private sector) and dispensary price (in the public sector) and the 'dispensed price') and the MWPP price taxonomy (MWPP stands for manufacturer price, wholesale price, pharmacy retail price net and pharmacy retail price gross. It can also be read as referring to the actors involved: manufacturer, wholesaler, pharmacy and patient.) (Vogler et al. 2019a) which defines four major price types that are common in the outpatient sector in countries with solidarity-based health systems (ex-factory price, wholesale price, pharmacy retail price net, pharmacy retail price gross). (Source: The author)

adequate amounts, in the appropriate dosage forms, with assured quality and adequate information, and affordable for the individual and the community (World Health Organization 2019).

In practice, unaffordability of medicines has been a major issue globally for many years. At least one-third of the world's population is estimated to lack regular access to essential medicines; in the poorest parts of Africa and Asia, this figure rises to over 50% (World Health Organization 2004; WHO 2011).

Evidence on the unaffordability of medicines used to address mainly **low- and middle-income countries** (LMIC) with a limited number of medicines in the private sector (full or partial coverage of expenses for medicines): Treatments for acute and chronic diseases were found to be unaffordable for patients in many of these countries (Cameron et al. 2009; Ewen et al. 2017; Mendis et al. 2007). In order to afford medicines, patients or their carers often take hard decisions such as running into debts, selling assets or refraining from other basic commodities such as food and are pushed into poverty (Niëns et al. 2010; Leive and Xu 2008; Li et al. 2012; Wagner et al. 2011).

In recent years, unaffordability of medicines has increasingly also become an issue for **high-income countries** (e.g. in Europe or the United States) given the market entry of new medicines (e.g. orphan medicines, cancer medicines, hepatitis C medication) with high price tags (Iyengar et al. 2016; Abboud et al. 2013; Kantarjian et al. 2013; Kelly and Smith 2014; World Health Organization 2018; Zaprutko et al. 2017). Even high-income countries whose publicly funded health-care systems usually cover the expenses of certain medicines have increasingly been struggling with ensuring access to medicines while not compromising the long-term sustainability of the solidarity-based health-care systems: in the European Union (EU), for instance, several councils during recent EU Presidencies have put the challenges of accessibility and affordability of (new) medicines on the agenda and discussed possible suggestions (Council of the European Union 2016, 2017; Vogler et al. 2018a).

Why Is There a Need for Pricing Policies?

Against this backdrop of the special character of medicines and the pharmaceutical market (no normal competitive consumer markets) and the importance of medicines to treat diseases, there is the need to ensure affordable prices, as high prices are a major barrier to accessibility.

Price control (price regulation) helps limit medicine prices and thus sustain them at more affordable levels. To do so, governments can employ a variety of different pricing policies. Some policies address **certain medicines and market segments** (e.g. new innovative medicines, off-patent medicines, reimbursable = funded medicines), and the pricing policies relate to different stages in the supply chain (e.g. at the level of the manufacturer, wholesaler, pharmacy or consumer).

There is a large body of evidence, mainly for high-income countries that have had long-term experience in several pricing policies that showed the **impact of price regulation in terms of containing prices and expenditure**. Studies have shown that unregulated prices (e.g. in the private sector) were, often considerably, higher than prices achieved through tenders or other pricing policies (Cameron et al. 2009; Babar 2015; Babar et al. 2018). Thus, in order to ensure affordable access to (essential) medicines, there is a need for pricing policies (preferably a combination of different pharmaceutical pricing policies), as also recommended by the WHO (see WHO Guideline on Country Pharmaceutical Pricing Policies (World Health Organization 2013)).

At the same time, also in the light of new developments in recent years, limitations of existing pricing policies have increasingly become clear and resulted in discussions about new models and avenues.

The aim of this chapter is to present limitations of existing policies (particularly those for new medicines) and possible new models.

Limitations of Existing Pricing Policies

As an introduction of this chapter on limitations of pricing policies, three key messages should be taken into consideration.

First, to reiterate what was stated at the beginning of the chapter, pricing policies are **actions by public authorities** (representing governments). They are not taken by private sector representatives. Price sector actors (e.g. pharmaceutical industry) can develop and implement strategies to achieve their objectives (e.g. designing a pricing strategy to maximize profits), but these approaches of private sector actors are strategies and plans and not policies. They are not within the scope of this chapter.

Second, there is **linkage between pricing and reimbursement** (i.e. coverage of expenditure by a third-party payer such as a social health insurance/national health service), particularly in countries with solidarity-based public health-care systems, which may be strong. In many countries, the scope of price control relates to the reimbursement market, that is, to those medicines that are, at least, partially funded by the state (Vogler et al. 2008, 2018b). As such, pharmaceutical pricing policies can also include reimbursement elements. Some of the pricing policies that will be presented in the following (e.g. value-based pricing, managed entry agreements) could be even classified as reimbursement policies.

Third, it is important to note that pricing policies have, as mentioned above, **positive impacts on affordable access to medicines**, even if in some cases the benefits may be lower than expected. Thus, a chapter on limitations of pricing policies might be misleading. To acknowledge the value of pricing policies, additional information on possible and shown benefits of these policies will also be presented in the following.

External Price Referencing

External price referencing (EPR) relates to 'the practice of using the price(s) of a medicine in one or several countries in order to derive a benchmark or reference price for the purposes of setting or negotiating the price of the product in a given country' (WHO 2016). Synonyms are external reference pricing, international price comparison, international price benchmark and international referencing pricing.

It is a frequently applied pricing policy, mainly used for on-patent medicines in the outpatient sector which are (co-)funded by the public payer (Leopold et al. 2012a; Toumi et al. 2014; Espin et al. 2014; Vogler et al. 2016a). EPR has been implemented in 26 of the 28 Member States of the European Union (all but Sweden and the United Kingdom) and in further countries such as Iceland, Norway, Switzerland and Turkey (Vogler et al. 2016a; Rémuzat et al. 2015). EPR is also used in some countries in Africa (e.g. Egypt, South Africa), in the Asia-Pacific region (e.g. Malaysia, Japan, South Korea), in Latin America (e.g. Brazil, Colombia, Mexico) and in Canada (Espin et al. 2014; Schneider and Vogler 2018). An increasing number of countries introduced EPR.

EPR contributes to **availability limitations**. To avoid lower benchmark prices determined through EPR, pharmaceutical companies are incentivized to launch medicines first in countries with higher prices and delay, or not launch, in lower-priced countries. Delays in market launches of medicines, often of considerable duration, were observed in countries that have lower price levels or smaller market volumes (Toumi et al. 2014; Vogler et al. 2016a; Rémuzat et al. 2015; Espin et al. 2011; Kanavos et al. 2010; Danzon and Epstein 2008; Danzon and Towse 2003; Danzon et al. 2005; Kyle 2007; Kanavos et al. 2017; Stargardt and Schreyögg 2006; Vogler et al. 2019b).

Another limitation of EPR is that its capacity to inform policy-makers about the price situation in other countries is distorted by the fact that 'real' prices are frequently not known, particularly for high-priced medicines. **Confidential** discounts granted by the industry to public payers are common for these medicines (Morgan et al. 2017; Vogler et al. 2012). By referencing to official list prices instead of real discounted prices, payers risk **overpaying** (Bouvy and Vogler 2013). In addition, the information asymmetry limits the negotiation power of public payers, as they are not on even level playing field with the pharmaceutical industry, which has the full picture of the prices in all countries where the medicine is marketed. There is no evidence for payers that the promise of getting 'the best deal' has been realized (Vogler and Paterson 2017) (see also section "Transparency-Based Pricing" on transparency-based pricing).

It should be acknowledged that EPR is not a simple policy, as it has been claimed by some. The performance of high-quality EPR requires a **robust methodological design** that provides for solutions for challenges (e.g. missing data because medicines are not yet marketed in some countries, exchange rate volatility) and capacity-building for those performing EPR (Vogler et al. 2016a; Kanavos et al. 2010). Access to trustworthy and yet easy-to-handle price data sources has to be identified and ensured (Vogler and Schneider 2019).

Despite these limitations, there is evidence that EPR has been able to lower medicine prices (WHO 2013; Håkonsen et al. 2009; Leopold et al. 2012b; Windmeijer et al. 2006; Merkur and Mossialos 2007; Filko and Szilagyiova 2009). EPR's effectiveness appears to be strongest immediately after its implementation, but it tends to 'fade out' after some time (Vogler et al. 2016a). However, this is an effect that might be seen by several other policies as well.

Value-Based Pricing

Value-based pricing (VBP) describes an approach in which the 'value' that a medicine offers determines the price. A clear and generally agreed definition of VBP is, however, missing (Garner et al. 2018). In a narrow interpretation (in the context of the English national health service [NHS]), VBP has been defined as '(the price) that ensures that the expected health benefits [of a new technology] exceed the health predicted to be displaced elsewhere in the NHS, due to their additional cost' (Claxton 2007). Applying a broader approach of interpretation, any policy linking the price of a medicine to its added therapeutic benefit could be summarized under the VBP policy. To assess 'value', pharmacoeconomic evaluations and health technology assessments (HTAs) are performed (for further details on HTA, see section "New Developments Related to Tools to Support Evidence-Based Pricing").

VBP has been criticized for being an **industry approach** or even being a 'marketing instrument' (Vogler 2019). In fact, it originates from an industry approach: in other sectors of the economy, it typically refers to a strategy a company can use to set the prices of its goods and services. More precisely, when a company sets a price based on a VBP approach, it calculates and tries to earn the differentiated worth of its product for a particular customer segment when compared to its competitors. Setting such a price requires (1) referring to a specific market segment, (2) identifying attributes that differentiate this product from the one of competitors and (3) understanding of how consumers value this differential or how much they are willing to pay for it. It has been argued that by setting their pricing strategy, companies do not need to value each feature of their product separately but rather identify feature differences and assess customers' valuation of these differentiated features. If comparators set low prices of their products, it is difficult for a company to apply a VBP approach and justify high prices (Dholakia 2016).

Pharmaceutical companies have been using a VPB approach in the new millennium. Public authorities have more or less adopted this terminology, although the same words clearly have different meanings for different stakeholders (Vogler et al. 2018a). Even if a VBP policy in the narrower sense has only been implemented in a few countries (e.g. Australia, New Zealand, Canada, Sweden), the value-based approach (in contrast to a cost-driven approach; see section "Cost-Plus Pricing") has been guiding governments, including public payers, across the globe, while they additionally apply further pricing policies.

From a company's perspective, it is important to understand the **willingness-to-pay** (WTP) of public payers, in order to propose a price that will be considered acceptable for public funding. As such, VBP offers opportunities to the industry for 'gaming', in particular in the choice of the comparators and the threshold (Kanavos et al. 2010). It has been argued that if public payers disclose their WTP, this could create an incentive for the development of products that generate increased added value (Bouvy and Vogler 2013; Godman and Gustafsson 2013) and could signal their public health priorities (e.g. related to research and development [R+D]) (Consultative Expert Working Group on Research and Development 2016; Franken et al. 2012). But in a VBP system with published cost-effectiveness thresholds, pharmaceutical companies have an incentive to price up to the threshold (Hughes 2011).

Using value-based assessments as the sole basis for pricing implies that need, prevalence and affordability are not taken into consideration (Garner et al. 2018). Furthermore, it has been argued that the VBP pricing model is not viable in many countries because it does not take into account affordability and total cost (WHO 2017). In theory, a new medicine with a price above the incremental cost-effectiveness ratio (ICER) threshold would not be reimbursed, but policy-makers may deviate in practice from the ICER threshold, and have done so in the past, in case of unmet medical need, rarity and severity of the disease treated and public pressure (Paris and Belloni 2013; Simoens et al. 2013).

In practical terms, the application of a VBP approach that is informed by HTA and pharmacoeconomic evaluations suffers from the limitation that high levels of **capacity and resources** are required. This is particularly an issue for less-resourced and smaller countries.

Cost-Plus Pricing

Cost-plus pricing is a policy that determines a medicine price by taking into account production costs, promotional expenses, investments into R+D, administration costs, overheads and profits. Prices are based on information of the costs incurred provided by the pharmaceutical company plus a profit margin considered 'reasonable'.

Cost-plus pricing is applied in some LMIC (e.g. Bangladesh, China, Iran, Pakistan, Sri Lanka, Vietnam) but it is no longer used in any EU Member State. Some other countries (e.g. India, Colombia) have also discontinued applying this pricing policy (WHO 2013; Nguyen et al. 2014). So, over the years, the number of countries that apply cost-plus pricing has decreased.

A major limitation of this pricing policy is that the pricing authorities depend on the data provided by the pharmaceutical company since access to independent **cost information** is very difficult and practically impossible for many governments. The cost-plus policy could give an incentive to pharmaceutical companies to a 'manipulation of costing data' (WHO 2013), and it might thus result in higher prices.

Differential Pricing

Differential pricing is a pricing policy that provides different prices for different countries, depending on their income level. It is also called tiered pricing, as well as, less frequently, equity pricing (Rovira and Can 2013) and minimum-level pricing (Mossialos and Dukes 2000).

Differential pricing has mainly been used in LMIC. It has usually been limited to few therapeutic areas (e.g. HIV/AIDS, malaria, tuberculosis) and product groups (vaccines). Purchasers are frequently international organizations such as United Nations (UN) agencies (e.g. UNICEF, PAHO and UNFPA) and programmes as well as initiatives such as the Global Alliance for Vaccines and Immunisation (GAVI) or UNITAID. In a few cases, particularly related to middle-income countries, national governments have been involved in differential pricing (Babar and Atif 2014). More recently, differential pricing has been implemented to increase access to medicines for non-communicable diseases, mainly as part of public-private partnerships (Access And Affordability Initiative 2018).

While it has been argued that differential pricing has been effective in ensuring patient access in low-income and least-developed countries in which medicines would otherwise have been unaffordable (Babar and Atif 2014; Yadav 2010; Moon et al. 2011), it has some major limitations. It is not fully clear **who decides on the methodology** and which principles and rules are to be taken into consideration.

In some cases, differential pricing was not performed as a government action (or an intervention of supranational institutions), but it was the pharmaceutical company to decide on the different price levels through differentiating markets by confidential discounts, for instance. But this is not differential pricing as a policy since, as explained in the introduction, a pricing policy is an action taken by a government authority, not by a private sector representative. When pharmaceutical companies aim to achieve optimal pricing (from a business perspective) by differentiating markets according to the purchaser's demand elasticity, this is the commercial strategy of 'price discrimination' (also called 'Ramsey pricing' after the economist Frank Plumpton Ramsey).

As a government action, differential pricing describes a cross-country policy of setting the price of a medicine in accordance with the ability-to-pay and/or economic situation of different countries involved, based on coordinated decisions taken by national governments or international organizations. As such, differential pricing requires an **agreement of principles, mechanisms and rules** of the involved countries. Common understanding of the procedures (e.g. the extent of markdowns or mark-ups to reflect different ability-to-pay levels of countries) has to be reached.

Achieving an agreement of the principles and mechanisms between involved countries is very difficult. A study (Vogler et al. 2016a) exploring the feasibility of introducing differential pricing as a collaborative policy of EU Member States, as a possible solution to address the challenge of ensuring access to medicines with high price tags, concluded that, at that time of the research (2015), differential pricing appeared to be an unrealistic option in the EU for political reasons since it would require high political commitment from all 28 Member States to agreeing on principles.

Furthermore, a common argument against the implementation of differential pricing in Europe is the existence of **parallel trade** (i.e. resale of goods between countries without the authorization of the owner of the intellectual property rights associated with those goods) in the European Union. Parallel traders generate profits through buying goods in one country at a relatively low price and subsequently reselling them in another country where the price is higher. The European Commission has a supportive position on parallel trade arguing that parallel imports increase price competition and that this in turn increases consumer welfare as the import of goods from a country with lower prices forces sellers in the country of destination to reduce prices (De Souza 2007). In a more general context, there is, however, concern that the effects of the differential pricing policy would be undermined by large-scale importation of medicines from lower-priced to higher-priced countries. In addition, EPR and differential pricing are considered by many as mutually exclusive policies, though more recent literature offered examples of combining them by including some differential pricing traits into EPR (e.g. EPR with adjustment of reference countries by purchasing power parities).

Another limitation concerns the issue of how to set the **starting price**, since differential pricing only provides an answer to ensuring fair pricing across countries once a price for one country has been determined. For doing this, other pricing policies are likely needed.

Finally, differential pricing is not an appropriate policy to lower medicine prices since its major aim is to improve access. Studies showed that generic competition was more effective in reducing prices than differential pricing (Moon et al. 2011; Waning et al. 2009).

Tendering

In a tendering procedure, 'tenders (offers) are requested, received and evaluated for the procurement of goods, works or services, and as a consequence of which an award is made to the tenderer whose tender/offer is the most advantageous' (WHO 2016). In many cases, it is the (lowest) price that makes a bid most advantageous, but other criteria such as supply conditions, payment terms, frequency of delivery or packaging can also be decisive (Vogler et al. 2010a).

Tendering can be applied in settings where competition is possible, with multiple suppliers for same or similar medicines (e.g. therapeutic equivalents). Thus, it is a form of competitive pricing.

Tendering is the key procurement method in the public sector in many countries, including many LMIC (Seiter 2010), to purchase essential medicines and further medicines in the public sector (e.g. programmes for specific medicines such as HIV/AIDS, tuberculosis, diabetes and oncology medicines). In high-income countries, tendering is mainly applied in the hospital sector: hospitals, hospital groups and hospital procurement agencies (at regional and national levels) tender for needed medicines (Vogler et al. 2010a). Use of tendering in the outpatient sector is less frequent, but some European countries (e.g. Denmark, Germany, the Netherlands) apply tendering (or tendering-like procedures) to purchase off-patent medicines in the outpatient sector (Dylst et al. 2011; Kanavos 2012).

Tendering is able to achieve lower prices due to competition. The price-reducing effect of competition has been shown, for instance, for HIV/AIDS medicines. In Brazil, the price of HIV/AIDS medicines confronted with generic competition was reduced by 82% over five years, while prices of medicines without generic competitors remained rather stable, falling 9% over the same period of time. In LMIC, generic competition resulted in a decrease of the price of the AIDS triple therapy from USD 10,000 per patient and year to USD 350 within one year (T'Hoen et al. 2001).

Given evidence on the high savings for patients and public payers as a result of low prices achieved through tendering, this policy is overall seen as a beneficial one. The major argument against tendering is that it may drive prices down to a low level that is no longer attractive for pharmaceutical companies, and they withdraw their products from the market. Thus, there is the concern that tendering resulting in low prices contributes to **shortages and non-availability of medicines**.

In order to mitigate the risk of availability limitations, it has been advised to do 'strategic procurement' (Ferrario et al. 2016) which may include a 'divide-the-pie' strategy instead of a 'winner-takes-it-all' principle that has the potential to drive prices to lower levels.

Managed Entry Agreements

A managed entry agreement (MEA) is defined as 'an arrangement between a [pharmaceutical] manufacturer and payer/provider that enables access to (coverage or reimbursement of) a health technology subject to specific conditions' (Klemp et al. 2011). An agreement covered by this umbrella term may be designed as a financial-based scheme (such as in the form of a flat discount, a price-volume agreement or capping of utilization in terms of doses or patients) or a performance-based scheme (e.g. so-called coverage with evidence development with preliminary reimbursement while additional data are gathered in the context of clinical care to further clarify the impact of the medicine, a risk-sharing agreement or 'pay-for-performance') (Carlson et al. 2010; Garrison et al. 2013; Ferrario and Kanavos 2013).

MEAs provide earlier accessibility of medicines through the publicly funded health-care systems, even if added therapeutic value has not yet been proven. Against this backdrop of a MEA's contribution to (earlier) access to medicines, there are several drawbacks.

One major criticism of a MEA is its **non-transparent character**. In practically all countries that apply MEAs, these arrangements are linked to confidentiality. For some countries, it is even unknown which medicines are covered by a MEA (Pauwels et al. 2017). In any case, the arrangements about agreed conditions, in particular the extent of the price, are kept confidential (Ferrario and Kanavos 2013, 2015; Ferrario et al. 2017). This contributes to an imbalance in the pharmaceutical sector, with information asymmetry between the pharmaceutical company (knowing the different arrangements of its products across the countries) and the public payer. As a result, the bargaining power of payers is weakened by this asymmetry since they have no alternative but to trust the industry's promise that they 'got the best deal' (Vogler and Paterson 2017).

Manufacturers may systematically ask for **higher departing prices** in expectation of a MEA (Gerkens et al. 2017). It has been argued that by agreeing to a MEA, public payers implicitly accept high (list) prices (Vogler et al. 2016b).

The pharmaceutical industry has an interest to keep officially communicated list prices high as countries will refer to them in their EPR application (Bouvy and Vogler 2013). Thus, the policy instrument of a MEA has major **implications on** price levels in **other countries**. Unless they use the instrument of a MEA themselves (and, on their turn, contribute to non-transparency), governments risk overpaying when referencing to the published list prices in other countries.

Another frequently mentioned limitation of a MEA is that it can incur **high administrative costs** (Carlson et al. 2010; Gerkens et al. 2017; Adamski et al. 2010). This is particularly an issue for performance-based MEAs that require time-intensive data collection and monitoring. Also, their methodological design and introduction might be challenging as well.

As soon as real-world data are available, a pricing and reimbursement decision can be taken based on evidence. However, excluding a medicine from reimbursement might still be difficult for a public payer since patient expectations have already been created, and pressure from media and the public might be exercised (Vogler et al. 2017). Thus, to manage a decision of a possible discontinuation, the application of MEA should be accompanied by the **disinvestment** strategy.

Furthermore, it should be noted that given the novelty of MEAs (they were developed through experimenting and learning by doing within the last 10–15 years, in some countries much more recently), there is a **lack of methodology guidelines** for MEAs (only some general principles for performance-based MEAs have been proposed) (Garrison et al. 2013; Lieven and Luca 2017).

More Recent Approaches and New Models

New Developments Related to Tools to Support Evidence-Based Pricing

As described in the section on the value-based pricing policy (section "Value-Based Pricing"), evidence to take informed decisions and tools to guide such processes of data collection, analysis, assessment and appraisal are key for policy-makers.

In this respect, **health technology assessment (HTA)** has been frequently mentioned. Representing one type of health technologies, medicines are among the key fields of application of HTA. It is important to note that HTA is a supportive tool and not a pricing policy on its own: though it cannot provide affordable access to medicines, it constitutes a powerful instrument to improve access to cost-effective medicines if performed properly.

HTA is an instrument for **prioritization** with the aim to help policy-makers obtain better value for money. The methods applied in HTA may differ, since the concept is not defined globally. A 2015 WHO global survey on the use of HTA in public sector decisions defined HTA rather broadly as 'a systematic approach to evaluate the properties, effects, and impacts of health technologies or intervention' (World Health Organization 2015). In several high-income and some middle-income countries, there are more specific definitions. A frequently quoted definition is one of the European HTA network EUnetHTA (European network for health technology assessment): EuNetHTA defines HTA as 'a multidisciplinary process that summarises information about the medical, social, economic and ethical issues related to the use of a health technology in a systematic, transparent, unbiased, robust manner. Its aim is to inform the formulation of safe, effective, health policies that are patient focused and seek to achieve best value' (Radaelli et al. 2014).

An HTA process consists of the components of 'assessment' and 'appraisal'. While assessment is the synthesis of available research evidence and is done by HTA experts (researchers), an HTA-based decision also has to include the **appraisal** of the evidence's impact and applicability for a specific context. This is to be done by appraisal committees, which are at the crossroad of research and policy. Appraisal committees facilitate the life of policy-makers by translating research results into political recommendations.

In recent years, there has been growing understanding that HTA has to include both assessment and appraisal. Processes and structures to ensure appraisal in local settings are also and in particular key when countries do not have the capacity to perform their own assessments but use clinical assessments of other countries. These have to be 'translated' in their national settings.

The EUnetHTA group in Europe identified a lack in **uptake of HTA**, meaning that several HTA reports produced by HTA bodies were not used in policy-making. In its current project phase (so-called Joint Action 3 from 2016 to 2020), EUnetHTA analysed the reasons for the low uptake in national case studies and provided recommendations. The implementation report identified the requirements to prepare HTA reports in their national language and to use a specified report structure as well as the timing (HTA reports were available with delays, while policy-makers already required the evidence earlier to decide on pricing and reimbursement) as major limitations. Based on these lessons learned, a permanent model of HTA cooperation was recommended based on a set of principles such as avoidance of replication and broad involvement of HTA agency in joint assessments (EUnetHTA 2018).

As HTA is a resource-intensive process, collaboration is one of the pathways for the future. There are, in principle, different approaches of (cross-country) collaboration in HTA (Beneluxa Initiative on Pharmaceutical Policy 2018):

- Reuse of HTA reports, with governments using parts of HTA reports of other countries.
- Joint writing of an HTA report: Authors of several countries join forces to write one report which will be used in all countries involved.
- Mutual recognition of HTA reports: In this case, large or even all parts of an HTA report of one country are adopted by other countries in a parallel process, and the results of the assessments would be then published at the same time.
- External referees: Experts of one or more HTA agencies of the same or other countries review the draft report, which would not involve active work in the HTA process itself.

More technically, advances have been made in processes of complex decision-making, and various methods of **multiple-criteria decision analysis** (MCDA) have been proposed either as an alternative to address shortcomings of HTA or to be included in the HTA process (Angelis and Kanavos 2016, 2017). It has been argued that the advantage of MCDA methodologies is that they allow for a systematic and explicit consideration of multiple factors that influence the decision, through identified criteria that each are assigned a weight to make their values and objectives explicit. An example of an approach to include MCDA in HTA (a three-step process) was reported from the Italian region Lombardy: First, the region selects health technologies, including medicines, for appraisal based on applications from stakeholders that include evidence on the impacts of the health technology in eight dimensions (general relevance, safety, efficacy, effectiveness, economic and financial impacts, impacts on equity, social/ethical impacts and organizational impacts) compared to current technologies (prioritization). In a second step, a full assessment of the prioritized technologies is performed. The third step is an appraisal of the assessed technologies grounded on the analysis of multiple criteria of each dimension (Radaelli et al. 2014).

In this context, ongoing discussion on **real-world evidence** (RWE) is also to be mentioned. RWE refers to evidence obtained from real-world data (RWD), which are observational data obtained outside the context of randomized controlled trials (RCTs) and generated during routine clinical practice, such as from pharmacovigilance reports, electronic health records, registries and medical or reimbursement claims databases.

For medicines with high uncertainty at the time of pricing and reimbursement decisions (and still high price tags), follow-up collection, analysis and consideration of RWE is of high relevance to review a pricing decision. This is, in principle, the nature of performance-based MEA. Italy has, for instance, a history of registries linked to pricing and reimbursement decisions: in 2014 it was reported that, in addition to 25 medicines under a MEA, registries were implemented for a large number of medicines (namely, 46) to manage their use (Jommi and Minghetti 2015). In other countries, however, RWD collection is much less used, mainly due to capacity limitations since it is very time-intensive (and requires a disinvestment strategy), as explained in the section on MEA (section "Managed Entry Agreements"). In the Netherlands, collection of RWE to inform the MEA did not work out as planned (from 2006 to 2012, for 49 MEAs in place, insufficient evidence was generated through the implemented outcome research studies within four years to reach grounded conclusions for a third of research questions defined at the beginning) (Makady et al. 2019). In any case, it would be important to share such RWD obtained in one country, in order to allow use by other countries.

Collaborative Approaches

High expectations are set on collaborations to improve affordable access to medicines, and several initiatives and projects have been established in recent years. Public attention focused on cross-country collaborations in the areas of joint negotiations and procurement such as the Valletta Declaration and the Beneluxa initiative, but there are several further aspects of collaborations. Three major dimensions to define collaborations in this field are the following:

- The scope of activities, that is, its position in the value chain: Some collaborations are procurement collaborations and/or cooperation mechanisms of joint pricing and reimbursement, whereas others aim to bridge between pre-launch activities (i.e. policies undertaken before the launch of a medicine in the market such as horizon scanning), peri-launch activities (policies undertaken around the launch such as HTA, pricing, procurement and reimbursement) and post-launch activities (policies undertaken after the launch of a medicine, e.g. monitoring of effectiveness and safety of new medicines in clinical practice and of prescribing behaviour).
- The sectorial and geographic dimension, that is, intra- or cross-country collaborations, with or without the involvement of a supranational institution.
- The status of how formal the collaboration has been established.

An important regional procurement collaboration is the Pan-American Health Organization (PAHO) Strategic Fund which is a technical collaboration mechanism for pooled procurement of essential medicines and strategic health supplies that save lives. More than 150 products of assured quality offered by more than 75 suppliers are available from the **PAHO Strategic Fund**. It is available to all countries in the PAHO region: by now, 33 Latin American and Caribbean countries signed agreements with the Strategic Fund. Signatory countries in need of medicines are invited to submit an official purchase request for a specific number of units. The PAHO Strategic Fund handles the procurement procedure: PAHO sends a quote from the provider that includes freight and insurance to the port of delivery that must be approved by the country who, in return, has to transfer the funds for the purchase to PAHO, according to the quotation, or request a line of credit from the capitalization account. In 2017, participating countries made over 437 purchase requests to the PAHO Strategic Fund for a total of more than USD 90 million; since 2004, there has been an 18-fold growth in its use (Pan American Health Organization 2017).

Further **regional pooled procurement initiatives** comprise the Southern African Development Community (SADC), the Pharmaceutical Procurement Service of the Organization of Eastern Caribbean States (OECS) and the Gulf Cooperation Council (GCC) (WHO 2007; Huff-Rousselle 2012).

In the **EU**, the '**Joint Procurement Agreement** (JPA) of medical countermeasures' entered into force in 2014. It is a mechanism to a joint procurement of, for example, laboratory tests, diagnostic tools for seasonal or pandemic influenza, vaccines, antivirals, decontamination products and personal protective equipment depending on the need triggered by a serious cross-border threat to health. The collaboration is on a voluntary basis, with the minimum number of five contracting parties to launch a specific procurement procedure (the European Commission and four EU Member States) (European Commission 2014). Some EU Member States expressed hope that the scope of JPA could be extended to high-priced medicines against cancer and multiple sclerosis and orphan medicines. But this appears to be not intended (Vogler et al. 2017).

As neither EU-wide joint procurement nor any joint pricing policies (e.g. EU-harmonized prices with differentially set markups and markdowns, in accordance with the income levels of countries (Vogler et al. 2016c); see also the section on differential pricing, section "Differential Pricing") seemed to be feasible in the short run, EU Member States started to seek cooperation between smaller groups of countries. Cross-country procurement initiatives in Europe are, for instance, the **Baltic Procurement Initiative** of the three Baltic countries Estonia, Latvia and Lithuania that jointly procured a few vaccines (Espín et al. 2016) and the **Nordic Procurement Initiative** of Denmark, Norway and Iceland that launched its call for a common tender in 2019 (AMGROS 2019). More recently established European collaborations are the **Valletta Declaration** that includes several Mediterranean countries and the **'Vysegrad collaboration'** of Eastern and South-Eastern European countries. Both collaborations aim to jointly procure medicines and also collaborate in other areas such as HTA. The **Beneluxa initiative** (Belgium, the Netherlands, Luxembourg, Austria, Ireland) is not a procurement initiative (though sometimes wrongfully labelled as such) but collaborates on joint pricing and reimbursement negotiations as well as in the areas of horizon scanning and HTA (Vogler and Fatima 2018).

The examples of the collaborations across European countries also highlight that collaborations are not limited to pricing and procurement but also address pre-launch activities. In addition, there have been initiatives in Europe to foster dialogue and collaboration between authorities of different areas **across the value chain** (i.e. the life cycle of a medicine). For instance, under the Dutch EU Presidency, a meeting brought together marketing authorization agencies, HTA bodies and pricing authorities and allowed gaining an improved understanding of different perspectives. At national level, the German marketing authorization and benefit assessment authorities signed an agreement in April 2016 to collaborate on joint scientific advice (i.e. a service of European and national regulators to pharmaceutical companies planning to apply for marketing authorization) (Vogler et al. 2018a).

Intra-country collaboration in pricing and procurement is particularly required in a fragmented in-patient pharmaceutical sector in many countries when hospitals procure the medicines they require. Each hospital negotiates individually with the pharmaceutical company and may also conclude different managed entry agreements that are kept confidential to the others (Vogler et al. 2011), even if they all use taxpayers' money. Countries reacted to this challenge, for example, by creating a central procurement agency to serve all public hospitals (e.g. Denmark, Norway) or by installing a central coordinating body that can be asked to negotiate for defined medicines on behalf of the hospitals and their owners such as provinces (e.g. in Sweden). In addition to the fragmentation of the hospital sector, pricing policies and management of procurement for the outpatient sector are often the responsibility of other bodies. This is, for instance, the case in Austria, and to bridge this divide, enhanced collaboration between social health insurance (responsible for reimbursement of outpatient medicines), the regions (responsible for financing medicines procured in the hospital sector) and the federal state (overall pricing policy framework) has been on the agenda of a long-term health reform project (Vogler et al. 2018a).

The formal collaborations in this field are supplemented by more informal initiatives. One of them is the **pharmaceutical pricing and reimbursement information (PPRI) network** of competent authorities for pricing and/or reimbursement of medicines from 47 countries (mainly from the European region). PPRI network member countries do not set joint prices, nor do they negotiate or procure jointly, but they share information on pharmaceutical pricing and exchange experiences of good and less successful practices (Vogler et al. 2014).

Transparency-Based Pricing

Intransparency has been identified as a major limitation to fair prices and thus affordable access to medicines, by researchers, civil society, national authorities (e.g. the Patented Medicine Prices Review Board in Canada (PMPRB 2015) and Latin American governments (Iunes et al. 2019)) and international institutions and bodies (e.g. the United Nations Secretary General's High-Level Panel on Access to Medicines (United Nations Secretary General's 2016) and the WHO in the course of the Fair Pricing Forum (WHO 2017)).

Two topics are usually addressed in the discussion related to transparency (and confidentiality):

- Transparency of research and development (R+D) costs (see also section "Delinkage and New Business Models")
- Price transparency

Price intransparency frequently relates to the confidential price deals made in MEA on high-priced medicines, usually in high-income countries. However, there is also a lack of price information (including the different price components resulting from add-ons such as wholesale and retail markups) in many countries globally, particularly those without medicine price regulation. There is evidence that medicine price control and advances in reimbursement coverage have contributed to uniform prices across a country and to improved price transparency (Mardetko et al. 2018).

In high-income countries, public payers often feel 'trapped' since they have to trust the pharmaceutical company, which has the complete overview of pricing conditions for its products, that they would get the 'best deal'. In a survey, Canadian policy-makers expressed power-related concerns about confidential negotiations, including the possibility that 'payers could be manipulated or "gamed" by manufacturers' (Morgan et al. 2013).

There is controversy with regard to the ability of price transparency to achieve fair prices. **Opponents** of price transparency have been arguing that confidential deals allow the pharmaceutical company to grant high discounts to lower-income countries, thus making medicines affordable to them (it has been argued that they could not do so in a transparent manner because this may lead to higher benchmark prices referred to by other countries applying EPR). However, as shown for Europe, countries of lower income (e.g. those in Central and Eastern Europe) lack access to some new medicines because they cannot afford their prices (Kaló et al. 2013). A price survey for oncology medicines in 15 European countries highlighted high cross-country variation of both list prices and discounted prices. It also showed that hospitals in Central and Eastern European countries were granted smaller, or no, discounts compared with the discounts in Western European countries (particularly Italy and Spain) for the same medicines (van Harten et al. 2016). This strongly challenges the argument of benefits of confidentiality (and price discrimination applied by the pharmaceutical industry). In addition, since there is empirical evidence globally that in some cases lower-income countries paid higher list prices (if adjusted by purchasing power parity) for new medicines than higher-income countries (Iyengar et al. 2016; Khatib et al. 2016; Machado et al. 2011), this would require more even larger discounts for lower-income countries to achieve fairness.

Thus, the arguments of price transparency opponents that confidentiality would lead to more affordable prices and access were not confirmed by empirical evidence. However, there is little empirical evidence on the consequences of price transparency in practice (e.g. impact studies on the disclosure of discounts or cross-sectorial studies) given the prevailing confidentiality. A study published a decade ago on discounts and 'real' discounted medicine prices for hospital medicines showed that, on average, Norway (the only country of the study with transparent pricing, at that time, and with centralized procurement for public hospitals) did better in terms of discounts and prices compared to four other European countries. On individual products, however, hospitals in the other countries could yield higher discounts (or received them cost-free, e.g. in Austria) (Vogler et al. 2010b, 2013a, b).

From a theoretical point of view, **information asymmetry** weakens the bargaining power of the party that has less information. Thus, it appears to be justified that transparency-based pricing will lead to more affordable price. Nonetheless, the pathway to more transparency will be a challenging one, since several suppliers and also purchasers might be opposed to it.

As for all other policies, transparency-based pricing might have some limitations, and possible drawbacks in the short run might be seen and have to be addressed in the course of implementation. Transparency-based pricing is not a pricing policy per se, but rather an approach to be applied while making progresses in universal health coverage (UHC). Transparency in pharmaceutical pricing should not only relate to price transparency but also to **transparency of further data of public interest** (e.g. R+D costs, findings of clinical research) and **transparent processes** (e.g. procedural issues of pricing committees: criteria for decision, timelines, involvement of experts and stakeholders, possibility to appeal, publication of prices and the rationale of decision) to ensure good governance.

In May 2019, the World Health Assembly (WHA) adopted a **resolution** on 'improving the transparency of markets for medicines, vaccines and other health products' in an effort to expand access. In this resolution, Member States are urged to enhance public sharing of information on net prices paid by governments and other purchasers for health products and greater transparency on pharmaceutical patents, clinical trial results and other determinants of pricing along the value chain from laboratory to patient (WHA 2019).

Delinkage and New Business Models

The pharmaceutical industry has been arguing that premium prices for new medicines are justified given their investments into R+D (so-called 'reward for innovation').

However, the **investment into R+D** is not known; published figures on costs to develop a new medicine vary considerably. The most frequently quoted figure is USD 2.6 billion published by the Tufts Institute (DiMasi et al. 2003). But considerably lower numbers were published by Light and Warburton (USD 180–231 million) (Light and Warburton 2011) and by the Drugs for Neglected Diseases initiative (DNDi), which is a public-private partnership (€100–150 million). The DNDi figures took into account the attrition in the field of R+D for infectious diseases and the inherent risk of failure; otherwise, DNDi reported costs of €30–40 million for the development of a new chemical entity (DNDi 2014).

In addition, as a second aspect to consider, the **share of public funding incurred in the R+D** of medicines should not be disregarded: several new medicines were initially developed based on government funding (e.g. in universities), and pharmaceutical companies then bought up successful start-ups. Based on available data, the share of government funding into health-related research was identified to amount to 30%, compared to 60% of the business sector and 10% of other sources, including private not-for-profit organizations and universities' own funds (Røttingen et al. 2013).

In reaction to the industry's motivation of high prices by R+D, the idea of 'delinkage', that is, to separate R+D costs and the price of the medicines (and other health products), has been called for (UNITAID 2016). Given the non-existence of a link between prices and (unknown) R&D costs, several experts do not consider the term 'delinkage' as the most appropriate one. Thus, it has been proposed to talk of new (business) models instead of 'delinkage'. Overall, it refers to a set of options that aim to change the way in which innovation is financed (World Health Organization 2011; Velásquez and Seuba 2011; Røttingen and Chamas 2012), since the current system is considered to be 'broken' (Moon et al. 2012; Outterson et al. 2015).

Proposals include expanding direct government funding of R+D, R+D subsidies and innovation inducement prizes (i.e. rewarding for the successful development of a new medicine by a cash prize) (Knowledge Ecology International (KEI) 2018; Jayadev and Stiglitz 2009; Love and Hubbard 2007; Agitha 2013). Some new mechanisms for funding R+D have been trialled to incentivize the development of new effective antibiotics (Outterson et al. 2015; The Review on Antimicrobial Resistance 2016; So and Shah 2014).

In this context, the debate on the 'new cost-plus pricing' policy as a possible reaction to address the high prices of new medicines should also be mentioned. As for R+D costs, production costs are frequently not known. However, as also confirmed by research, production costs can be low or even very low for medicines for which high prices are charged (for instance, manufacturing costs for 12-week courses of direct-acting antivirals to cure hepatitis C virus were estimated to be USD 21–63 for ribavirin, USD 10–30 for daclatasvir, USD 68–136 for sofosbuvir, USD 100–210 for faldaprevir and USD 130–270 for simeprevir (Hill et al. 2014)). Bringing up the argument of production costs, the advocates of this 'new cost-plus policy' do not aim to reinstall a cost-plus pricing policy that solely relies on costing data, but have argued to use production costs as a threshold, while further pricing policies remain.

Further new models have been debated in the recent times, as proposal of how to ensure access to new medicines and maintain the long-term sustainability of health-care systems. While they all address the challenge of high medicine prices, not all of them are necessarily pricing policies (e.g. amortization and the 'Netflix' models are rather funding policies).

Conclusions

There is evidence that price regulation contributes to fairer medicine prices and thus more affordable access to medicines.

There are different pricing policies to control medicine prices, and different policies target different types of medicines. For new medicines, frequently new pricing policies are external price referencing, managed entry agreements and value-based pricing (or elements of it).

All policies have their benefits but also their limitations. Some of the limitations can be addressed through methodological advances, (real-world) data collection and supportive tools (e.g. HTA). In addition, new pathways appear necessary. In this respect, collaborative approaches and consideration of more transparency appear to be very promising. Since there is a lack of evidence on the impact of some of the newer policies, or policy elements, it is suggested to evaluate and review the implementation of pricing policies.

References

WHO Collaborating Centre for Pharmaceutical Pricing and Reimbursement Policies. Glossary of pharmaceutical terms. Update 2018. Vienna: 2018. Available from: https://ppri.goeg.at/ppri-glossary (accessed 3 February 2019).

WHO, HAI. Measuring medicine prices, availability, affordability and price components. 2nd Edition. Geneva: World Health Organization, Health Action International, 2008.

Vogler S, Schneider P, Zimmermann N. Preparing price studies – Key methodological decisions. In: Vogler S, editor. Medicine Price Surveys, Analyses and Comparisons. London: Elsevier; 2019a.

World Health Organization. Essential medicines 2019. Available from: https://www.who.int/topics/essential_medicines/en/ (accessed 2 May 2019).

World Health Organization. Equitable access to essential medicines: a framework for collective action. 2004 Contract No.: 8.

WHO. The World Medicines Situation. Access to Essential Medicines as Path of the Right to Health. Geneva: World Health Organization, 2011. Available from: http://apps.who.int/medicinedocs/documents/s18772en/s18772en.pdf (accessed 2 May 2019).

Cameron A, Ewen M, Ross-Degnan D, Ball D, Laing R. Medicine prices, availability, and affordability in 36 developing and middle-income countries: a secondary analysis. The Lancet. 2009;373(9659):240–9.

Ewen M, Zweekhorst M, Regeer B, Laing R. Baseline assessment of WHO's target for both availability and affordability of essential medicines to treat non-communicable diseases. PLOS ONE. 2017;12(2):e0171284.

Mendis S, Fukino K, Cameron A, Laing R, Filipe Jr A, Khatib O, et al. The availability and affordability of selected essential medicines for chronic diseases in six low-and middle-income countries. Bulletin of the World Health Organization. 2007;85(4):279–88.

Niëns LM, Cameron A, Van de Poel E, Ewen M, Brouwer WB, Laing R. Quantifying the impoverishing effects of purchasing medicines: a cross-country comparison of the affordability of medicines in the developing world. PLoS medicine. 2010;7(8):1056.

Leive A, Xu K. Coping with out-of-pocket health payments: empirical evidence from 15 African countries. Bulletin of the World Health Organization. 2008;86(11):849-56C.

Li Y, Wu Q, Xu L, Legge D, Hao Y, Gao L, et al. Factors affecting catastrophic health expenditure and impoverishment from medical expenses in China: policy implications of universal health insurance. Bulletin of the World Health Organization. 2012;90:664–71.

Wagner AK, Graves AJ, Reiss SK, LeCates R, Zhang F, Ross-Degnan D. Access to care and medicines, burden of health care expenditures, and risk protection: Results from the World Health Survey. Health policy. 2011;100(2):151–8.

Iyengar S, Tay-Teo K, Vogler S, Beyer P, Wiktor S, de Joncheere K, et al. Prices, Costs, and Affordability of New Medicines for Hepatitis C in 30 Countries: An Economic Analysis. PLoS Med. 2016;13(5):e1002032.

Abboud C, Berman E, Cohen A, Cortes J, DeAngelo D, Deininger M, et al. The price of drugs for chronic myeloid leukemia (CML) is a reflection of the unsustainable prices of cancer drugs: from the perspective of a large group of CML experts. Blood. 2013;121(22):4439–42.

Kantarjian HM, Fojo T, Mathisen M, Zwelling LA. Cancer drugs in the United States: Justum Pretium—the just price. Journal of Clinical Oncology. 2013;31(28):3600–4.

Kelly RJ, Smith TJ. Delivering maximum clinical benefit at an affordable price: engaging stakeholders in cancer care. The lancet oncology. 2014;15(3):e112-e8.

World Health Organization. Technical report: pricing of cancer medicines and its impacts: a comprehensive technical report for the World Health Assembly Resolution 70.12: operative paragraph 2.9 on pricing approaches and their impacts on availability and affordability of medicines for the prevention and treatment of cancer. 2018.

Zaprutko T, Kopciuch D, Kus K, Merks P, Nowicka M, Augustyniak I, et al. Affordability of medicines in the European Union. Plos one. 2017;12(2):e0172753.

Council of the European Union. Council conclusions on Encouraging Member States-driven Voluntary Cooperation between Health System. 16 June 2017. Available from: http://data.consilium.europa.eu/doc/document/ST-10381-2017-INIT/en/pdf (accessed 1 March 2019).

Council of the European Union. Council conclusions on strengthening the balance in the pharmaceutical systems in the EU and its Member States. 17 June 2016. Available from: https://www.consilium.europa.eu/en/press/press-releases/2016/06/17/epsco-conclusions-balance-pharmaceutical-system/ (accessed 1 March 2019).

Vogler S, Paris V, Panteli D. Ensuring access to medicines: How to redesign pricing, reimbursement and procurement? Policy Brief 30. Copenhagen: World Health Organization, 2018a.

Babar Z-U-D. Pharmaceutical Prices in the 21st Century: Springer; 2015.

Babar Z-U-D, Hussain R, Hasan SS. Medicine Prices in Asia-Pacific Countries. In: Vogler S, editor. Medicine Price Surveys, Analyses and Comparisons (in print)2018.

World Health Organization. WHO Guideline on Country Pharmaceutical Pricing Policies. Geneva: 2013.

Vogler S, Habl C, Leopold C, Rosian-Schikuta I, de Joncheere K, Lyager Thomsen T. PPRI Report. Vienna: Pharmaceutical Pricing and Reimbursement Information, 2008.

Vogler S, Haasis MA, Dedet G, Lam J, Bak Pedersen H. Medicines reimbursement policies in Europe. Copenhagen: World Health Organization, 2018b.

WHO Collaborating Centre for Pharmaceutical Pricing and Reimbursement Policies. Glossary of pharmaceutical terms. Update 2016. Vienna: 2016. Available from: http://whocc.goeg.at/Literaturliste/Dokumente/MethodologyTemplate/Glossary_Update2016_final.pdf (accessed 5 January 2018).

Leopold C, Vogler S, Mantel-Teeuwisse AK, de Joncheere K, Leufkens HG, Laing R. Differences in external price referencing in Europe-A descriptive overview. Health policy. 2012a;104(1):50–60.

Toumi M, Rémuzat C, Vataire A-L, Urbinati D. External reference pricing of medicinal products: simulation-based considerations for cross-country coordination. Final Report. Available from: https://www.redaccionmedica.com/contenido/images/erp_reimbursement_medicinal_products_en-1.pdf (accessed 28 November 2017). European Commission, 2014.

Espin J, Rovira J, Ewen M, Laing R. Mapping External Reference Pricing Practices for Medicines. Health Action International and the Andalusian School of Public Health, 2014.

Vogler S, Lepuschütz L, Schneider P, Stühlinger V. Study on enhanced cross-country coordination in the area of pharmaceutical product pricing. Available from: http://ec.europa.eu/health/systems_performance_assessment/docs/pharmaproductpricing_frep_en.pdf (accessed 6 September 2017). Luxembourg: Gesundheit Österreich Forschungs- und Planungs GmbH; Publications Office of the European Commission, 2016a.

Rémuzat C, Urbinati D, Mzoughi O, El Hammi E, Belgaied W, Toumi M. Overview of external reference pricing systems in Europe. Journal of Market Access & Health Policy. 2015;3.

Schneider P, Vogler S. Practice of External Price Referencing (EPR). In: Vogler S, editor. Medicine Price Surveys, Analyses and Comparisons (in print)2018.

Espin J, Rovira J, de Labry AO. Working paper 1: External price referencing – review series on pharmaceutical pricing policies and interventions. Available from: http://www.haiweb.org/medicineprices/24072012/ERPfinalMay2011.pdf (accessed 28 December 2017). Geneva: World Health Organization and Health Action International, 2011.

Kanavos P, Nicod E, Espin J. Short-and Long-Term Effects of Value-Based Pricing vs. External Price Referencing. Available from: http://whocc.goeg.at/Literaturliste/Dokumente/FurtherReading/Short- and long-term effect of value-based pricing.pdf (accessed 28 December 2017). London: 2010.

Danzon PM, Epstein AJ. Effects of regulation on drug launch and pricing in interdependent markets: Emerald Group Publishing Limited; 2008.

Danzon PM, Towse A. Differential pricing for pharmaceuticals: reconciling access, R&D and patents. Int J Health Care Finance Econ. 2003;3(3):183–205.

Danzon PM, Wang YR, Wang L. The impact of price regulation on the launch delay of new drugs—evidence from twenty-five major markets in the 1990s. Health economics. 2005;14(3):269–92.

Kyle MK. Pharmaceutical price controls and entry strategies. The Review of Economics and Statistics. 2007;89(1):88–99.

Kanavos P, Fontrier A-M, Gill J, Efthymiadou O, Boekstein N. The Impact of External Reference Pricing within and across Countries. London: London School of Economics, 2017.

Stargardt D-VT, Schreyögg J. Impact of Cross-Reference Pricing on Pharmaceutical Prices. Applied Health Economics and Health Policy. 2006;5(4):235–47.

Vogler S, Schneider P, Zimmermann N. Evolution of Average European Medicine Prices: Implications for the Methodology of External Price Referencing. PharmacoEconomics Open. 2019b:1–7.

Morgan S, Vogler S, Wagner AK. Payers' experiences with confidential pharmaceutical price discounts: a survey of public and statutory health systems in North America, Europe, and Australasia. Health Policy. 2017;121(4):354–62.

Vogler S, Zimmermann N, Habl C, Piessnegger J, Bucsics A. Discounts and rebates granted to public payers for medicines in European countries. Southern Med Review. 2012;5(1):38–46.

Bouvy J, Vogler S. Background Paper 8.3 Pricing and Reimbursement Policies: Impacts on Innovation. In: World Health Organization, editor. Priority Medicines for Europe and the World 2013 Update. Geneva World Health Organization; 2013.

Vogler S, Paterson KR. Can Price Transparency Contribute to More Affordable Patient Access to Medicines? PharmacoEconomics – Open. 2017;1(3):145–7

Vogler S, Schneider P. Assessing Data Sources for Medicine Price Studies. International Journal of Technology Assessment in Health Care. 2019;35(2):106–15.

WHO. WHO Guideline on Country Pharmaceutical Pricing Policies. Available from: http://apps.who.int/medicinedocs/documents/s21016en/s21016en.pdf(accessed 19 November 2017). Geneva: World Health Organization,, 2013.

Håkonsen H, Horn AM, Toverud E-L. Price control as a strategy for pharmaceutical cost containment—What has been achieved in Norway in the period 1994–2004? Health policy. 2009;90(2):277–85.

Leopold C, Mantel-Teeuwisse AK, Seyfang L, Vogler S, de Joncheere K, Laing RO, et al. Impact of External Price Referencing on Medicine Prices–A Price Comparison Among 14 European Countries. Southern Med Review. 2012b;5(1):34–41.

Windmeijer F, De Laat E, Douven R, Mot E. Pharmaceutical promotion and GP prescription behaviour. Health economics. 2006;15(1):5–18.

Merkur S, Mossialos E. A pricing policy towards the sourcing of cheaper drugs in Cyprus. Health policy. 2007;81(2):368–75.

Filko M, Szilagyiova P. Case 3: The Slovak experience in the international price benchmarking for prescription drugs. Value in Health. 2009;12(7):A229.

Garner S, Rintoul A, Hill SR. Value-Based Pricing: L'Enfant Terrible? PharmacoEconomics. 2018;36(1):5–6.

Claxton K. Oft, Vbp: Qed? Health economics. 2007;16(6):545–58.

Vogler S. Fair prices for medicines? Exploring competent authorities' and public payers' preferences on pharmaceutical policies. Empirica. 2019.

Dholakia UM. A Quick Guide to Value-Based Pricing. Harvard Business Review, 2016. Avaiable from: https://hbr.org/2016/08/a-quick-guide-to-value-based-pricing (accessed 8 June 2019).

Godman B, Gustafsson LL. A new reimbursement system for innovative pharmaceuticals combining value-based and free market pricing. Applied health economics and health policy. 2013;11(1):79.

Consultative Expert Working Group on Research and Development. Follow-up of the report of the Consultative Expert Working Group on Research and Development: Financing and Coordination (CEWG). Available from: http://www.who.int/phi/cewg/en/ (accessed 26 June 2016). 2016.

Franken M, le Polain M, Cleemput I, Koopmanschap M. Similarities and differences between five European drug reimbursement systems. International Journal of Technology Assessment in Health Care. 2012;28(4):349.

Hughes DA. Value-Based Pricing. Incentive for Innovation or Zero Net Benefit? Pharmacoeconomics. 2011;29(9):731–5.

WHO. Fair Pricing Forum. 2017 Meeting Report. Available from: http://www.who.int/medicines/access/fair_pricing/FairPricingForum2017MeetingReport.pdf?ua=1 (accessed 29 October 2017). Geneva: World Health Organization, 2017.

Paris V, Belloni A. Value in Pharmaceutical Pricing. OECD Health Working Papers, No. 63. Paris: OECD Publishing, 2013.

Simoens S, Picavet E, Dooms M, Cassiman D, Morel T. Cost-effectiveness assessment of orphan drugs: a scientific and political conundrum. Applied health economics and health policy. 2013;11(1):1.

Nguyen TA, Knight R, Roughead EE, Brooks G, Mant A. Policy options for pharmaceutical pricing and purchasing: issues for low-and middle-income countries. Health Policy and Planning. 2014;30:267–80.

Rovira J. Can EU citizens afford their medicines? The financial crisis and access to medicines in Europe. Presentation. Brussels: High Level Meeting. The European Parliament, 2013.

Mossialos E, Dukes G. Affordably priced new drugs for poor populations: Approaches for a global solution. The International journal of risk & safety in medicine. 2000;14(1):1–29.

Babar ZUD, Atif M. Differential pricing of pharmaceuticals: a bibliometric review of the literature. Journal of Pharmaceutical Health Services Research. 2014;5(3):149–56.

Access And Affordability Initiative. Access accelerated. Available from: https://accessaccelerated.org/initiative/access-and-affordability-initiative/ (accessed 19 May 2018). 2018.

Yadav P. Differential pricing of pharmaceuticals: Review of current knowledge, new findings and ideas for action – A study conducted for the UK Department for International Development (DFID). Zaragoza: MIT Zaragoza International Logistics Program, 2010.

Moon S, Jambert E, Childs M, von Schoen-Angerer T. A 'win-win solution?': A critical analysis of tiered pricing to improve access to medicines in developing countries. Globalization and Health. 2011;7:39.

De Souza N. Competition in Pharmaceuticals: the challenges ahead post AstraZeneca. Competition policy newsletter. 2007(1):39–43.

Waning B, Kaplan W, King AC, Lawrence DA, Leufkens HG, Fox MP. Global strategies to reduce the price of antiretroviral medicines: evidence from transactional databases. Bulletin of the World Health Organization. 2009;87(7):520–8.

Vogler S, Habl C, Leopold C, Mazag J, Morak S, Zimmermann N. PHIS Hospital Pharma Report. Available from: http://whocc.goeg.at/Literaturliste/Dokumente/BooksReports/PHIS_Hospital Pharma_Report.pdf (accessed 3 April 2018). Vienna: Pharmaceutical Health Information System (PHIS); commissioned by the European Commission and the Austrian Federal Ministry of Health, 2010a.

Seiter A. A practical approach to pharmaceutical policy. Washington DC: World Bank Publications, 2010.

Dylst P, Vulto A, Simoens S. Tendering for outpatient prescription pharmaceuticals: What can be learned from current practices in Europe? Health Policy. 2011;101(2):146–52.

Kanavos P. Tender systems for outpatient pharmaceuticals in the European Union: Evidence from the Netherlands and Germany. Available from: http://www.progenerika.de/wp-content/uploads/2013/02/Anlage-2_Tendering-Report-EMINET-13OCT2012-FINAL.pdf (accessed 1 March 2018). London: EMINET, January. 2012.

T'Hoen E, Moon S, Pecoul B. Pills and pocketbooks. 2001.

Ferrario A, Kanavos P, Humbert T, Iwamoto K, Bak Pedersen H. Challenges and opportunities in improving access to medicines through efficient public procurement in WHO European Region. 2016 9289052155.

Klemp M, Frønsdal KB, Facey K. What principles should govern the use of managed entry agreements? International Journal of Technology Assessment in Health Care. 2011;27(01):77–83.

Carlson JJ, Sullivan SD, Garrison LP, Neumann PJ, Veenstra DL. Linking payment to health outcomes: A taxonomy and examination of performance-based reimbursement schemes between healthcare payers and manufacturers. Health Policy. 2010;96(3):179–90.

Garrison LP, Towse A, Briggs A, de Pouvourville G, Grueger J, Mohr PE, et al. Performance-based risk-sharing arrangements—good practices for design, implementation, and evaluation: report of the ISPOR good practices for performance-based risk-sharing arrangements task force. Value in Health. 2013;16(5):703–19.

Ferrario A, Kanavos P. Managed entry agreements for pharmaceuticals: The European experience. EMINet, 2013.

Pauwels K, Huys I, Vogler S, Casteels M, Simoens S. Managed Entry Agreements for oncology drugs: lessons from the European experience to inform the future. Frontiers in Pharmacology. 2017;8:171.

Ferrario A, Arāja D, Bochenek T, Čatić T, Dankó D, Dimitrova M, et al. The Implementation of Managed Entry Agreements in Central and Eastern Europe: Findings and Implications. PharmacoEconomics. 2017;35(12):1271–85.

Ferrario A, Kanavos P. Dealing with uncertainty and high prices of new medicines: A comparative analysis of the use of managed entry agreements in Belgium, England, the Netherlands and Sweden. Social Science & Medicine. 2015;124(1):39–47.

Gerkens S, Neyt M, San Miguel L, Vinck I, Thiry N, Cleemput I. How to improve the Belgian process for managed entry agreements? An analysis of the Belgian and international experience. Brussels: Belgian Health Care Knowledge Centre (KCE), 2017.

Vogler S, Zimmermann N, Ferrario A, Wirtz VJ, de Joncheere K, Pedersen HB, et al. Pharmaceutical policies in a crisis? Challenges and solutions identified at the PPRI Conference. Journal of Pharmaceutical Policy and Practice. 2016b;9(1):1.

Adamski J, Godman B, Ofierska-Sujkowska G, Osinska B, Herholz H, Wendykowska K, et al. Risk sharing arrangements for pharmaceuticals: potential considerations and recommendations for European payers. BMC health services research. 2010;10:153.

Vogler S, Paris V, Ferrario A, Wirtz VJ, de Joncheere K, Schneider P, et al. How Can Pricing and Reimbursement Policies Improve Affordable Access to Medicines? Lessons Learned from European Countries. Applied Health Economics and Health Policy. 2017:1–15.

Lieven A, Luca P. Dynamic outcomes based approaches to pricing and reimbursement of innovative medicines. 2017.

World Health Organization. 2015 Global Survey on Health Technology Assessment by National Authorities (accessed 5 February 2018). Geneva: 2015.

EUnetHTA. EUnetHTA WP7: Implementation report. European network for health technology assessment, November 2018.

Beneluxa Initiative on Pharmaceutical Policy. HTA 2018. Available from: http://www.beneluxa.org/hta (accessed 16 July 2019).

Angelis A, Kanavos P. Value-based assessment of new medical technologies: towards a robust methodological framework for the application of multiple criteria decision analysis in the context of health technology assessment. Pharmacoeconomics. 2016;34(5):435–46.

Angelis A, Kanavos P. Multiple Criteria Decision Analysis (MCDA) for evaluating new medicines in Health Technology Assessment and beyond: The Advance Value Framework. Social Science & Medicine. 2017;188:137–56.

Radaelli G, Lettieri E, Masella C, Merlino L, Strada A, Tringali M. Implementation of EUnetHTA core model® in Lombardia: the VTS framework. International Journal of Technology Assessment in Health Care. 2014;30(1):105–12.

Jommi C, Minghetti P. Pharmaceutical pricing policies in Italy. Pharmaceutical prices in the 21st century: Springer; 2015. p. 131–50.

Makady A, van Veelen A, De Boer A, Hillege H, Klungel O, Goettsch W. Implementing managed entry agreements in practice: The Dutch reality check. Health Policy. 2019;123(3):267–74.

Pan American Health Organization. PAHO Strategic Fund. 2017. Available from: http://www.paho.org/hq/index.php?option=com_content&view=article&id=12163&Itemid=42005&lang=en (accessed 22 July 2019).

WHO. Multi-Country Regional Procurement of Medicines. World Health Organization,, 2007.

Huff-Rousselle M. The logical underpinnings and benefits of pooled pharmaceutical procurement: a pragmatic role for our public institutions? Social Science & Medicine. 2012;75(9):1572–80.

European Commission. Medical Countermeasures that could be procured in common under the joint procurement agreement. Accessible at: http://ec.europa.eu/health/preparedness_response/docs/jpa_note_scope_en.pdf (accessed 1 March 2019). Luxembourg: 2014.

Vogler S, Lepuschütz L, Schneider P, Stühlinger V. Study on enhanced cross-country coordination in the area of pharmaceutical product pricing. Luxembourg: Gesundheit Österreich Forschungs- und Planungs GmbH; Publications Office of the European Commission, 2016c.

Espín J, Rovira J, Calleja A, Azzopardi-Muscat N, Richardson E, Palm W, et al. How can voluntary cross-border collaboration in public procurement improve access to health technologies in Europe? Policy Brief. 2016;21. Available from: https://www.eu2017.mt/Documents/Programmes/PB21.pdf (accessed 1 March 2019).

AMGROS. First Common Nordic Tendering Procedure Launched. 26 April 2019. Available from: https://amgros.dk/en/knowledge-and-analyses/articles/first-common-nordic-tendering-procedure-launched/.

Vogler Sabine, Suleman Fatima. Research study on impact and benefits of cross border collaboration in WHO European Region. Presentation at the International Conference "Facing the Challenges: Equity, Sustainability and Access". Lisbon: 28 November 2018. Available from: http://www.infarmed.pt/documents/15786/2835945/Sabine+Vogler_Fatima+Suleman.pdf/ec485707-043e-404e-b5a1-74c4f0d59390 (accessed 21 July 2019).

Vogler S, Zimmermann N, Mazag J. Procuring medicines in hospitals: results of the European PHIS survey. EJHP Practice. 2011(2):20–1.

Vogler S, Leopold C, Zimmermann N, Habl C, de Joncheere K. The Pharmaceutical Pricing and Reimbursement Information (PPRI) initiative–experiences from engaging with pharmaceutical policy makers. Health Policy and Technology. 2014;3(2):139–48.

PMPRB. Strategic Plan 2015–2018. Ottawa: Patented Medicine Prices Review Board 2015.

Iunes RF, Uribe MV, Torres JB, Garcia MM, Dias CZ, Alvares-Teodoro J, et al. Confidentiality agreements: a challenge in market regulation. International Journal for Equity in Health. 2019;18(1):11.

United Nations Secretary General's High-Level Panel on Access to Medicines. Report of the United Nations Secretary General's High-Level Panel on Access to Medicines. Promoting innovation and access to health technologies. September 2016.

WHO. Fair Pricing Forum. 2017 Meeting Report. Geneva: World Health Organization, 2017. Available from: http://www.who.int/medicines/access/fair_pricing/FairPricingForum2017MeetingReport.pdf?ua=1 (accessed 1 March 2019).

Mardetko N, Kos M, Vogler S. Review of studies reporting actual prices for medicines. Expert review of pharmacoeconomics & outcomes research. 2018;19(2).

Morgan SG, Thomson PA, Daw JR, Friesen MK. Canadian policy makers' views on pharmaceutical reimbursement contracts involving confidential discounts from drug manufacturers. Health Policy. 2013;112(3):248–54.

Kaló Z, Annemans L, Garrison LP. Differential pricing of new pharmaceuticals in lower income European countries. Expert review of pharmacoeconomics & outcomes research. 2013;13(6):735–41.

van Harten WH, Wind A, de Paoli P, Saghatchian M, Oberst S. Actual costs of cancer drugs in 15 European countries. The Lancet Oncology. 2016;17(1):18–20.

Khatib R, McKee M, Shannon H, Chow C, Rangarajan S, Teo K, et al. Availability and affordability of cardiovascular disease medicines and their effect on use in high-income, middle-income, and low-income countries: an analysis of the PURE study data. The Lancet. 2016;387(10013):61–9.

Machado M, O'Brodovich R, Krahn M, Einarson TR. International drug price comparisons: quality assessment. Revista Panamericana de Salud Publica. 2011;29(1):46–51.

Vogler S, Habl C, Leopold C, Mazag J, Morak S, Zimmermann N. PHIS Hospital Pharma Report. Vienna: Pharmaceutical Health Information System (PHIS); commissioned by the European Commission and the Austrian Federal Ministry of Health, 2010b.

Vogler S, Zimmermann N, Leopold C, Habl C, Mazag J. Discounts and Rebates Granted for Medicines for Hospital Use in Five European Countries. The Open Pharmacoeconomics & Health Economics Journal 2013a;5:1–10.

Vogler S, Zimmermann N, Habl C, Mazag J. The role of discounts and loss leaders in medicine procurement in Austrian hospitals – a primary survey of official and actual medicine prices. Cost Effectiveness and Resource Allocation. 2013b;11(1):15.

WHA. Improving the transparency of markets for medicines, vaccines, and other health products. Resolution. Geneva: World Health Assembly, 28 May 2019.

DiMasi JA, Hansen RW, Grabowski HG. The price of innovation: new estimates of drug development costs. Journal of health economics. 2003;22(2):151–85.

Light DW, Warburton R. Demythologizing the high costs of pharmaceutical research. BioSocieties. 2011;6(1):34–50.

DNDi. An innovative approach to R&D for neglected patients: Ten years of experience and lessons learned by DNDi. Drugs for Neglected Diseases (DNDi), 2014.

Røttingen J-A, Regmi S, Eide M, Young AJ, Viergever RF, Årdal C, et al. Mapping of available health research and development data: what's there, what's missing, and what role is there for a global observatory? The Lancet. 2013;382(9900):1286–307.

UNITAID. An economic perspective on delinking the cost of R+D from the price of medicines. Discussion paper. Geneva: World Health Organization, 2016.

World Health Organization. Global strategy and plan of action on public health, innovation and intellectual property. Geneva: 2011.

Velásquez G, Seuba X. Rethinking global health: A binding convention for R&D for pharmaceutical products. South Center Research Papers. 2011;42:29.

Røttingen J-A, Chamas C. A New Deal for Global Health R&D? The Recommendations of the Consultative Expert Working Group on Research and Development (CEWG). PLoS Med. 2012;9(5):e1001219.

Moon S, Bermudez J, t Hoen E. Innovation and Access to Medicines for Neglected Populations: Could a Treaty Address a Broken Pharmaceutical R& System? PLoS Med. 2012;9(5):e1001218.

Outterson K, Powers JH, Daniel GW, McClellan MB. Repairing the broken market for antibiotic innovation. Health affairs. 2015;34(2):277–85.

Knowledge Ecology International (KEI). Delinkage.org. Available from: http://delinkage.org/ (accessed 21 April 2018).

Jayadev A, Stiglitz J. Two ideas to increase innovation and reduce pharmaceutical costs and prices. Health Affairs. 2009;28(1):w165-w8.

Love J, Hubbard T. Bid Idea: Prizes to Stimulate R& (and) D for New Medicines, The. Chi-Kent L Rev. 2007;82:1519.

Agitha T. Alternative incentive models delinking R&D costs from pharmaceutical product price. Journal of Intellectual Property Rights 2013;18(5):491–8.

The Review on Antimicrobial Resistance. Tackling drug-resistent infections globally: Final Report and Recommendations. London: 2016.

So AD, Shah TA. New business models for antibiotic innovation. Upsala Journal of Medical Sciences. 2014;119(2):176–80.

Hill A, Khoo S, Fortunak J, Simmons B, Ford N. Minimum Costs for Producing Hepatitis C Direct-Acting Antivirals for Use in Large-Scale Treatment Access Programs in Developing Countries. Clinical Infectious Diseases. 2014;58(7):928–36.

6

Pharmacy Practice and Policy Research in Pakistan: A Review of Literature Between 2014 and 2019

Iram Malik, Muhammad Atif, Shane L. Scahill, and Zaheer-Ud-Din Babar

Introduction

Globally, there is no single representative policy directing pharmacy practice, and different nations show divergences in ongoing pharmaceutical policy and practice (International Pharmaceutical Federation 2000; Wiedenmayer et al. 2006). Pharmaceutical care (PC), clinical pharmacy, social and administrative pharmacy and pharmacy practice are terms that have been largely used interchangeably to explain facets of pharmacy

---

Electronic Supplementary Material: The online version of this chapter (https://doi.org/10.1007/978-981-15-2724-1_6) contains supplementary material, which is available to authorized users.

I. Malik • M. Atif (✉)
Department of Pharmacy, The Islamia University of Bahawalpur, Bahawalpur, Punjab, Pakistan

S. L. Scahill
School of Pharmacy, University of Auckland, Auckland, New Zealand

Z. Babar (ed.), *Global Pharmaceutical Policy*,
https://doi.org/10.1007/978-981-15-2724-1_6

practice (Scahill et al. 2017). However, these terms are used in an ambiguous fashion, and they signify different things to different people (Scahill et al. 2017). Pharmacy practice and policy research is obligatory to strengthen the field of pharmacy practice and the overall healthcare system, especially within developing countries (Babar and Jamshed 2008). Pharmacy practice and policy research, which is predominantly linked to social and administrative pharmacy (Babar and Jamshed 2008), is an element of health services research that involves the assessment and evaluation of pharmacy practice to assist with a well-versed understanding of medicines, helps move towards evidence-based practices and aids policymakers in developing and commissioning new services (Koshman and Blais 2011; Fakeye et al. 2017a). This encompasses the areas related to drug distribution, drug selection, drug regulation, drug safety, efficacy and quality, pharmaco-epidemiology, access to medicines, pharmacoeconomics, pharmacovigilance (PV) and PC (Desselle 2005; Babar and Jamshed 2008). In this regard, the International Social Pharmacy Workshop (ISPW) has provided a basis for the expansion of the research and practice network throughout the world, and their focus has been on research directed toward all the sub-disciplines (Scahill et al. 2017).

According to a report in 2010, approximately US$240 billion is invested annually into health-related research globally (Macleod et al. 2014). Healthcare research requires workforce development with the building of capacity and capability to grow and sustain professional performance and knowledge (Sarwar et al. 2018b). Thus, it is crucial to develop an interest in pharmacists to engage with high-quality and impactful practice-based research (Sultana et al. 2016). That is, any identifiable advantage to, or constructive influence on, the community, economy, health, quality of life, policy or services, surroundings or academia should help with engagement and outcomes (Cruz Rivera et al. 2017) of practice-based research (Sultana et al. 2016). Considering the need to set forth an evidence-based process of documentation of practices related to patient care and treatment outcomes, the American College of Clinical Pharmacy (ACCP) has encouraged pharmacists to engage

Z. Babar
Centre for Pharmaceutical Policy and Practice Research,
University of Huddersfield, Huddersfield, UK
e-mail: z.babar@hud.ac.uk

with research (Yee and Haas 2014). Likewise, Australia's National Translational Research Collaborative (NTRC) is supporting high-quality research to deliver up-to-date practice-based evidence to support ongoing pharmacy practice and quality use of medicines (International Pharmaceutical Federation 2017).

In accordance with global trends, the higher education department in Pakistan implemented the Department of Pharmacy Practice in 2014 (Hashmi and Saleem 2017). However, the implementation has been stifled by a lack of qualified pharmacy practice scholars and practitioners in the country (Hashmi and Saleem 2017). Only 5% of pharmacists in Pakistan are involved in teaching and/or research (Azhar et al. 2011). These individuals face barriers to conducting pharmacy practice and policy research including a persistent lack of documentation, time shortage, lack of financial support, inadequate pharmacist training and skills, and inadequate levels of collaboration with other healthcare professionals (Azhar et al. 2016; Malik et al. 2019b).

Research scholars in Pakistan experience a lack of cooperation from hospital management to support research carried out to overcome system imperfections. Additionally, most of the healthcare centres across Pakistan do not promote pharmacoeconomic research, even though costs associated with healthcare service provision are increasing in Pakistan as they are globally, and there are no evidence-based control measures available which could be instituted (Ahmed et al. 2018; Malik et al. 2019b).

The rising population in Pakistan, coupled with an allocation of only 2.8% of gross domestic product (GDP) to health, indicates that the healthcare system is gradually deteriorating (Inamullah et al. 2017). In concert with the absence of a fully developed disease surveillance system, it is difficult for researchers to efficiently undertake research into endemic diseases in Pakistan, and consequently challenges arise in the effective implementation of healthcare policy (Ahmed et al. 2018).

Research into pharmacy practice particularly in the community setting is conventionally difficult in Pakistan. This is due to the very limited number of drug stores (0.02%) that operate with a qualified pharmacist and the reluctance of that limited number of pharmacists to become involved in research (Aslam 2019; Saini et al. 2005). This further impedes the expansion of pharmacy practice and policy research in Pakistan.

Recognizing this, the Ministerial Standing Committee on Scientific and Technological Cooperation of the Organization of Islamic Cooperation

(COMSTECH) conducted an international workshop on "Integrating Clinical Pharmacy Education, Practice and Research: Bridging the Gap" in 2016 and established a set of targets to improve the existing situation of pharmacy practice in Pakistan (Khan 2016). Despite this workshop, there continues to be a reticence by Pakistani regulators to direct resource towards the strengthening of infrastructure and direction for pharmacy practice research (Ahmed et al. 2018). In Pakistan, most of the pharmacy practice research prior to the introduction of the Department of Pharmacy Practice was centred on the validation, protection, extension and progression of pharmacy roles and services provided, especially in hospital settings (Azhar et al. 2009, 2010; Rahim and Usmani 2012; Aslam and Ahmed 2011; Khan et al. 2011; Din Babar 2006). The authors are not aware of any research that has been undertaken in terms of pricing, access and affordability of medicines in Pakistan (Din Babar 2006). Besides this, there is a dearth of research in the various domains of pharmaceutical policy and practice and particularly using advanced methodologies, i.e. qualitative methods, clinical trials and action research (Abbas and Khan 2014; Babar and Jamshed 2008). In short, both the quantity and quality of practice-based research have been less than optimal.

In Pakistan, the practice evidence to policy linkage is delicate, owing to disconnection between researchers, practitioners and policymakers (Ahmad et al. 2017; World Health Organization 2016). Evidence-based policy is best developed through considering local research data; however, while devising policies in developing countries, insight is usually taken from research data and success stories of developed nations. This does not take into account the local context and the realities of health service delivery and the economic differences in the country (Ahmad et al. 2017). Realizing the need to work through this problem, the National Health Vision Pakistan 2016–2025 has adopted the mission "Health Information Systems and Research" to provide evidence-based healthcare to the Pakistani population and subsequently attain sustainable development goals (Ryan et al. 2007).

While recently wide-ranging pharmacy practice studies have been coming out of Pakistan, the overall typology and impact of their findings has not been accessed to date. Considering this, systematic reviews are required to enable the current available body of research to influence and inform healthcare policymakers to allow them to understand the impact of findings on professional practices and subsequent patient outcomes. Furthermore, the quality of available literature needs to be thoroughly evaluated as a body of knowledge to ensure that policy is set based on robust evidence. Founded on this, the systematic review outlined in this chapter set out to (1) assess the typology and quality of pharmaceutical policy and practice studies conducted within the last five years in Pakistan, (2) summarize the expected impact of published studies on policy and (3) change the discourse around pharmacy practice and policy research in Pakistan. The findings are intended to provide a roadmap for future innovation in pharmaceutical policy and pharmacy practice research and are expected to contribute towards realigning pharmacy practice and healthcare policy in Pakistan.

Methods

The systematic review was conducted according to the guidelines described in the Preferred Reporting Items for Systematic Reviews and Meta-Analyses: The PRISMA Statement (Moher et al. 2009).

Research Strategy

A broad search strategy combining Medical Subject Headings (MeSH) searches and free-text terms was used to identify the relevant literature (i.e. originating from Pakistan) regarding pharmacy practice and policy published from 1 January 2014 to 30 September 2019. Searches were performed using the following electronic databases: PubMed, Medline, Scopus, ScienceDirect and SpringerLink. A systematic search was conducted by using the keywords (pharmaceutical policy OR practice); AND (evidence OR impact OR rational OR rational use of medicines); AND (community pharmacy OR community pharmacies OR pricing OR access to medicines OR generic medicines). Other relevant studies were searched through three Internet search engines (Google, Google Scholar and Google Images) using the same keywords. Reference lists of relevant articles were also checked to identify further publications through manual searching. Specific journals in the relevant domains were searched to identify further relevant articles.

Inclusion and Exclusion Criteria for Selection of Studies

Initially, records were downloaded into EndNote (version X7.3.1), and duplicates were removed. Only studies published in English and containing the keywords were selected. In the first round, title/abstract screening was performed independently by two researchers from the group. Relevant studies that fell into any of the following domains were included:

A. Community pharmacy studies
B. Pharmacovigilance
C. Pharmaceutical policy
D. Practice
E. Medicine pricing
F. Rational use
G. Medicine access

Studies that were not related to the search criteria were excluded. Inclusion and exclusion criteria for the studies are outlined in Table 6.1. The systematic review flow diagram is shown in Fig. 6.1 following the PRISMA guidelines.

Table 6.1 Inclusion and exclusion criteria for studies

Inclusion criteria
Studies published in electronic databases as scientific literature
Full-text studies
Studies representing the principal objectives of this meta-analysis published during 2014–2019
All studies published in English
Studies showing quality evaluation criteria >75%
Exclusion criteria
Pilot studies, letters, commentaries and viewpoints, editorials, review articles and animal clinical trials
Research that did not address the goal of this meta-analysis
Research not stating clear outcomes

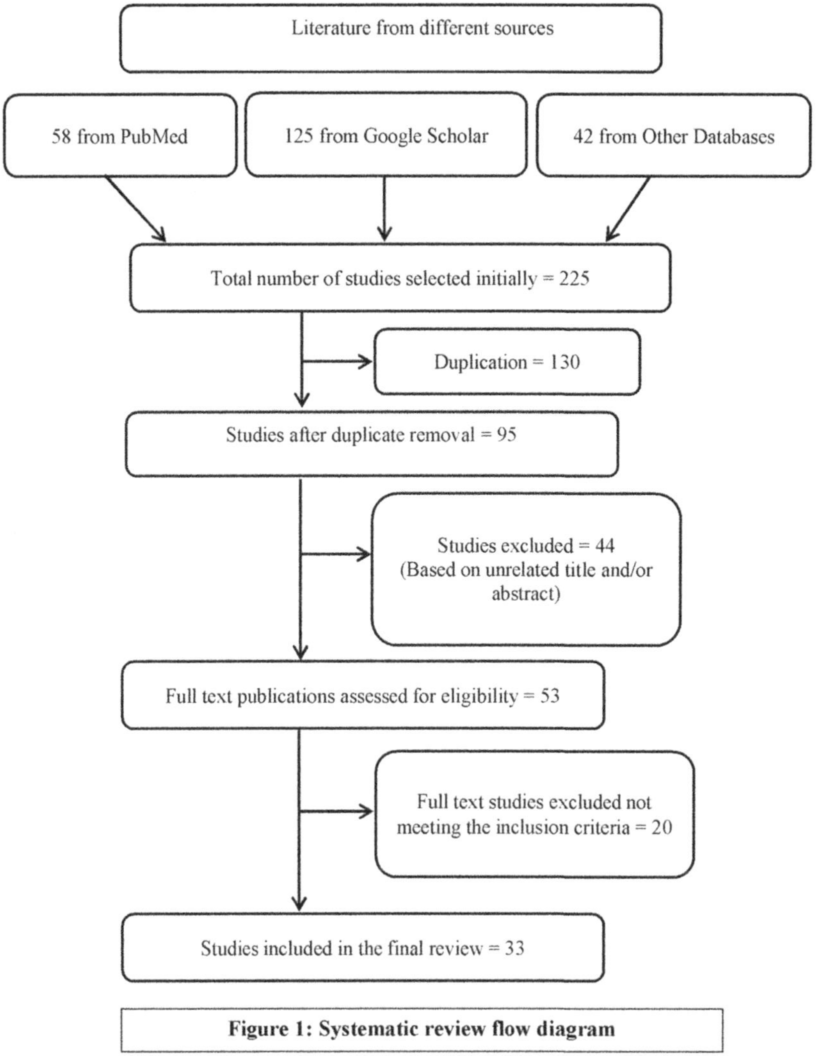

Fig. 6.1 Systematic review flow diagram

Risk of Bias (Quality) Assessment

The studies were evaluated and analysed for quality using a standard quality testing protocol for quantitative and qualitative studies developed by Kmet et al. (2004). Two independent reviewers evaluated and scored selected studies on the basis of 14 items for quantitative and 10 items for qualitative studies (each item with a maximum score of 2). Detail of the scoring process is provided elsewhere (Kmet et al. 2004). Inconsistencies highlighted by the reviewers were resolved in peer panel meetings. Only studies having quality scores of greater than 75% were included in this review. Detailed quality scoring processes and outcomes of the individual studies are provided in Supplementary File 1.

Data Extraction and Analysis

The following information from the selected articles was then extracted and examined by the researchers, IM and MA and ZB: (1) first author, (2) year of publication, (3) name of the journal, (4) study objective, (5) study design, (6) study setting, (7) sample size and (8) main findings of the study. A spreadsheet to record this information was completed for all selected articles and subsequently tabulated (Supplementary File 2).

The elements of pharmacy practice and policy research documented in the literature were used as a reference/starting point for the thematic analysis of the selected papers (Babar and Jamshed 2008; Desselle 2005). According to Ryan and Bernard (2003), themes are taken to reflect the theoretical underpinnings, arguments and conceptual connections of terms on which the problem statement, concepts and/or analysis of an article are based (Ryan and Bernard 2003). Based on this, themes were extracted after understanding the fundamental concepts within each article. All papers were coded independently by each author into categories. Multi-objective articles were classified into the category that was more closely aligned with the main subject matter stated within the paper. The resulting sets of classifications were compared, and highly compatible classifications were grouped into final themes in a group discussion. Where there was any non-consensus or disagreement, the discussion and outcome were moderated by a senior author (MA).

Results

As provided in the PRISMA diagram (Fig. 6.1), the initial literature search from 2014 to 2019 resulted in a total of 225 potentially relevant citations. Of these, 130 were duplicates which were omitted. Out of the 95 remaining articles, 44 were excluded based on titles and/or abstracts being irrelevant. Subsequently, 53 studies were carefully examined to assess eligibility, and 20 articles were excluded at this stage for failing to present pertinent information. In the final grouping, 33 articles met the inclusion criteria and were selected for this review.

Characteristics of the Selected Studies

The main characteristics of the 33 studies are provided in Supplementary File 2. Among the quantitative studies, nineteen studies utilized prospective cross-sectional study designs (Shakeel et al. 2014; Umair Khan et al. 2015; Riaz et al. 2016a, b; Asif et al. 2017; Inamullah et al. 2017; Sarwar et al. 2017, 2018a, b, c; Aziz et al. 2018a, b; Husnain et al. 2018; Rehman et al. 2018; Syed et al. 2018; Saeed et al. 2019a; Atif et al. 2019e), two were retrospective cross-sectional studies (Atif et al. 2016b; Sarwar et al. 2018a), one used both retrospective and prospective cross-sectional study techniques (Atif et al. 2016c), two were simulated cross-sectional studies (Aziz et al. 2019b; Khan et al. 2019), and one was a descriptive study (Malik et al. 2019a). A qualitative study design was adopted in six studies (Hashmi et al. 2017; Hussain et al. 2018; Aziz et al. 2019a; Asghar et al. 2019; Atif et al. 2019a, d). The remaining two studies applied mixed-method designs (qualitative and quantitative) (Umair Khan et al. 2015; Atif et al. 2019b). Most of the studies, that is, twelve (Aziz et al. 2018a, b; Husnain et al. 2018; Rehman et al. 2018; Sarwar et al. 2018a, b, c; Syed et al. 2018), were published in 2018. Out of the 21 remaining studies, ten were published in 2019 (Atif et al. 2019b, d; Aziz et al. 2019a, b; Khan et al. 2019; Saeed et al. 2019a), four each in 2016 (Atif et al. 2016b, c; Riaz et al. 2016a, b) and 2017 (Asif et al. 2017; Hashmi et al. 2017; Inamullah et al. 2017; Sarwar et al. 2017), two in 2015 (Jamshed et al. 2015; Umair Khan et al. 2015) and one in 2014 (Shakeel et al. 2014).

Twenty-two studies were published in journals with stated impact factors (range, 0.44–3.44). Three studies were published in *PLOS One* (Aziz et al. 2018b; Saeed et al. 2019a; Sarwar et al. 2018c); and two studies each were published in *BMC Health Services Research* (Riaz et al. 2016b; Hashmi et al. 2017), *Infection and Drug Resistance* (Atif et al. 2019b; Sarwar et al. 2018b), *International Journal of Environmental Research and Public Health* (Aziz et al. 2018b; 2019a), *Journal of Pharmaceutical Policy and Practice* (Atif et al. 2016c; Sarwar et al. 2017), *Pharmacy* (Rehman et al. 2018; Syed et al. 2018) and *BMJ Open* (Saqib et al. 2018; Atif et al. 2019d).

Through the rigorous thematic content analysis previously outlined, seven research domains were identified: drug utilization pattern and irrational practices ($n = 13$) (Atif et al. 2016b, c, 2019b, e; Sarwar et al. 2017, 2018a; Riaz et al. 2016a, b; Husnain et al. 2018; Aziz et al. 2018a, b; Asghar et al. 2019; Malik et al. 2019a); knowledge, attitude and perception of healthcare professionals towards PV and adverse drug reaction reporting ($n = 4$) (Shakeel et al. 2014; Umair Khan et al. 2015; Syed et al. 2018; Hussain et al. 2018); community pharmacy practices ($n = 4$) (Aziz et al. 2018b, 2019a, b; Khan et al. 2019); perceptions about the emerging role of the pharmacists and current practice ($n = 5$) (Inamullah et al. 2017; Hashmi et al. 2017; Rehman et al. 2018; Sarwar et al. 2018b; Atif et al. 2019a); access to medicines ($n = 4$) (Saeed et al. 2019b; Sarwar et al. 2018c; Saqib et al. 2018; Atif et al. 2019d); the concept of generic medicines (Jamshed et al. 2015; Asif et al. 2017) ($n = 2$); and practice-based research ($n = 1$) (Sarwar et al. 2018c). The key focus of the pharmacy practice and policy-related Pakistani studies published in the last five years is summarized in Fig. 6.2.

Discussion

This chapter set out to understand the literature published on pharmacy practice and policy research in Pakistan over the past five years. A thematic synthesis of the literature identified seven domains which demonstrate the research focus, and each is addressed in this section. These include the following:

Domain 1: Drug utilization pattern and irrational practices

- Alarming irrational use of medicines
- Rising antibiotic abuse
- Common inappropriate medication related practices
- Inadequate medication related knowledge among patients
- Unavailability of appropriate pack sizes of antibiotics

Domain 2: Pharmacovigilance and adverse drug reaction reporting

- Undergraduate pharmacy students and working pharmacist had positive attitudes and better knowledge towards pharmacovigilance and ADR reporting as compared to medical students
- Unavailability of reporting forms, ignorance about pharmacovigilance center and lack of knowledge are major barriers towards ADR reporting

Domain 3: Community pharmacy practices

- Patient dissatisfaction regarding community pharmacy services and quality of counseling
- Rural pharmacy practice is facing multiple challenges
- Absence of qualified pharmacy professionals at communty pharmacy i.e. 90.4%
- Poor management of minor and chronic illness in community pharmacies

Domain 4: Emerging role of pharmacists

- Public positively perceived role of pharmacist as healthcare professional
- Healthcare professionals were willing to accept pharmacist as well-rounded professional and wanted them to provide extended pharmacy services
- Pharmacists' urged but face barriers to provide extended pharmacy services
- Pharmacists' had positive perceptions but poor practices regarding antimicrobial stewardship

Domain 5: Access to medicines

- High prices of medicines
- Unaffordable standard treatment i.e. above a single day wage.
- Availability of both originator brand and low price generic far below WHO global targets of 80%, especially in public centers
- Poor availability and affordability of anti-cancer medicines, especially biologics
- Unavailability of many essential and life-saving medicines is attributable to active pharmaceutical ingredient and raw material availability issues, lack of traditional distribution system and pricing issue.

Domain 6: Concept of generic medicines

- Merely 23.3% – 51.5% generic prescribing
- Pharmacy students had positive perception about generic medicines but lacked a thorough understanding of the concepts of generic medcines and bioequivalence

Domain 7: Practice-based research

- Pharmacists acknowledged the importance of research in raising pharmacy practice bar and seemed willing and motivated to be involved in research
- Pharmacists' participation in practice based research is hindered by time constraints followed by lack of incentives and lack of support

Fig. 6.2 Key focus of pharmacy practice and policy research in Pakistan (2014–2019)

- Drug utilization patterns and irrational practices
- Pharmacovigilance and adverse drug reaction reporting
- Community pharmacy practices

- Emerging role of pharmacists
- Access to medicines
- The concept of generic medicines
- Practice-based research

It is interesting to see the umbrella of pharmacy practice and policy research extending from the traditional pharmacists' role of dispensing, distribution and administration to emerging research areas such as PC, PV and medication therapy management (MTM) (Okonta et al. 2012; Fakeye et al. 2017b). Despite the introduction of the Department of Pharmacy Practice in 2014 and increasing trends towards pharmacy practice research in Pakistan over the past five years, this is the first systematic review that has focused on pharmacy practice and policy research in this context. Therefore, the rationale behind this review was to document a typology and outline the quality of pharmacy practice and policy research in Pakistan to gain a deeper understanding of future research direction, policy requirements and the need for change in practice and attitudes towards this. The key research domains of pharmacy practice and policy research that emerged from this review are diverse and provide a very important picture of what has been undertaken and the gaps that continue to exist. That is the significant contribution of this work. Compared to the research undertaken prior to the introduction of contemporary pharmacy practice, Pakistani research in this area has improved significantly in both volume and quality, especially for community pharmacy research.

In terms of advanced methodologies, the body of knowledge outlined in this review highlights the use of mixed methods, while qualitative and cross-sectional simulated study designs are gaining momentum. Although the standard of pharmacy practice and policy research is improving in Pakistan, there is a scarce literature exploring the impact of pharmacy research and policy and pharmacoeconomics which are the emerging fields of pharmacy practice. This is likely due to a lack of access to a broad range of patient data and lack of well-founded relationships and alliances with other healthcare professionals, especially medical doctors (Fakeye et al. 2017b).

Domain 1: Drug Utilization Pattern and Irrational Practices

Since the existence of mankind, traditional and conventional medicines have been essential for reducing mortality and morbidity from a range of diseases (Mohamad Azmi et al. 2013). Nonetheless, the irrational use of medicines is known to create a high-risk environment for ineffective treatment, proliferation of chronic conditions, increased treatment cost and financial burden (Akl et al. 2014). In the case of antibiotics, unsupervised and unrestricted sale and subsequent inappropriate use raise significant concerns about antimicrobial resistance (Atif et al. 2019b; Asghar et al. 2019) and the need for appropriate stewardship (Atif et al. 2019a). According to the World Health Organization (WHO), more than 50% of all medicines are irrationally prescribed, dispensed or sold, especially in developing countries (Ofori-Asenso et al. 2016; World Health Organization 2004).

Similarly, irrational drug use practices in Pakistan are alarmingly high as many studies included in this review have demonstrated poor prescribing and deviations from the expected norms for patient care and health facility INRUD indicators (Aziz et al. 2018a; Riaz et al. 2016a, b; Atif et al. 2016b, c). The main factors contributing to inappropriate and suboptimal use of medicines from the Pakistani literature include medicine overuse (2.3–4.63 per prescription encounter) (Aziz et al. 2018a; Riaz et al. 2016a, b; Atif et al. 2016b, c), high prevalence in use of antibiotics (39.6–51.5% per prescription encounter) (Atif et al. 2016c, 2019b; Riaz et al. 2016b) and injectable medicines (0–27.1% per prescription encounter) (Atif et al. 2016c; Riaz et al. 2016b), prescribing of medicines outside of clinical practice guidelines, unavailability of key medicines (only 72.4–82%) and prescription of originator brands (OBs) rather than generics (only 23.3–51.5% generic) (Aziz et al. 2018a; Riaz et al. 2016a, b; Atif et al. 2016b, c).

Additionally, inappropriate dose and duration of treatment, unavailability of appropriate pack sizes of medicines, lack of standard treatment guidelines, poorly governed pharmacy and therapeutics committees, lack of knowledge and awareness among healthcare providers and the public about rational medicine use (Atif et al. 2019b, 2016c; Riaz et al. 2016b;

Sarwar et al. 2018a; Malik et al. 2019a), short consultation and dispensing times (Atif et al. 2016c, Riaz et al. 2016b), prescription errors (both omission and commission), non-compliance and drug interaction-related errors further contribute to irrational use (Aziz et al. 2018a; Husnain et al. 2018).

Overuse of inappropriate self-medication practices by the public and other inappropriate medication-related practices also contribute to the vulnerability of Pakistanis to the irrational use of medicines (Husnain et al. 2018; Aziz et al. 2018b; Atif et al. 2019e). Among inappropriate medication use practices, use of bottle caps to measure liquid dosage forms, use of hot water to reconstitute suspensions, use of leftover medicines and medicine sharing were highly prevalent in the Pakistani population (Husnain et al. 2018). According to an estimate, a number of essential medicines sold in Pakistan are supplied without prescription (Aziz et al. 2018b), and this is very concerning. This precarious situation seems to pose a huge challenge for the promotion of rational use of medicines in Pakistan (Aziz et al. 2018a; Riaz et al. 2016a, b; Atif et al. 2016b, c), as well as the specific overuse of antimicrobials (Atif et al. 2019b; Sarwar et al. 2018a) and inappropriate medication-related practices (Atif et al. 2019b, e; Husnain et al. 2018). Irrational prescribing, dispensing and sale of medicines without prescriptions from doctors in community pharmacies signifies the lack of a regulated healthcare infrastructure and less than optimal implementation of national drug policies. Overuse of risk-prone self-medication and inappropriate medication-related practices demonstrate significant issues with regard to health literacy, affordability of and access to healthcare facilities and poor community pharmacy practices in Pakistan (Atif et al. 2019b).

Pakistan has been struggling with the irrational use of medicines since the early 1990s. In order to improve the situation, the first National Essential Medicines List (NEML) of Pakistan was made available in 1994 (revised in 1995, 2000, 2003, 2007, 2013 and 2018) (Atif et al. 2019c), as the concept of essential medicines is a significant platform for the promotion of the rational use of medicines in developing nations (Atif et al. 2017; World Health Organization 2004; Government of Pakistan 2018). A National Medicine Policy (NMP) also exists in official documentation form and was last modified in 1997 (World Health Organization 2014). The Pakistani healthcare system is driving alignment of its laws and policies with obligations required through international agreements which guarantee access to high-quality essential medicines in accordance with international best practice (Government of Pakistan 2018). However, unfortunately due to many other factors, irrational use continues to occur at alarming rates.

The literature suggests that the situation demands collective drive and performance of institutions, healthcare professionals and patients to promote rational use of medicines in Pakistan. Moreover, effective regulation, clear clinical guidance, training, education and management would be minimum requirements for progress to occur. The pharmacists' critical role in both hospital and community settings needs to be promoted, owing to their capability in improving the current scenario by performing patient-oriented services, developing and implementing surveillance systems in hospitals and, for example, providing drug information relating to antimicrobial stewardship (AMS) to promote more rational prescribing among doctors in Pakistan (Sarwar et al. 2018a; Riaz et al. 2016b).

However, according to one report, hospital pharmacists in Pakistan are restricted to procurement and dispensing (Atif et al. 2017), and there are 0.06 pharmacists to cater the needs of 10,000 people in Pakistan. This is well below the targeted benchmark, that is, five pharmacists per 10,000 person population (Rashid 2015). Considering this patient-pharmacist workforce imbalance, the appointment of pharmacists in hospitals as well as in the private healthcare setting is an absolute necessity and is highly recommended if Pakistan is to improve the quality use of medicines. Pakistan also needs effective implementation of policies to monitor medication sales and to regulate the unnecessary sales of prescription medicines not prescribed by a doctor (Atif et al. 2019b; Aziz et al. 2018b). Public education about rational medication use and limits and regulation on medicine advertisements with promotion of community pharmacy services must be implemented to cope with overuse of self-medication and other inappropriate medication use practices (Atif et al. 2019b; Husnain et al. 2018).

Domain 2: Pharmacovigilance and Adverse Drug Reaction Reporting

Adverse drug reactions (ADRs) are a significant public health concern leading to real economic burden on healthcare systems and society as a whole (Kongkaew et al. 2008). It is accepted globally that efficient PV systems to detect, record, report, prevent and manage ADRs are of vital importance and result in improved drug safety. Although PV is well established in developed nations, it is virtually non-existent in many developing countries, and this includes Pakistan (Iffat et al. 2014). Regardless of witnessing the aftermath of the "Fake Drug Crisis (2012)" (Nishtar 2012), research conducted in 2016 has shown that Pakistani healthcare professionals had suboptimal knowledge about this important concept and PV-related practices were non-existent (Atif et al. 2016a).

Thus far, Pakistan has a limited accountability system for medicines, and the actual number of deaths related to ADRs is not known due to an unrecognized and underdeveloped system of PV (Mahmood et al. 2011). Recently, Pakistan became a full member of the Uppsala Monitoring Centre after the implementation of the National Pharmacovigilance Centre in 2017 and multiple regional PV centres in 2018 (Mahmood et al. 2011; Syed et al. 2018; Hussain and Hassali 2019). With regard to this programme, healthcare professionals working in public sector hospitals have demonstrated a good knowledge of PV and show positive attitudes towards ADR reporting, even though the majority of them have never reported any ADRs (Syed et al. 2018; Malik et al. 2018). It was reported that in Pakistan with a population of over 200 million people, the ADR reporting rate was very low in comparison with the WHO standards (over 200 reports per 1,000,000 inhabitants per year) (Syed et al. 2018).

In contrast to the findings of working healthcare professionals, studies focusing on medical students had shown that more than 55% of students did not know the term pharmacovigilance (Iffat et al. 2014). Although the Drug Regulatory Authority of Pakistan (DRAP) has introduced a PV system, only 12.61% of medical students were knowledgeable about the existence of ADR reporting systems in any healthcare facility, and just over one-quarter (27.49%) of respondents were familiar with the DRAP form for reporting of ADRs (Iffat et al. 2014). This lack of knowledge may be due to lack of time and interest by students and lack of training and courses on ADRs and PV in their curricula (Iffat et al. 2014; Umair Khan et al. 2015). In comparison with the medical students, pharmacy students reflected sound knowledge and understanding of ADRs (Shakeel et al. 2014). Shakeel et al. reported that about 98.37% of pharmacy students have knowledge of ADRs and PV. Furthermore, 89.79% of these students understand the role of pharmaceutical companies and the Ministry of Health in ADR reporting, and just under half (44.77%) have information about the availability of DRAP forms for reporting ADRs (Shakeel et al. 2014). This enhanced knowledge compared with medical students may be due to the difference in their curricula (Umair Khan et al. 2015). Although the majority of medical students were not familiar with PV, they showed positive attitudes toward ADR reporting. Close to 60% (59.88%) of medical and dental students emphasized the need to include ADR in their curriculum (Iffat et al. 2014).

Numerous factors have been reported to influence the underreporting of ADRs in Pakistan including an ignorance about PV, complex ADR reporting forms, uncertainty about assigning ADR causality, lack of training of healthcare professionals on PV and lack of awareness about detection, communication and spontaneous monitoring of ADRs (Iffat et al. 2014; Syed et al. 2018). The studies highlighted the need to devise an appropriate ADR reporting system along with effective training programmes not only for students but also for already registered and working healthcare professionals. Implementation of PV rules and regulation is required in order to improve drug safety and the health-related quality of life of Pakistani people.

Domain 3: Community Pharmacy Practices

Community pharmacies are of utmost importance for the provision of optimum primary healthcare services as the traditional role of medication dispensing is replaced by a more patient-oriented clinical approach (Aziz et al. 2018b). Among the range of services provided in community pharmacy, the most common role is the supply and use of medicines within a quality framework. Furthermore, the importance of community pharmacies in minimizing the cost of treatment for individuals and society at large, counselling to improve medication adherence, management of minor ailments, emergency contraception, referral for medical advice and initiating smoking cessation therapies has also been reported (Birenbaum 1982; Azhar et al. 2009; Munroe et al. 1997). Although pharmacy practice is a well-established discipline around the globe, some variations exist in the practices among different countries (Aslam et al. 2012). The literature is scarce regarding the standard of community pharmacy practice in developing countries as in Pakistan the standard of these services has not yet been evaluated (Smith 2009; Rabbani et al. 2001). In accordance with the Good Pharmacy Practice (GPP) guidelines published by the International Pharmaceutical Federation (FIP) and WHO in 2011, patient counselling services have been implemented to some degree in Pakistan, but there is still significant room for improvement to meet international standards across the country (Aziz et al. 2018b). According to a study conducted in 2018, less than one-third (29.4%) of simulated patients were counselled about their medication (Aziz et al. 2018b). Lack of knowledge of working staff and absence of pharmacists at these counselling and drug sale points were the main reasons for this (Aziz et al. 2018b).

In Pakistan, community pharmacies are generally owned by non-pharmacists (businessmen), and the owners follow conventional business planning and management approaches (Khan et al. 2019). Khan et al. reported that 9.6% of the pharmacies run under the supervision of a pharmacist. Similarly, another study reports that there are 8102 registered pharmacists in Pakistan, but it is estimated there are 45,000–50,000 wholesale and retail drug outlets (Haq et al. 2017). Additionally, despite a massive influx of females into the pharmacy profession, their underrepresentation as community pharmacists due to assorted reasons leads to further shortages in the pharmacist workforce (Malik 2019). Considering the status quo, clearly not each of the drug retail outlets in the country can be staffed by a registered pharmacist. Thus, in the absence of pharmacists, most of these pharmacies are managed by staff with inadequate knowledge and no professional qualifications which means that patient-oriented activities are likely to be compromised (Shet et al. 2015; Asghar et al. 2019).

Patient views are valuable indicators of service provision and outcomes when evaluating health services management and healthcare delivery systems (Aziz et al. 2018b). Studies exploring patients' perceptions and their expectations were included in this review as an indicator to capture the extent to which community pharmacy practices in Pakistan are patient centric (Aziz et al. 2018b, 2019a). In this regard, many customers were discontent with the dispensing and counselling practices of community pharmacies in Pakistan (Aziz et al. 2019a). According to the findings of these studies, patients were not pleased with the qualifications held by pharmacy staff and the knowledge of those counselling them (Aziz et al. 2018b, 2019a). However, according to a study conducted in urban areas of Pakistan, many patients were very satisfied with instructions given about their medications (Aziz et al. 2018b). In comparison with the findings of urban areas, dissatisfaction with short counselling times, inappropriate packing of medicines, improper labelling and inadequate drug storage facilities revealed far worse pharmacy practices in rural areas (Aziz et al. 2019a). Although the WHO produced guidelines for sound storage practices in 2003 (Organization 2003), improper storage practices coupled with unlawful dispensing have been reported in Pakistan (Aziz et al. 2019a). The Ministry of Health officials and other regulatory authorities can strengthen pharmacy practice services by implementing appropriate policies, ensuring the presence of registered pharmacists and encouraging pharmacy staff training to provide maximum benefits to Pakistani patients.

Domain 4: Emerging Role of Pharmacists

The past few decades have been witness to a transition of roles within the professional pharmacy practice (Malik et al. 2019b). Worldwide, the count-and-pour system replaced the customary compounding role and more recently has been transformed to the delivery of PC. Acceptance of PC in the early 1990s has evolved to embrace diverse services at the community level (Hepler and Strand 1990; Hepler 1993, 1996). Likewise, recently the scenario in Pakistan witnessed a transition of perceived roles of the community pharmacist from customary compounding and dispensing to provision of services ranging from patient education and counselling to antimicrobial stewardship and extended pharmacy services (EPS) (Sarwar et al. 2018b; Rehman et al. 2018; Inamullah et al. 2017; Hashmi et al. 2017; Atif et al. 2019a; Malik et al. 2019b).

A study has revealed that the public positively perceives the role of the pharmacist as a healthcare professional in Pakistan. Likewise, healthcare professionals were ready to accept the pharmacist as a well-rounded health professional and want them to deliver clinical services (Inamullah et al. 2017). Another study regarding extended pharmacy services reported a handful of pharmacists being unaware of PC, but they were willing to accept and provide enhanced clinical services if equipped with the requisite skills and training (Hashmi et al. 2017). The study also reported a range of barriers such as inadequate personal knowledge, poor community awareness and acceptance, insufficient physician-pharmacist collaboration and poor salary structures which need to be addressed to allow provision of EPS (Hashmi et al. 2017). In view of the emerging concept of innovative PC services and EPS, the Pakistani government needs to play its role in addressing the challenges faced by community pharmacies to ensure the delivery of EPS to contribute to improved public health. Moreover, a set of targeted strategies and health system modifications are needed to realize the full potential of community pharmacists in Pakistan and ensure ongoing capacity and capability to deliver (Sadek et al. 2016).

In combating the issue of antimicrobial stewardship (AMS), programmes are known to optimize the treatment of infectious diseases and minimize adverse events linked to antibiotic overuse (Rehman et al. 2018). In accordance with international recommendations in 2015, a national antimicrobial resistance surveillance system was implemented in Pakistan (World Health Organization 2017), with the AMS programme being initiated by the Medical Microbiology and Infectious Diseases Society of Pakistan across public and private institutions (Medical Microbiology and Infectious Diseases Society of Pakistan 2014). However, the AMS programme failed to get established and flourish, probably due to the lack of AMS teams in real terms. In this regard, a survey conducted in 2018 showed that only a few private and public hospitals have functioning stewardship activities in place (Khan 2018).

Community pharmacists' participation in collaborative interdisciplinary teams would play a crucial role in the development and successful implementation of AMS programmes in Pakistani community settings (Atif et al. 2019a). This is the case as pharmacists are then in direct contact with patients and are in an ideal position to provide medicine information to patients (Sarwar et al. 2018b; Malik et al. 2019b). This is expected to help prevent the major contributing factors to antimicrobial resistance such as self-medication, substandard and spurious availability of medicines, inappropriate prescriptions and unlimited and uncontrolled access to over-the-counter (OTC) sale of antimicrobials in drug stores (Rehman et al. 2018). Fortunately, pharmacists are recognizing their role in this regard, as a study focused on exploring the perceptions and practices of community pharmacists towards AMS has revealed positive perceptions regarding AMS with more than 80% of participating pharmacists agreeing that AMS is crucial to high-quality patient care (Rehman et al. 2018; Sarwar et al. 2018b). However, despite the attitude being good, practices relating to AMS were discouraging. A study revealed that well less than half (39.8%) of pharmacist participants put their efforts in to avoid or minimize the spread of infections within the community (Rehman et al. 2018). Another recent study depicted that dispensing practices were not followed by community pharmacists and very few patients were instructed about the antibiotics they were purchasing (Atif et al. 2019a). In order to reduce the threat of antimicrobial resistance and the associated economic burden and morbidity in Pakistan, revival of AMS programmes is required alongside the formation of collaborative interdisciplinary teams and increased participation of pharmacists in AMS awareness campaigns (Sarwar et al. 2018b; Rehman et al. 2018; Atif et al. 2019a).

Domain 5: Access to Medicines

Availability and affordability are considered as key prerequisites for worldwide access to medicines in any country (Sachs and McArthur

2005; Alefan et al. 2018). Nevertheless, inadequate access to medicines in concert with uncontrolled prices is one of the foremost health-related issues in developing nations, and Pakistan hasn't escaped this (Saeed et al. 2019a). This review has found that the overall availability of medicines in Pakistan is far below the optimal benchmark set by the WHO global action plan, that is, 80% availability of essential medicines by 2025. Pakistan has been facing this issue for the past two decades, and a study in 2006 exposed for the first time the worst possible situation of medicine unavailability with originator brands (OBs) being completely unavailable, and only 3.3% of lowest-priced generics (LPGs) were available at public healthcare centres (Kiani et al. 2006). In contrast to this, another health facility survey conducted in 2014 reported significant improvements in the availability of both OBs (28.8%) and LPGs (30.7%) (Shahnaz 2014). This is likely due to the establishment of DRAP in 2012 and the subsequent implementation and procurement of the NEML system (Saeed et al. 2019b). Another recent study reported a significant reduction in the availability of OBs (6.8%), while the availability of LPGs (35.3%) showed slight improvements. This is heartening, but the overall availability of essential medicines in both private and public health facilities is disappointing (Saeed et al. 2019b).

It would appear that the major reason behind the extremely poor availability of medicines in Pakistan may be due to the unceasing deadlock between manufacturers and DRAP regarding the establishment of reasonable pricing which may have resulted in lower stocks and the shortage of essential medicines (Saeed et al. 2019b). A recent study affirmed that alongside the low pricing issue, raw material shortages and lack of traditional distribution systems were the other two prominent reasons of short supply of life-saving and essential medicines in the country (Atif et al. 2019d). Moreover, in Pakistan, the amount allocated for medicines in the public healthcare centres is below the critical threshold of $2 per capita per year advocated by the WHO to prevent stock-outs (World Health Organization 2002). Besides this, inefficient budget management further exacerbates this issue in Pakistan (Zaidi et al. 2013). Multiple factors contribute to inefficient budget management of pharmaceuticals including inadequate demand prediction, poor procurement systems and tracking, medicine pilferage and unavailability or lack of active participation by pharmacists and non-active and ineffective pharmacy and therapeutics committees (Zaidi et al. 2013; Saeed et al. 2019b).

According to the literature, prices for all the surveyed medicines in comparison to international reference prices have shown significant variation from 0.48–2.96 in 2014 to 0.42–60.63 in 2019, and the cost of standard treatments has risen from "below a single daily wage" in 2014 to "above a single daily wage" in 2019 (Saeed et al. 2019b; Shahnaz 2014). Regardless of the establishment of DRAP in 2012 and introduction of comprehensive drug pricing policies in 2015, the gradual increase in medicine prices over the past few years seems attributable to multiple factors. These include devaluation of the Pakistani rupee, poor implementation and regulation of pharmaceuticals by the appropriate authorities, value-based pricing, anticipated benefits to multinational pharmaceutical companies and a disproportionate focus on profitability over affordability (Saeed et al. 2019b).

For the first time, Sarwar et al. and Saqib et al. report significant non-availability and un-affordability of anticancer medicines in Pakistan that may expose patients to inequities in healthcare alongside increased morbidity and mortality (Sarwar et al. 2018c; Saqib et al. 2018). The lack of affordability of anticancer medicines is driven by protracted periods before patents run out on OBs and ignorance regarding the availability of health insurance schemes (Saqib et al. 2018).

In this regard, the Ministry of National Health Services, Regulation and Coordination had been providing medicines free of charge via public healthcare centres and adopting policies that help to support the poor (Zaidi et al. 2013). Nonetheless, the low availability of medicines in public premises may force patients to purchase their medicines from retail drug stores, where they pay out of their own pockets (Kiani et al. 2006). Recently, DRAP has notified of a further 9–15% increase in the prices of life-saving and other medicines (Shabbir Hussain 2019) that may actively encourage a reasonable level of availability but further decrease in affordability of medicines, in Pakistan. Given the overall picture surrounding medicine availability and affordability, there is a need to act and take steps to promote generic prescribing, strengthen and systematize procurement processes and budget management strategies, improve pricing policies and monitoring systems, re-examine the national essential medicine policy and continue research into medicine availability and affordability for the betterment of the health system and the population.

Domain 6: The Concept of Generic Medicines

Generic medicines have been influential in reducing the cost associated with originator branded drugs and therefore improving the international affordability of medicines, particularly in developing nations (Jamshed et al. 2009). The perennial problem has been that the uptake in use of generic medicines has been well below what is expected to assist the health system and its patients as a whole. The extent of generic medicine use varies across countries in the developing world, and the domestic availability of generics in real terms and their quality and optimal use still remain largely unknown to a great extent (Jamshed et al. 2009). The WHO advocates for a policy of 100% generic prescribing to ensure access to medicines, but recent Pakistani studies have confirmed that this shift is difficult with a minimal number of drugs being prescribed by the generic name (Aziz et al. 2018a; Atif et al. 2016c; Riaz et al. 2016b). This finding highlights the need to implement policies that promote generic prescribing to improve availability and access and curtail economic pressure through greatly increased affordability.

In 1972, the Generic Drug Act was introduced in Pakistan to forbid the use of originator brand names and promote prescribing by generic names on prescriptions. This legislation was in place until 1975, and generic marketing and prescribing was revoked by the government at this point due to intensified promotional activities and failure to bring down medicine prices (Jamshed et al. 2013). The Pakistani government needs to reconsider the implementation of a revised generic prescribing policy to promote the availability and use of high-quality generic medicines that are cost-effective (Atif et al. 2017).

Studies included in this review point toward Pakistani pharmacy and medical students having inadequate knowledge of generic medicines and the concept of bioequivalence (Asif et al. 2017; Jamshed et al. 2015). This is likely to influence their prescribing behaviour as future doctors and their clinical recommendations as future practicing pharmacists. To overcome this knowledge deficit among pharmacy and medical students before they graduate and step into practice, it is vital that the topics of generic medicines and bioequivalence are strengthened in the curricula (Al-Tamimi et al. 2016; Chisholm and Hawkins 1996).

A study from Karachi in Pakistan indicated that pharmacist participants had a sound knowledge of generic medicines and their full-time availability within pharmacies improved the perceptions of patients as well as other healthcare professionals with respect to generic medicines (Jamshed et al. 2010). Barriers to proper practice of generic substitution might be obscured system of medicine distribution, absence of generic substitution regulations and lack of marketing and subsequent unawareness of the importance of utilizing generic medicines (Kaplan et al. 2012). Furthermore, the full use of generic medicines is discouraged by poor confidence of healthcare professionals and the public in generics and lack of incentive schemes on generic prescribing and substitution for healthcare professionals (Cameron and Laing 2010).

Generic medicines are approved to be bioequivalent to originator branded drugs in terms of safety, strength and quality by the US Food and Drug Administration (FDA) (Jamshed et al. 2009). Taking into account this legislation, the registration process in Pakistan had been revisited and was reformed after the establishment of the DRAP Act, to ensure safety, efficacy and quality of drugs (Imaduddin 2014). DRAP has formulated an outline for post-marketing surveillance of medicines in alliance with the United States Pharmacopoeia Promoting the Quality of Medicines (USP-PQM) (Hussain and Hassali 2019). Unfortunately, no recent Pakistani studies have been undertaken which compare the quality and safety of OBs and generic medicines. Although the use of generics is accepted by general physicians in Pakistan, they still hesitate to practice generic prescribing due to perceived concerns around safety and reliability (Sharif et al. 2016). To counter such misconceptions and ensure improved quality of generic drugs, future comparative bio-dissolution studies should be instituted for generic products in the case that bioavailability studies are not feasible (Anand et al. 2011). Besides this, future interventional studies using generic medicines should be conducted to provide an evidence-based platform for healthcare professionals, institutions and regulators to institute policy.

Domain 7: Practice-Based Research

Practice-based research has beneficial impacts on pharmacists with regard to multiple aspects such as information gathering and evidence-based practices and improved proficiency and provision of patient-oriented services (Sarwar et al. 2018c). Traditionally, pharmacists have been hesitant to participate in research compared with some other primary healthcare professionals (Awaisu and Alsalimy 2015). However, this trend has been changing over the past few decades, and pharmacy organizations are advocating and supporting practice-based research throughout the world (Simpson et al. 2001; Sultana et al. 2016). Even though the trend has changed and pharmacists' willingness to participate in research and their positive attitude towards research has improved, several studies from around the globe have reported barriers to pharmacy practice research. Among these, major barriers to pharmacist involvement in pharmacy practice-based research included lack of access to patient data, lack of time, inadequate training in research methodologies, lack of financial support and institutional review board challenges (Bakken et al. 2009; Sultana et al. 2016; Fakeye et al. 2017a; Simpson et al. 2001). A recent Pakistani study found that pharmacists' participation in research was mostly hindered by time constraints, then followed by lack of incentives and lack of support (Sarwar et al. 2018c). Regardless of the multiple barriers identified, pharmacists acknowledged the importance of research in raising the standards of pharmacy practice and seemed willing and motivated to be involved in research (Sarwar et al. 2018c). Nevertheless, their interest in research does not correspond to their actual skills to undertake research.

By addressing the barriers identified in the literature, there is the potential to improve the policy and practice research outputs in Pakistan. Considering the importance of research, the WHO and FIP have included "potential to be a researcher" as one of the traits of a well-rounded pharmacist in their "seven-star" notion (Ibrahim et al. 2012; Wiedenmayer et al. 2006; International Pharmaceutical Federation 2000; Ryan et al. 2007). Given the increasing amount of medical research knowledge

(Sultana et al. 2016), pharmacists' engagement in research is highly recommended worldwide to strengthen pharmacist-provided services and improve patient care (Sultana et al. 2016).

Likewise, in Pakistan where a lack of evidence-based research is one of the reasons for substandard healthcare delivery (Shaikh and Rabbani 2004; World Health Organization 2016), pharmacists can play a considerable role engaging in research due to their direct participation in delivery of optimal care to patients. The issue of time constraint for involvement in research could be resolved through minimizing the burden of pharmacists and improving the ratio of pharmacists in Pakistan. Regarding the lack of funds and support, the government of Pakistan, taking into consideration the need to improve the state of evidence-based research, has allocated 91 billion rupees to the Higher Education Commission (HEC) to stimulate this activity (Memon 2017). According to one estimate, the HEC will utilize a total of 2.2 billion rupees to promote health-related research (Memon 2017). The HEC is also formulating attractive strategies for encouraging research such as the National Research Program for Universities and National Awards for Outstanding Researchers and providing online access to research through the HEC digital library (Memon 2017). The National Health Vision Pakistan 2016–2025 has also emphasized the need to facilitate information collection, surveillance and research in Pakistan (World Health Organization 2016).

Although pharmacists have positive attitudes, perception and willingness to participate in practice-based research and the government of Pakistan seems keen to promote healthcare research, a multidisciplinary approach is still required to overcome the barriers faced by pharmacists attempting to engage in research. Moreover, the Pakistani government also needs to promote evidence-based research through easy access to hospitalized patient data to aid broad surveys and procurement of data to aid pharmacoeconomic research. There is also a need for the government of Pakistan to be open to research being undertaken which may show the imperfections in the existing healthcare system and allow for controversial topics to be addressed through research which deals with these issues head-on.

Conclusion

This systematic review provides an update of pharmacy practice and policy-related research since the introduction of the concept of pharmacy practice in Pakistan, which focuses on structuring the professional responsibilities of pharmacists. Studies have demonstrated research in drug utilization patterns and irrational practices; knowledge, attitudes and perceptions of healthcare professionals towards PV and adverse drug reaction reporting; community pharmacy practices; perceptions about the emerging role of the pharmacists and current pharmacy practices; access to medicines; the concept of generic medicines; and also practice-based research. While the majority of the literature focused on traditional pharmacy practice research domains, a lack of literature was apparent on the impact of pharmacy practice and policy, pharmacoeconomics and the emerging pharmacists' role in Pakistan, that is, PC, PV and medication therapy management.

What was encouraging was the emerging trends and awareness of the terms PV, extended pharmacy services, antibiotic stewardship programmes and practice-based research, the use of advanced study designs and the exploration of patients' views. This review only selected those manuscripts that demonstrated a high degree of rigor based on preset criteria. However, it is important to highlight that many of the published studies were not sufficiently robust to be included. Hence, future studies must employ more robust study designs to support the good literature found and help drive pharmacy practice and policy research forward in Pakistan. Without this evidence, it is difficult to engage key local and international stakeholders to push forward with what the future should look like for pharmacy services in Pakistan.

References

Abbas, A. & Khan, N. 2014. Clinical trials involving pharmacists in Pakistan's healthcare system: A leap from paper to practice. *Pharmacy*, 2, 244–247.

Ahmad, H., Khalid, M. & Hudebia, A. B. 2017. Healthcare System Of Pakistan. *Int J Advanced Res Public*.

Ahmed, A., Tanveer, M., Siddiqui, A. & Khan, G. M. 2018. Bridging the Gap for Clinical Pharmacist in Developing Countries like Pakistan. *J Coll Physic Surg Pak,* 28, 229–232.

Akl, O. A., El Mahalli, A. A., Elkahky, A. A. & Salem, A. M. 2014. WHO/INRUD drug use indicators at primary healthcare centers in Alexandria, Egypt. *J Taibah Uni Med Sci,* 9, 54–64.

Al-Tamimi, S. K., Hassali, M. A., Shafie, A. A. & Aa, A. L. 2016. The need to incorporate generic medicines topic in the curriculum of Yemeni pharmacy colleges. *Int J Pharm Pract,* 24, 72–3.

Alefan, Q., Amairi, R. & Tawalbeh, S. 2018. Availability, prices and affordability of selected essential medicines in Jordan: a national survey. *BMC Health Serv Res,* 18, 787.

Anand, O., Yu, L. X., Conner, D. P. & Davit, B. M. 2011. Dissolution Testing for Generic Drugs: An FDA Perspective. *The AAPS Journal,* 13, 328.

Asghar, S., Atif, M., Mushtaq, I., Malik, I. & Hayat, K. 2019. Factors associated with inappropriate dispensing of antibiotics among non-pharmacist pharmacy workers. *Res Soc Admin Pharm.*

Asif, U., Saleem, Z., Yousaf, M., Saeed, H., Hashmi, F. K. & Hassali, M. A. 2017. Exploring the knowledge and attitude of medical and pharmacy students about generic medicine in Lahore, Pakistan. *J Generic Med,* 14, 22–28.

Aslam, F. 2019. Role of Community Pharmacies in Rational use of Medicines: A Scenario in Pakistan. *J Pharm Pract Comm Med,* 5.

Aslam, N. & Ahmed, K. Z. 2011. Clinical Pharmacy Clerkship in Pakistan: A leap from paper to practice.

Aslam, N., Bushra, R. & Khan, M. U. 2012. Community pharmacy practice in Pakistan. *Arch Pharm Pract,* 3, 297.

Atif, M., Ahmad, M., Saleem, Q., Curley, L. & Qamar-Uz-Zaman, M. 2017. Pharmaceutical policy in Pakistan. *Pharmaceutical Policy in Countries with Developing Healthcare Systems.* Springer.

Atif, M., Arslan, B., Quratulain, S., Zainab, A., Aminah, N., Sonia, A., Azeem, M., Sarwar, M. R. & Chioma, S. 2016a. Knowledge, attitude, and practices of health care professionals regarding pharmacovigilance in Pakistan. *Value in Health,* 19, A278.

Atif, M., Asghar, S., Mushtaq, I. & Malik, I. 2019a. Community pharmacists as antibiotic stewards: A qualitative study exploring the current status of Antibiotic Stewardship Program in Bahawalpur, Pakistan. *J Inf Public Health.*

Atif, M., Asghar, S., Mushtaq, I., Malik, I., Amin, A., Babar, Z.-U.-D. & Scahill, S. 2019b. What drives inappropriate use of antibiotics? A mixed methods study from Bahawalpur, Pakistan. *Infect Drug Resist,* 12, 687–699.

Atif, M., Azeem, M., Sarwar, M. R., Shahid, S., Javaid, S., Ikram, H., Baig, U. & Scahill, S. 2016b. WHO/INRUD prescribing indicators and prescribing trends of antibiotics in the Accident and Emergency Department of Bahawal Victoria Hospital, Pakistan. *SpringerPlus,* 5, 1928–1928.

Atif, M., Malik, I., Dawoud, D., Gilani, A., Ahmed, N. & Babar, Z.-U.-D. 2019c. Essential Medicine List, Policies, and the World Health Organization. *In:* BABAR, Z.-U.-D. (ed.) *Encyclopedia of Pharmacy Practice and Clinical Pharmacy.* Oxford: Elsevier.

Atif, M., Malik, I., Mushtaq, I. & Asghar, S. 2019d. Medicines shortages in Pakistan: a qualitative study to explore current situation, reasons and possible solutions to overcome the barriers. *BMJ Open,* 9, e027028.

Atif, M., Rasheed, W., Mushtaq, I., Malik, I., Kanwal, S. & Qamar-Uz-Zaman, M. 2019e. Medication Related Knowledge and Practices Among Patients Attending Pharmacies in Bahawalpur, Pakistan: a Cross-Sectional Study *Lat. Am. J. Pharm,* 38, 1404–15

Atif, M., Sarwar, M. R., Azeem, M., Umer, D., Rauf, A., Rasool, A., Ahsan, M. & Scahill, S. 2016c. Assessment of WHO/INRUD core drug use indicators in two tertiary care hospitals of Bahawalpur, Punjab, Pakistan. *J Pharm Policy Pract,* 9, 27–27.

Awaisu, A. & Alsalimy, N. 2015. Pharmacists' involvement in and attitudes toward pharmacy practice research: A systematic review of the literature. *Res Social Adm Pharm,* 11, 725–48.

Azhar, S., Hassali, M. & Ibrahim, M. 2010. Doctors' perception and expectations of the role of the pharmacist in Punjab, Pakistan. *Trop J Pharm Res,* 9.

Azhar, S., Hassali, M. A., Ibrahim, M. I. M., Ahmad, M., Masood, I. & Shafie, A. A. 2009. The role of pharmacists in developing countries: the current scenario in Pakistan. *Human Resources for Health,* 7, 54.

Azhar, S., Hassali, M. A. & Ibrahim, M. M. 2011. Perceptions of hospital pharmacist's role in Pakistan's healthcare system: a cross-sectional survey. *Tropical Journal of Pharmaceutical Research,* 10.

Azhar, S., Kousar, R., Khan, S. A. & Murtaza, G. 2016. Evolving Scenario Of Pharmaceutical Care In Pakistan And Other Countries: Health Impact Assessment In Public Health Practice. *Acta poloniae pharmaceutica,* 73, 1101.

Aziz, M., Ji, W., Masood, I., Farooq, M., Malik, M., Chang, J., Jiang, M., Atif, N. & Fang, Y. 2018a. Patient Satisfaction with Community Pharmacies Services: A Cross-Sectional Survey from Punjab; Pakistan. *International journal of environmental research and public health,* 15, 2914.

Aziz, M. M., Jiang, M., Masood, I., Chang, J., Shan, Z., Raza, M. A., Ji, W., Yang, C. & Fang, Y. 2019a. Patients' Anticipation for the Pharmacies of

Rural Communities: A Qualitative Study from Pakistan. *Int J Environ Res Public Health,* 16, 143.

Aziz, M. M., Masood, I., Yousaf, M., Saleem, H., Ye, D. & Fang, Y. 2018b. Pattern of medication selling and self-medication practices: A study from Punjab, Pakistan. *PLoS One,* 13, e0194240.

Aziz, M. M., Yang, S., Masood, I., Zhu, S., Raza, M. A., Ji, W., Anwar, N., Saeed, A. & Fang, Y. 2019b. An assessment of counseling quality provided by community pharmacies to type 2 diabetic adult patients for oral therapy: a simulated patient study from Pakistan. *Endocrine J,* EJ18-0429.

Babar, Z. U. & Jamshed, S. 2008. Social pharmacy strengthening clinical pharmacy: why pharmaceutical policy research is needed in Pakistan? *Pharm World Sci,* 30, 617–9.

Bakken, S., Lantigua, R. A., Busacca, L. V. & Bigger, J. T. 2009. Barriers, enablers, and incentives for research participation: a report from the Ambulatory Care Research Network (ACRN). *J Am Board Fam Med,* 22, 436–45.

Birenbaum, A. 1982. Reprofessionalization in pharmacy. *Soc Sci Med,* 16, 871–878.

Cameron, A. & Laing, R. Cost savings of switching private sector consumption from originator brand medicines to generic equivalents. World health report, 2010.

Chisholm, M. A. & Hawkins, D. W. 1996. Analysis of Pharmacotherapy Recommendations Provided by Doctor of Pharmacy Clerkship Students. *J Pharm Teach,* 5, 3–12.

Cruz Rivera, S., Kyte, D. G., Aiyegbusi, O. L., Keeley, T. J. & Calvert, M. J. 2017. Assessing the impact of healthcare research: A systematic review of methodological frameworks. *PLoS Med,* 14, e1002370.

Desselle, S. P. 2005. The birth of research in social & administrative pharmacy: a sincere welcome to subscribers, readers, and authors. *Research in Social and Administrative Pharmacy,* 1, 1–4.

Babar, Z.-U. 2006. Pakistan's National University of Pharmaceutical Sciences. *Am J Pharmaceutica Edu,* 70, 123–123.

Fakeye, T. O., Adisa, R., Olukotun, R. T. & Morawo, P. K. 2017a. Hospital and community pharmacists' perception of the scope, barriers and challenges of pharmacy practice-based research in Nigeria. *Pharmacy Practice (Granada),* 15.

Fakeye, T. O., Adisa, R., Olukotun, R. T. & Morawo, P. K. 2017b. Hospital and community pharmacists' perception of the scope, barriers and challenges of pharmacy practice-based research in Nigeria. *Pharmacy practice,* 15, 881–881.

Government of Pakistan 2018. National Essential Medicines List 2018. Islamabad.

Haq, N. U., Riaz, S. & Nasim, A. 2017. Pharmacy without pharmacist: Body without soul. *Arch Pharm Pract,* 8, 84–84.

Hashmi, F. K., Hassali, M. A., Khalid, A., Saleem, F., Aljadhey, H., Babar, Z. U. D. & Bashaar, M. 2017. A qualitative study exploring perceptions and attitudes of community pharmacists about extended pharmacy services in Lahore, Pakistan. *BMC Health Serv Res,* 17, 500–500.

Hashmi, F. K. & Saleem, F. 2017. Pharmacy practice in Pakistan: The Catch-22 continues. *Research in social & administrative pharmacy: RSAP,* 14, 213.

Hepler, C. D. 1993. Pharmaceutical care and specialty practice. *Pharmacother,* 13, 64S–69S.

Hepler, C. D. 1996. Pharmaceutical care. *Pharm World Sci,* 18, 233–5.

Hepler, C. D. & Strand, L. M. 1990. Opportunities and responsibilities in pharmaceutical care. *Am J Hosp Pharm,* 47, 533–43.

Husnain, S. Z., Bukhari, N. I., Hussain, K. & Saleem, Z. 2018. Inappropriateness of medication use and associated health risks: A cross-sectional study from Pakistan. *Trop J Pharm Res,* 17, 715–721.

Hussain, R. & Hassali, M. A. 2019. Current status and future prospects of pharmacovigilance in Pakistan. *J Pharm Policy Pract,* 12, 14.

Hussain, R., Hassali, M. A., Hashmi, F. & Farooqui, M. 2018. A qualitative exploration of knowledge, attitudes and practices of hospital pharmacists towards adverse drug reaction reporting system in Lahore, Pakistan. *J Pharm Policy Pract,* 11, 16.

Ibrahim, A. H., Jose, D. & Jegan, R. 2012. Pharmacists in the Wider Public Health Workforce-A Review. *Arch Pharm Pract,* 3, 166.

Iffat, W., Shakeel, S., Naseem, S., Imam, S. & Khan, M. 2014. Attitudinal survey to assess medical and dental students' belief of ADR reporting in Pakistan. *Int J Pharm Pharm Sci,* 6, 279–283.

Imaduddin. 2014. Govt promoting sale of effective, quality of generic drugs: NA told. *Business Recorder.*

Inamullah, K., Najm Ul Hassan, K., Momina, N., Kishwar, S. & Ossam, C. 2017. Analyzing The Perception Level Of General Public & Other Health Care Professionals About The Pharmacist & Its Role In The Community Of Abbottabad & Rawalpindi, Pakistan. *Int J Basic Med Sci Pharm,* 7.

International Pharmaceutical Federation 2000. International Pharmaceutical Federation (FIP) Statement of Policy on good pharmacy education and practice. The Hague, The Netherlands.

International Pharmaceutical Federation 2017. Research, development and evaluation strategies for pharmaceutical education and the workforce: a global report. *In:* BADER, L. R. & BATES, I. (eds.). The Netherlands

Jamshed, S., Babar, Z. U. D., Ibrahim, M. I. M. & Hassali, M. A. A. 2009. Generic Medicines As A Way To Improve Access And Affordability: A Proposed Framework For Pakistan. *J Clin Diagnostic Res,* 3, 1596–1600.

Jamshed, S., Hassali, M., Ibrahim, M., Shafie, A. & Babar, Z. 2010. Knowledge, perception and attitude of community pharmacists towards generic medicines in Karachi, Pakistan: a qualitative insight. *Trop J Pharm Res,* 9.

Jamshed, S. Q., Ibrahim, M. I., Hassali, M. A., Sharrad, A. K., Shafie, A. A. & Babar, Z. U. 2015. Understanding and perceptions of final-year Doctor of Pharmacy students about generic medicines in Karachi, Pakistan: a quantitative insight. *Adv Med Educ Pract,* 6, 359–66.

Jamshed, S. Q., Malik, M. A., Löfgren, H. & Gilani, A.-H. 2013. The pharmaceutical industry, intellectual property rights and access to medicines in Pakistan. *The New Political Economy of Pharmaceuticals.* Springer.

Kaplan, W. A., Ritz, L. S., Vitello, M. & Wirtz, V. J. 2012. Policies to promote use of generic medicines in low and middle income countries: a review of published literature, 2000–2010. *Health policy,* 106, 211–224.

Khan, A., Iqbal, Q., Haider, S., Khalid, A., Hassali, M. A. & Saleem, F. 2019. Acute Diarrheal Management in Adults: A Simulated Client Study at Community Pharmacies of Quetta City, Pakistan. *J Pharm Pract Comm Med,* 5.

Khan, E. A. 2018. Situation Analysis Report on Antimicrobial Resistance in Pakistan. Center for Disease Dynamics, Economics & Policy.

Khan, G. M. Integrating Clinical Pharmacy Education, Practice & Research: Bridging the Gap. 2016.

Khan, T., Ahmed, K. M. & Anwar, M. 2011. A perspective for clinical pharmacy curriculum development and validation in Asian developing nations. *J Young Pharm,* 3, 151–154.

Kiani, A., Qadeer, A., Mirza, Z., Khanum, A., Tisocki, K. & Mustafa, T. 2006. Prices, availability and affordability of medicines in Pakistan. Geneva: Health Action International (HAI).

Kmet, L. M., Lee, R. C. & Cook, L. S. 2004. Standard quality assessment criteria for evaluating primary research papers from a variety of fields. Alberta Heritage Foundation for Medical Research Edmonton.

Kongkaew, C., Noyce, P. R. & Ashcroft, D. M. 2008. Hospital admissions associated with adverse drug reactions: a systematic review of prospective observational studies. *Ann Pharmacother,* 42, 1017–25.

Koshman, S. L. & Blais, J. 2011. What is pharmacy research? *The Canadian journal of hospital pharmacy,* 64, 154.

Macleod, M. R., Michie, S., Roberts, I., Dirnagl, U., Chalmers, I., Ioannidis, J. P., Al-Shahi Salman, R., Chan, A. W. & Glasziou, P. 2014. Biomedical research: increasing value, reducing waste. *Lancet,* 383, 101–4.

Mahmood, K. T., Amin, F., Tahir, M. & Haq, I. U. 2011. Pharmacovigilance-A need for best patient care in Pakistan. A review. *J Pharm Sci Res,* 3, 1566.

Malik, I. 2019. Lack of female pharmacist leadership and struggling pharmacy profession: A call to action. *Res Soc Admin Pharm.*

Malik, I., Atif, M., Riaz, F., Asghar, S. & AHMAD, N. 2019a. Pediatric Antibiotic Pack Size Compliance With the Dosage Regimen: A Descriptive Study. *Ther Innov Regul Sci,* 2168479019853770.

Malik, I., Ikram, H. & Rafiq, S. 2019b. 71st anniversary of pharmacy profession in Pakistan: Why pharmacists' are still flying under the radar? *Res Social Adm Pharm.*

Malik, M., Amin, A. & Hussain, A. 2018. A Descriptive Cross-Sectional Study Exploring Perceptions and Attitude of Pharmacists towards Adverse Drug Reporting in Pakistan. *Int J Pharmacovigil,* 3, 1–7.

Medical Microbiology and Infectious Diseases Society of Pakistan. 2014. *Antibiotic Stewardship Initiative In Pakistan (ASIP)* [Online]. Available: http://www.mmidsp.com/wp-content/uploads/2014/02/ANTIBIOTIC-STEWARDSHIP-INITIATIVE-IN-PAKISTAN.pdf.

Memon, A. R. 2017. Research publications and education in Pakistani medical universities: Avoiding predatory journals and improving the quality of research. *J Pak Med Assoc,* 67, 830–833.

Mohamad Azmi H, Asrul Akmal S & Chua GN 2013. *A National Survey On The Use Of Medicines (NSUM) By Malaysian Consumers,* Malaysia, Quality Use of Medicines: Pharmaceutical Services Division

Moher, D., Liberati, A., Tetzlaff, J. & Altman, D. G. 2009. Preferred reporting items for systematic reviews and meta-analyses: the PRISMA statement. *Ann Internal Me,* 151, 264–269.

Munroe, W. P., Kunz, K., Dalmady-Israel, C., Potter, L. & Schonfeld, W. H. 1997. Economic evaluation of pharmacist involvement in disease management in a community pharmacy setting. *Clin ther,* 19, 113–123.

Nishtar, S. 2012. Pakistan's deadly cocktail of substandard drugs. *The Lancet,* 379, 1084–1085.

Ofori-Asenso, R., Brhlikova, P. & Pollock, A. M. 2016. Prescribing indicators at primary health care centers within the WHO African region: a systematic analysis (1995–2015). *BMC Public Health,* 16, 724.

Okonta, J. M., Okonta, E. O. & Ofoegbu, T. C. 2012. Barriers to Implementation of Pharmaceutical Care by Pharmacists in Nsukka and Enugu metropolis of Enugu State. *J Basic Clin Pharm,* 3, 295–8.

Organization, W. H. 2003. Guide to Good Storage Practices for Pharmaceuticals. *WHO Technical Report Series,*. World Health Organization.

Rabbani, F., Cheema, F., Talati, N., Siddiqui, S., Syed, S., Bashir, S., Zuberi, L., Shamim, A. & Mumtaz, Q. 2001. Behind the counter: pharmacies and dispensing patterns of pharmacy attendants in Karachi. *J Pak Med Assoc,* 51, 149.

Rahim, N. & Usmani, S. 2012. Physicians' opinion about the role of pharmacist in the health care system of Pakistan. *Int J,* 3, 257–60.

Rashid, H. 2015. Impact of the drug regulatory authorityPakistan: An evaluation. *New Visions Public Affairs,* 7, 50–61.

Rehman, I., Asad, M., Bukhsh, A., Ali, Z., Ata, H., Dujaili, J., Blebil, A. & Khan, T. 2018. Knowledge and practice of pharmacists toward antimicrobial stewardship in Pakistan. *Pharmacy,* 6, 116.

Riaz, H., Godman, B., Bashir, S., Hussain, S., Mahmood, S., Waseem, D., Malik, F. & Raza, S. A. 2016a. Evaluation of drug use indicators for non-communicable diseases in Pakistan. *Acta Poloniae Pharmaceutica ñ Drug Res,* 18, 19.

Riaz, H., Godman, B., Bashir, S., Hussain, S., Mahmood, S., Waseem, D., Malik, F. & Raza, S. A. 2016b. Evaluation of drug use indicators for non-communicable diseases in Pakistan. *Acta Poloniae Pharmaceutica ñ Drug Research,* 18, 19.

Ryan, G. W. & Bernard, H. R. 2003. Techniques to identify themes. *Field methods,* 15, 85–109.

Ryan, K., Bissell, P., Anderson, C., Traulsen, J. M. & Sleath, B. 2007. Teaching social sciences to undergraduate pharmacy students: an international survey. *Pharmacy Education,* 7.

Sachs, J. D. & McArthur, J. W. 2005. The millennium project: a plan for meeting the millennium development goals. *The Lancet,* 365, 347–353.

Sadek, M. M., Elnour, A. A., Al Kalbani, N. M. S., Bhagavathula, A. S., Baraka, M. A., Aziz, A. M. A. & SHEHAB, A. 2016. Community pharmacy and the extended community pharmacist practice roles: The UAE experiences. *Saudi Pharm J,* 24, 563–570.

Saeed, A., Saeed, H., Saleem, Z. & Fang, Y. 2019a. Evaluation of prices, availability and affordability of essential medicines in Lahore Division, Pakistan: A cross-sectional survey using WHO/HAI methodology. *PloS one,* 14, e0216122.

Saeed, A., Saeed, H., Saleem, Z., Fang, Y. & Babar, Z.-U.-D. 2019b. Evaluation of prices, availability and affordability of essential medicines in Lahore

Division, Pakistan: A cross-sectional survey using WHO/HAI methodology. *PLOS ONE,* 14, e0216122.

Saini, B., Brillant, M., Filipovska, J., Gelgor, L., Mitchell, B., Rose, G. & Smith, L. 2005. Recruitment and retention of community pharmacists in pharmacy practice research. Faculty of Pharmacy, University of Sydney Sydney, Australia.

Saqib, A., Iftikhar, S. & Sarwar, M. R. 2018. Availability and affordability of biologic versus non-biologic anticancer medicines: a cross-sectional study in Punjab, Pakistan. *BMJ open,* 8, e019015.

Sarwar, M. R., Atif, M., Scahill, S., Saqib, A., Qamar-Uz-Zaman, M. & Babar, Z. 2017. Drug utilization patterns among elderly hospitalized patients on poly-pharmacy in Punjab, Pakistan. *J Pharm Policy Pract,* 10, 23–23.

Sarwar, M. R., Iftikhar, S. & Saqib, A. 2018a. Availability of anticancer medicines in public and private sectors, and their affordability by low, middle and high-income class patients in Pakistan. *BMC cancer,* 18, 14.

Sarwar, M. R., Saqib, A., Iftikhar, S. & Sadiq, T. 2018b. Knowledge of community pharmacists about antibiotics, and their perceptions and practices regarding antimicrobial stewardship: a cross-sectional study in Punjab, Pakistan. *Infection and drug resistance,* 11, 133–145.

Sarwar, M. R., Saqib, A., Riaz, T., Aziz, H., Arafat, M. & Nouman, H. 2018c. Attitude, perception, willingness, motivation and barriers to practice based research: A cross-sectional survey of hospital pharmacists in Lahore, Punjab, Pakistan. *PloS one,* 13, e0203568–e0203568.

Scahill, S. L., Atif, M. & Babar, Z. U. 2017. Defining pharmacy and its practice: a conceptual model for an international audience. *Integrated pharmacy research & practice,* 6, 121–129.

Shabbir Hussain. 2019. DRAP approves 15% increase in medicine prices. *THE EXPRESS TRIBUNE.*

Shahnaz, G. 2014. Pharmaceutical Situation Assessment – LEVEL II Health Facilities Survey in Pakistan. Pakistan: Ministry of National Health Services, Regulation and Coordination

Shaikh, B. T. & Rabbani, F. 2004. The district health system: a challenge that remains. *East Mediterr Health J,* 10, 208–14.

Shakeel, S., Iffat, W., Anjum, F., Bushra, R., Ibrahim, S. & Shafiq, S. 2014. Emerging need of pharmacovigilance: perspectives of future pharmacist in Pakistan. *Int J Pharm Teach Pract,* 5, 966–969.

Sharif, H., Sharif, S. & Zaighum, I. 2016. Reasons of brand switching and preference in prescription medicines: A comparison between physicians and pharmacists of Karachi. *Pharm Innovat,* 5, 99.

Shet, A., Sundaresan, S. & Forsberg, B. C. 2015. Pharmacy-based dispensing of antimicrobial agents without prescription in India: appropriateness and cost burden in the private sector. *Antimicrob Resist Infect Control,* 4, 55.

Simpson, S. H., Johnson, J. A., Biggs, C., Biggs, R. S., Kuntz, A., Semchuk, W., Taylor, J. G., Farris, K. B. & Tsuyuki, R. T. 2001. Practice-based research: lessons from community pharmacist participants. *Pharmacotherapy,* 21, 731–9.

Smith, F. 2009. The quality of private pharmacy services in low and middle-income countries: a systematic review. *Pharm World Sci,* 31, 351–61.

Sultana, K., Al Jeraisy, M., Al Ammari, M., Patel, R. & Zaidi, S. T. 2016. Attitude, barriers and facilitators to practice-based research: cross-sectional survey of hospital pharmacists in Saudi Arabia. *J Pharm Policy Pract,* 9, 4.

Syed, A., Azhar, S., Raza, M. M., Saeed, H. & Jamshed, S. Q. 2018. Assessment of Knowledge, Attitude and Barriers towards Pharmacovigilance among Physicians and Pharmacists of Abbottabad, Pakistan. *Pharmacy,* 6.

Umair Khan, M., Ahmad, A., Ejaz, A., Ata Rizvi, S., Sardar, A., Hussain, K., Zaffar, T. & Q Jamshed, S. 2015. Comparison of the knowledge, attitudes, and perception of barriers regarding adverse drug reaction reporting between pharmacy and medical students in Pakistan. *J Edu Evaluation Health Prof,* 12, 28–28.

Wiedenmayer, K., Summers, R. S., Mackie, C. A., Gous, A. G., Everard, M., Tromp, D. & Organization, W. H. 2006. Developing pharmacy practice: a focus on patient care: handbook. Geneva: World Health Organization.

World Health Organization. 2002. WHO Drug Information.

World Health Organization 2004. The World Medicines Situation. Geneva, Switzerland: World Health Organization,.

World Health Organization 2014. PHARMACEUTICAL SITUATION ASSESSMENT – LEVEL II Health Facilities Survey in PAKISTAN Islamabad.

World Health Organization 2016. National Health Vision Pakistan 2016–2025. Country Planning Cycle Database.

World Health Organization 2017. Joint external evaluation of IHR core capacities of the Islamic Republic of Pakistan: mission report: 27 April-6 May 2016 World Health Organization,.

Yee, G. C. & Haas, C. E. 2014. Standards of practice for clinical pharmacists: the time has come. *Pharmacotherapy,* 34, 769–70.

Zaidi, S., Bigdeli, M., Aleem, N. & Rashidian, A. 2013. Access to essential medicines in Pakistan: policy and health systems research concerns. *PloS one,* 8, e63515.

7

Promoting Access to Cancer Medicines in Mexico: *Seguro Popular* Key Policy Components

Daniela Moye-Holz, Anahí Dreser, Octavio Gómez-Dantés, and Veronika J. Wirtz

Abbreviations

25%ile	25% interquartile range
75%ile	75% interquartile range
approx.	Approximately
CAUSES	Universal Catalogue of Health Services, *Catálogo Universal de Servicios de Salud*

D. Moye-Holz (✉)
Department of Community and Occupational Medicine, University Medical Center Groningen, University of Groningen, Groningen, The Netherlands

A. Dreser • O. Gómez-Dantés
National Institute of Public Health (Instituto Nacional de Salud Pública), Cuernavaca, Morelos, Mexico

V. J. Wirtz
Department of Global Health, University of Boston School of Public Health, Boston, MA, USA

Z. Babar (ed.), *Global Pharmaceutical Policy*,
https://doi.org/10.1007/978-981-15-2724-1_7

CBMCIS	Basic Medicines Scheme and Catalogue of Health Inputs, *Cuadro Básico de Medicamentos y Cátalogo de Insumos del Sector Salud*
CCNPMIS	Coordinating Commission for the Price Negotiation of Medicines and Other Health Inputs, *Comisión Coordinadora para la Negociación de Precios de Medicamentos e Insumos de Salud*
CENETEC	National Center for Technological Excellence in Health, *Centro Nacional de Excelencia Tecnológica en Salud*
CNPSS	National Commission for Social Protection in Health, *Comisión Nacional de Protección Social en Salud*
COFEPRIS	Federal Commission for the Protection Against Sanitary Risks, *Comisión Federal para la Protección Contra Riesgos Sanitarios*
CSG	National Health Council, *Consejo de Salubridad General*
FPGC	Fund for the Protection Against Catastrophic Expenditure, *Fondo de Protección Contra Gastos Catastróficos*
FSPSS	System of Social for Health Trust, *Fideicomiso del Sistema de Protección Social en Salud*
IMSS	Mexican Institute for Social Security, *Instituto Mexicano del Seguro Social*
IRP	International reference prices
ISSSTE	Social Security Institute for Civil Servants, *Instituto de Seguridad y Servicios Sociales de los Trabajadores del Estado*
LMIC	Low- and middle-income countries
max	Maximum
min	Minimum
MoH	Ministry of Health
MPR	Median price ratio
MRP	Maximum retail price
NCD	Non-communicable diseases
PEMEX	Mexican Oil Company, *Petróleos Mexicanos*
popl.	Population
REPSS	Social Protection in Health State Regimes, *Régimenes Estatal de Protección Social en Salud*
SEDENA	Defence Ministry, *Secretaría de la Defensa Nacional*

SEMAR	Navy Ministry, *Secretaría de la Marina*
SP	People's Health Insurance, *Seguro Popular*
STG	Standard treatment guidelines
UHC	Universal health coverage
WHO	World Health Organization
WHO-EML	World Health Organization Model List of Essential Medicines

Introduction

Effective cancer care requires a wide array of essential services, including preventive, diagnostic, therapeutic and palliation services (Knaul et al. 2011). Access to effective treatment, including pharmaceutical treatment, is essential for the control of cancer (Shulman et al. 2016; Strasser-Weippl et al. 2015). Pharmaceutical treatment for cancer demands different types of medicines, including chemotherapeutic agents, hormones and palliative remedies (Knaul et al. 2011; Shulman et al. 2016).

Essential medicines are those that satisfy the priority healthcare needs of the population and should be available at all times and at a price the population can afford (Gray et al. 2015). Following this definition and due to the growing cancer burden, the concept of essential medicines includes an increasing number of cancer medicines in an effort to guarantee access to cancer treatment and effective control (Hogerzeil et al. 2013; Robertson et al. 2016; WHO 2004).

Cancer has become a leading cause of mortality worldwide and a major cause of disability (World Health Organization 2019), particularly in low- and middle-income countries (LMIC). As a result, access to cancer control services is becoming part of the healthcare packages offered in LMICs moving towards universal health coverage (UHC). Since essential medicines are key components of any well-functioning health system and UHC strategy (Wirtz et al. 2017), countries moving towards UHC must include cancer treatment and cancer medicines in their essential packages of health services.

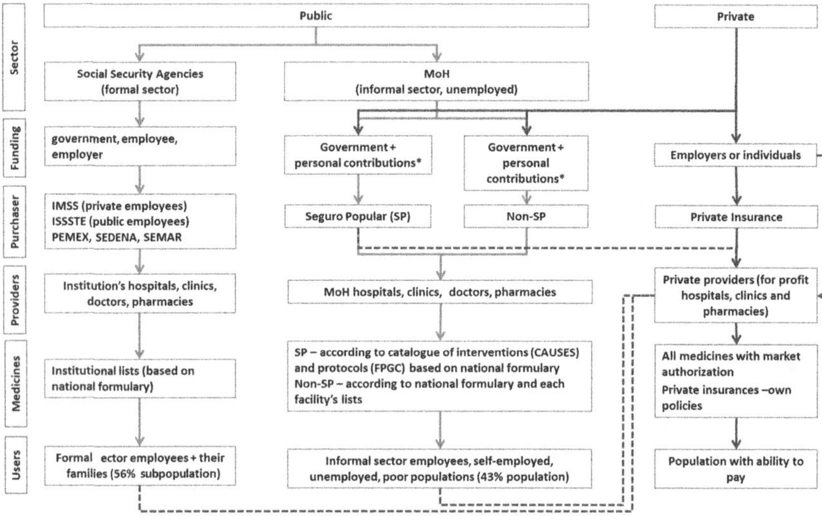

Fig. 7.1 The health system of Mexico
IMSS - Mexican Social Security Institute; ISSSTE - Social Security Institute for Civil Servants; MoH - Ministry of Health; PEMEX - Mexican Oil Company (Petróleos Mexicanos); SEDENA - Defence Ministry (army); SEMAR - Navy Ministry; SP - Popular Health Insurance; CAUSES - Universal Health Services Catalogue; FPGC - Fund Against Catastrophic Expenditure; popl. - population; approx. - approximately
*Personal contributions—a type of copayment according to level of income
**The sum of the percentages is higher than the 100% of the population, because users may enjoy/use more than one health coverage scheme (e.g. IMSS + private sector user (paying out-of-pocket or through private insurance))
Source: Author's (Moye-Holz 2019) based on Gomez-Dantes (Gómez Dantés et al. 2011) and Gonzalez-Block (González-Block 2017)

Mexico, in the search for UHC, has gone through various health reforms, the last of which expanded access to cancer treatment. At the turn of the century, the Mexican health system had a public and private sector (Fig. 7.1). The public sector included the Ministry of Health (MoH) and various social security agencies: the Mexican Institute for Social Security (IMSS), the Social Security Institute for Civil Servants (ISSSTE) and other minor social security agencies (PEMEX, SEDENA and SEMAR). Social security agencies were (and still are) financed through employer, employees and government contributions and provided comprehensive healthcare in their own clinics and hospitals to the salaried workers and their families. The MoH was financed mostly with federal and state contributions and provided healthcare in its own facilities to the uninsured population.

In 2003, the Mexican Congress approved a reform to the General Health Law creating the System of Social Protection in Health (*Sistema de Protección Social en Salud* or *SPSS*) (Secretaría de Salud 2003). The insurance component of this system is *Seguro Popularde Salud* (SP) or Popular Health Insurance, a public insurance scheme whose objective is to provide financial protection in health to the non-salaried population. For each individual enrolled in SP, the state has to mobilize enough resources (through federal and state contributions and affiliate contributions based on income level) to guarantee access to a package of essential services (Universal Catalogue of Essential Health Services or *Catálogo Universal de Servicios Esenciales de Salud* (CAUSES)) and a package of high-cost interventions (including neonatal intensive care, treatment for HIV/AIDS and several cancers, etc.) financed with resources from an independent fund (Fund for the Protection Against Catastrophic Expenses or *Fondo de Protección Contra Gastos Catastróficos* (FPGC)). By 2018, 53.5 million people (informal sector workers, self-employed and unemployed individuals and those living outside the labour market) were enrolled in SP.

The purpose of this chapter is to analyse Mexico's experience in expanding access to essential cancer medicines through SP in order to increase cancer care coverage and reach UHC. This chapter describes the burden of cancer in Mexico and the way in which several public policies have confronted this burden. It also describes the key components of SP and the way in which they have increased access to cancer care and medicines. It uses as reference the World Health Organization (WHO) Access to Medicines Framework (World Health Organization 2004), which includes selection, financing, price and affordability of medicines, as well as procurement and supply. Finally, it discusses the main achievements and challenges that Mexico faces to guarantee universal access to cancer medicines.

Information presented in this chapter derives from a document analysis (publicly available data and governmental documents), a scoping literature review and a survey conducted in 2017 (Moye-Holz 2019). The survey reported on availability, prices and affordability of medicines, together with opinions from health professionals on access to cancer medicines in health facilities (Moye-Holz 2019).

Burden of Cancer in Mexico

Mexico's burden of disease is characterized by the predominance of non-communicable diseases (NCD), particularly diabetes, cardiovascular diseases and cancer. Cancer is responsible for approximately 13% of all deaths (Reynoso-Noverón and Mohar 2014; Reynoso-Noverón and Alejandro 2000). Leukaemia (acute lymphoblastic leukaemia) is the leading cause of mortality attributed to cancer in children (Shalkow 2018; Secretaría de Salud 2015); breast and cervical cancer are the leading causes of mortality and disability due to cancer in women (Reynoso-Noverón and Alejandro 2000); and colorectal cancer, lung cancer and prostate cancer are the leading causes of mortality and disability due to cancer in men (Reynoso-Noverón and Alejandro 2000). Figure 7.2 shows

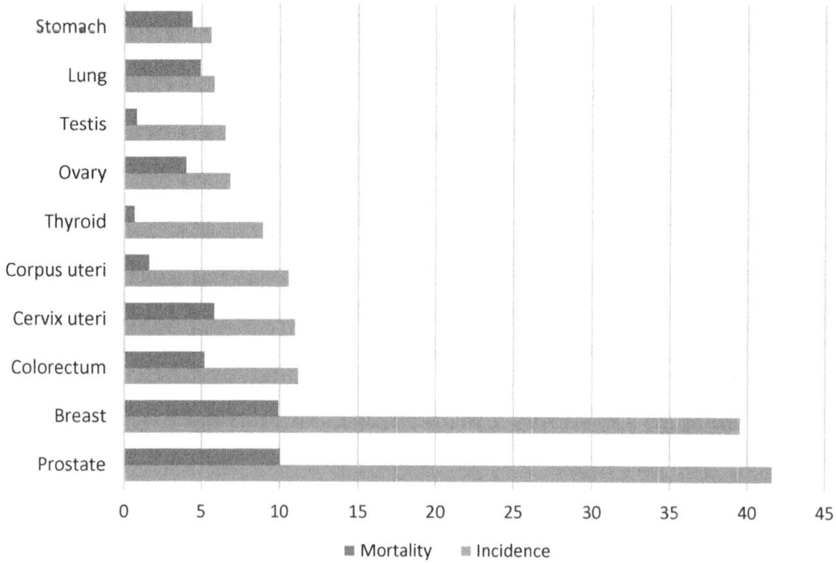

Fig. 7.2 Estimated age-standardized cancer incidence and mortality rates in Mexico in 2018 (both sexes, all ages). (Source: Author's based on data from the International Agency for Research on Cancer (International Agency for Research on Cancer 2019))

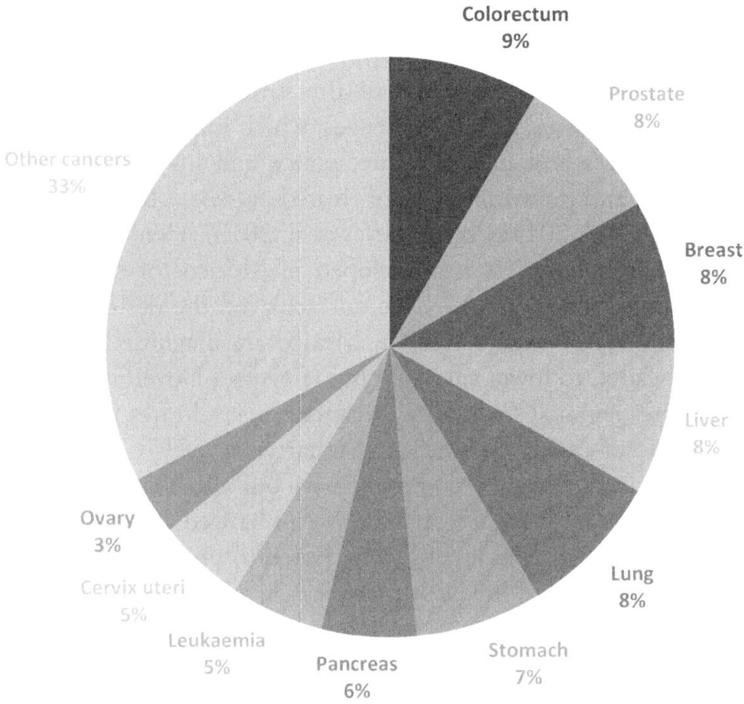

Fig. 7.3 Estimated number of deaths attributed to cancer in Mexico in 2018 (all cancers, both sexes, all ages). (Source: Author's based on data from the International Agency for Research on Cancer (International Agency for Research on Cancer 2019))

the 2018 estimated age-standardized incidence and mortality rates for Mexico for both sexes and all ages. It is noteworthy that the incidence of lung and stomach cancer is similar to their respective mortality. Figure 7.3 shows the estimated number of deaths due to cancer in Mexico in 2018.

Key Cancer Policies in Mexico

Since 1970, a series of national programmes have been developed to promote early detection, prevention, diagnosis, treatment and palliation of mainly female cancers (breast cancer, ovary cancer and cervical cancer), prostate cancer and cancer in children (Hernández-Peña et al. 1997;

Secretaria de Salud 2013, 2014, 2019a). Cancer has been recognized as a national priority and goals were established for its detection and treatment.

However, the implementation of the various national cancer programmes has faced a series of challenges, which include insufficient provision of services and infrastructure, scarce and low-quality detection interventions and poor follow-up of treated patients (Torres-Mejía et al. 2013; Bright et al. 2011; Pérez-Cuevas et al. 2013). Hence, despite some notable achievements, efforts developed in Mexico for the prevention and early detection of cancer have not achieved the desired outcomes. More than 70% of cancer cases in Mexico are diagnosed in advanced stages, associated to lower survival rates (Reynoso-Noverón et al. 2016). Furthermore, regional inequality in cancer survival rates is a distinctive characteristic of cancer in Mexico (Mohar et al. 2015). Therefore, the need to guarantee not only comprehensive but also timely treatment to all cancer patients in Mexico has been emphasized (Reynoso-Noverón and Mohar 2014), a goal intrinsically related to pharmaceutical policies and the organization of the health system.

Access to Medicines in Mexico

Regarding access to medicines in the public health sector, the Mexican government has promoted equitable access to high-quality treatments. Mexico does not have an official national pharmaceutical policy document (Moye-Holz et al. 2017), but a series of administrative bodies and regulations provide the framework for national pharmaceutical policies, as described in Box 7.1.

Seguro Popular's Key Components to Promote Access to Cancer Medicines

SP includes several components directed to promote access to medicines. Following the WHO Access to Medicines Framework (World Health Organization 2004), these components address four main areas: selection, financing, pricing and healthcare and delivery services, including procurement and supply. Figure 7.4 presents an overview of key SP components within each of these four components.

Box 7.1 Policies and administrative bodies related to access to medicines in Mexico

Administrative bodies related to access to medicines	Key policy instruments and regulations
National Health Council (Consejo de Salubridad General or CSG) updates and reviews the national formulary every year following national regulations (Rivas and Rico n.d.) that define and standardize the assessment of medicines and health technologies based on scientific, clinical, economic and epidemiological evidence (Consejo de Salubridad General 2011; Ríos et al. 2013; Barraza-Lloréns and Campos-Hernández 2007). The CSG is also responsible for defining the list of diseases, treatment protocols, list of medicines and devices to be financed by the FPGC.	Basic Medicines Scheme and Catalogue of Health Inputs **(Cuadro Básico de Medicamentos y Cátalogo de Insumos del Sector Salud or CBMCIS)**. The national formulary serves as a reference and provides a comprehensive list of medicines and health devices that may be covered and procured by public institutions and facilities in Mexico (Ríos et al. 2013; Moïse and Docteur 2008).
Federal Commission for the Protection Against Sanitary Risks (Comisión Federal para la Protección Contra Riesgos Sanitarios or COFEPRIS). This regulatory body is in charge of registering pharmaceuticals and guaranteeing their quality; it has also participated in efforts to foster generics penetration in the Mexican market.	National pharmacopoeia
National Center for Technological Excellence in Health (Centro Nacional de ExcelenciaTecnológica en Salud or CENETEC) is in charge of producing information to improve the management, assessment and use of health-related technologies, including medicines. Additionally, CENETEC is also in charge of developing the national standard treatment guidelines (STG) (Centro Nacional de Excelencia Tecnológica en Salud 2018, 2017) used by all public institutions.	National standard treatment guidelines (STG)

(*continued*)

Box 7.1 (continued)

Coordinating Commission for the Price Negotiation of Medicines and Other Health Inputs (Comisión Coordinadora para la Negociación de Precios de Medicamentos e Insumos de Salud or CCNPMIS). The CCNPMIS was created in 2008 to end the variance in procurement prices of single-sourced medicines in the public sector. The CCNPMIS negotiates directly with the pharmaceutical companies the procurement prices of single-sourced (often patented) products included in the national formulary (Moye-Holz et al. 2017; Gómez-Dantés et al. 2012).	Price negotiation procedures

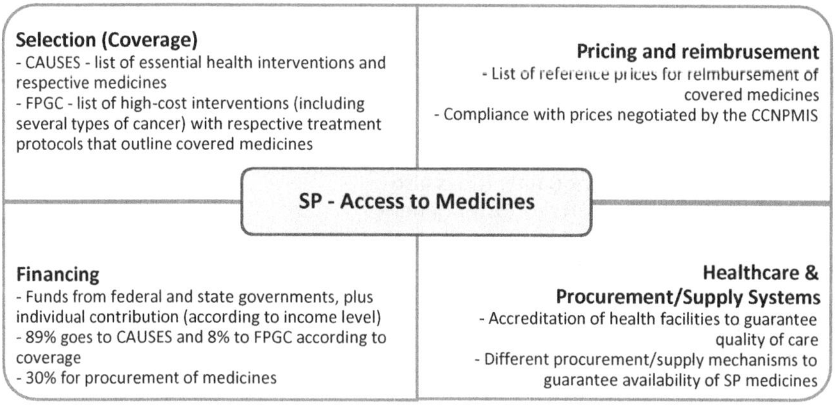

Fig. 7.4 Key components of Seguro Popular to promote access to medicines CAUSES, Catálogo Universal de Servicios de Salud (Universal Catalogue of Health Services); FPGC, Fondo de Protección Contra Gastos Catastróficos (Fund Against Catastrophic Expenditure); CCNPMIS, Comisión Coordinadora para la Negociación de Precios de Medicamentos y otros Insumos para la Salud (Coordinating Commission for the Price Negotiation of Medicines); SP, Seguro Popular de Salud (People's Health Insurance) (Moye-Holz 2019)

Selection of Cancer Medicines and Standard Treatment Guidelines

By 2016, through FPGC, SP provided access to treatment of 66 costly interventions (Secretaria de Salud 2018). Of the 66 diseases covered by FPGC, 33 are cancers, both in patients under and above 18 years of age (Table 7.1) (Reynoso-Noverón et al. 2016). However, by presidential decree in 2006, the FPGC also provides health coverage to all paediatric cancers (Secretaría de Salud 2014).

The National Health Council (*Consejo de Salubridad General* or *CSG*) is responsible for defining the list of diseases, treatments protocols, medicines and devices to be financed by FPGC. The criteria used to define the diseases covered by FPGC are their contribution to the burden of disease, safety and cost-effectiveness of their treatment and social acceptability of the interventions (González-Block 2017). The diseases covered by FPGC should follow treatment protocols, which include treatment guidelines, interventions, medicines and other resources necessary for the treatment of each disease. CSG develops and updates treatment guidelines taking into consideration medical and technological advances through the revision of national and international clinical guidelines and scientific evidence (Consejo de Salubridad General 2017).

In 2016, 90 cancer medicines were covered through FPGC. As outlined in Table 7.2, SP covers little more than 45% (90/185) of all the cancer medicines listed in the national formulary. Of the medicines covered by SP, 77% are generic medicines and 23% are patented medicines. Cancer medicines represent 28.3% (90/296) of the total number of medicines covered by SP through FPGC. SP covers more than 90% of the cancer medicines listed in the WHO Model List of Essential Medicines (WHO-EML) (World Health Organization 2015).

Financing of Cancer Medicines Through *Seguro Popular*

The National Commission for Social Protection in Health *(Comisión Nacional de Protección Social en Salud* or *CNPSS*) carries out all financial and administrative procedures of SP through the Social Protection in

Table 7.1 Cancers covered by SP through FPGC

Group	Intervention	Subcategory
Cancer for population < 18yo	Central nervous system tumours	Astrocytoma
		Ependymoma
		Medulloblastoma
		Neuroblastoma
		Others
	Renal tumours	Wilms' tumour
		Others
	Leukaemia	Acute lymphoblastic leukaemia
		Acute myeloblastic leukaemia
		Chronic leukaemia
		Myelodysplastic syndromes
	Hepatic tumours	Hepatocellular carcinoma
		Hepatoblastoma
	Bone tumours	Osteosarcoma
		Ewing's sarcoma
	Lymphomas	Non-Hodgkin's lymphoma
		Hodgkin's lymphoma
	Eye tumours	Retinoblastoma
	Sarcoma	Soft tissue sarcoma
	Germ cell tumours	Gonadal and extragonadal tumour
	Carcinomas	Several
	Histiocytosis	Malignant histiocytosis
Cancer in populations > 18yo	Malignant ovary tumour	Epithelial malignant ovary tumour
		Germ cell malignant ovary tumour
	Prostate cancer	Malignant prostate tumour
	Testicular cancer	Seminoma or non-seminoma
	Cervical cancer	Cervical cancer
	Breast cancer	Breast cancer
	Colorectal cancer	Colon malignant tumour
		Malignant tumour of the sigmoid-rectal junction
		Rectal malignant tumour
	Non-Hodgkin's lymphoma	Follicular
		Diffuse

Source: CAUSES (2016)

Health State Regimes (*Régimenes Estatales de Protección Social en Salud* or *REPSS*) (González-Block et al. 2016). REPSS are public decentralized bodies responsible for the supervision at the state level of the delivery of health services to those enrolled in SP, management of financial resources

Table 7.2 Medicines included in the national formulary and with SP-FPGC coverage (2016)

Formulary	Total number of medicines included	Number of cancer medicines included	Generic cancer medicines	Patented cancer medicines	Cancer medicines included in WHO-EML (2015)
National	2005	185	91/185 (+ 24 unknown)	70/185	45/48
SP(FPGC)	296	90	70/90	20/90	45/48

SP, Seguro Popular de Salud (People's Health Insurance); *FPGC*, Fondo de Protección Contra Gastos Catastróficos (Fund Against Catastrophic Expenditure); *WHO-EML*, World Health Organization Model List of Essential Medicines

and payment to providers (accredited health facilities) (Chemor Ruiz et al. 2018). Through REPSS, CNPSS allocates 89% of SP financial resources to cover all provision of services included in CAUSES, where only 30% of those funds can be used for the procurement of medicines (Servan-Mori et al. 2015). Through a health trust, CNPSS allocates 8% of SP resources to FPGC (Lozano and Garrido 2015; Sistema de Protección Social en Salud 2016, 2017). The remaining resources (3% of the total resources) are allocated in a fund for health infrastructure and to meet unexpected service demands (González-Block et al. 2016).

State outpatient facilities and general hospitals receive an annual budget to provide the services included in CAUSES, while national, regional and state high-specialty hospitals are reimbursed for the treatment of interventions covered by FPGC. Health facilities are reimbursed per case, which is first notified by the health facility and then validated by CNPSS (González-Block 2017; Orozco-Núñez et al. 2016). Patients with diseases or in need of medicines not covered by SP pay out-of-pocket. Patients pay either the total cost of medicines to the health facility or a copayment based on their level of income. Health facilities, when possible, absorb the remaining costs (Moye-Holz 2019).

In 2016 and 2017, 15.1% and 10.5% of all cases paid by the FPGC, respectively, were cancers, representing 48.5% and 33.9% of the total funds paid by this fund, respectively (Table 7.3).

Table 7.3 Cases of cancer financed by FPGC

Year	Validated interventions		Validated amount (Mexican pesos, in millions)		Paid interventions		Paid amount (Mexican pesos, in millions)	
	Total	Cancer (%)	Total	Cancer (%)	Total	Cancer(%)	Total	Cancer(%)
2016	243,913	34,760 (14.2%)	13,691.3	5475.9 (40%)	214,216	32,252 (15.1%)	10,330.1	5016 (48.5%)
2017	240,999	25,853 (10.7%)	12,720.3	4332.7 (34.1%)	239,229	25,176 (10.5%)	12,574.8	4260.4 (33.9%)

Source: SPS results reports (Sistema de Protección Social en Salud 2016, 2017)

Pricing of Cancer Medicines

SP reimburses health facilities for high-cost interventions based on tabulators (Seguro Popular 2019). The tabulator fixes maximum prices for all interventions, which are non-negotiable, although they are adjusted for inflation. Table 7.4 shows the price tabulator for breast cancer care, as an example. In the case of breast cancer, more than half of the treatment costs are attributable to pharmaceutical treatment.

Furthermore, SP has established guidelines on how medicines and other health inputs should be procured by health facilities and later reimbursed by SP (O'she Cuevas 2016). In these guidelines, SP lists all medicines and health devices it covers with their corresponding maximum reimbursement or reference price. The maximum reference prices of medicines are only applicable to generic medicines. For patented medicines, SP follows the prices set by the Coordinating Commission for the Price Negotiation of Medicines and Other Health Inputs (*Comisión Coordinadora para la Negociación de Precios de Medicamentos e Insumos de Salud* or *CCNPMIS*). The price negotiated by CCNPMIS is the price by which all public facilities should procure negotiated patented medicines (Moye-Holz et al. 2017; Gómez-Dantés et al. 2012; OECD 2016). During all negotiation rounds since 2010, approximately 13–15% of the total of negotiated medicines have been cancer medicines. They represent the second largest therapeutic group of

Table 7.4 Example of price tabulator for breast cancer treatment (2017)

Health service	Periodicity	Tabulator (in MXP)
Diagnosis	1×	$6119
Radiotherapy (as many as needed)	1×	$12,000
Surgery (optional)	1×	$13,968
Chemotherapy (stages 0–IIIC)	1×	$403,549
Annual follow-up (including aromatase inhibitors)	5×	$18,096
Aesthetic breast reconstruction	1×	$6905
Chemotherapy (stage IV and stage IV sarcomas)	1×	$280,787
Monoclonal antibodies	1–5×	$168,888
Palliative care	1×	$20,637

Source: Tabulators for SP (Comisión Nacional de Protección Social en Salud 2017); periodicity is the number of times a service is provided

negotiated medicines, only preceded by infectious diseases (Secretaría de Salud 2019b; Moye-Holz et al. 2019).

Reimbursement prices of cancer medicines set by SP are comparable, in general, to international reference prices (IRPs) (Table 7.5). However, some individual medicines were 2 to 12 times higher than IRPs (see Annex 1). In 2017, a price survey was conducted in Mexico in 21 accredited public facilities providing cancer care, which included 31 cancer medicines covered by SP (Moye-Holz 2019). When comparing the prices of the survey against the reference prices listed by SP, the surveyed prices were overall comparable to the prices listed by SP (O'she Cuevas 2016).

Procurement and Supply of Cancer Medicines

Patients affiliated to SP can receive healthcare, including medicines, at health facilities that have undergone an accreditation process for both CAUSES and FPGC interventions. SP affiliates in need of any interventions covered by the FPGC can receive care at the MoH facilities or other public or private facilities that have undergone an accreditation process that is disease based (González-Block 2017). The purpose of this process is to guarantee that the facilities have in place the resources and infrastructure needed to provide a specific intervention according to SP protocols and quality standards. SP has set guidelines that health facilities need to meet in order to get accreditation (García 2016). SP adopted a portability character which allows patients unrestricted access to healthcare at any accredited facility regardless of their location. In 2017, there were a total of 356 facilities that were accredited to provide FPGC interventions for SP. Only 57 are accredited to provide cancer care to children (see Annex 2). Some public reports indicate that there are around 41 private facilities and only 2 IMSS facilities with SP accreditation for FPGC interventions across the country (approximately 15% of all accredited facilities (González-Block 2017; Secretaría de Salud 2019c).

The procurement of medicines and other inputs in these accredited facilities must follow the federal procurement law and related state laws, which regulate public procurement of goods and services in the public

Table 7.5 Prices of cancer medicines according to SP reference prices and the negotiation of prices by CCNPMIS expressed as median ratios

		Comparison SP prices with IRP (2017)		Comparison SP prices with MRP (2017)		Comparison with 2017 survey prices with SP prices	
Mechanism	Cancer medicines included	Cancer medicines included	Ratio $/ IRP	Cancer medicines included	Ratio $/ MRP	Cancer medicines included	Ratio $/SP$
SP reference price	70 generic 20 patented	51 generic	0.92	NA	NA	25 generic	1.04 (0.1–1.39)
CCNPMIS	2016: 230 meds, approx. 30 oncology meds	10 patented	0.66	11 patented	0.42	6 patented	1.00 (0.80–1.35)

SPS, Seguro Popular de Salud (People's Health Insurances); *CCNPMIS*, Comisión Coordinadora para la Negociación de Precios de Medicamentos y otros Insumos (Coordinating Commission for the Price Negotiation of Medicines); *IRP*, international reference price; *MRP*, maximum retail price (i.e. maximum price a patented medicine can have in the Mexican market)—only patented medicines. This table reports median prices of cancer medicines

Sources: SP guidelines (O'she Cuevas 2016), national formulary (Comisión Interinstitucional del Cuadro Básico y Catálogo de Insumos del Sector Salud 2016) and 2017 survey (Moye-Holz 2019)

sector (de la Unión and de Diputados 2010). In public health facilities, a procurement committee should be in place to guarantee compliance with the regulation and guard the selection, procurement and supply of medicines (Granados-Cosme et al. 2011). In the public sector, there are several models for the procurement of medicines and other goods, which are described in the following sections.

Conventional Procurement Model

The conventional procurement model is based on tender procedures. Planning, forecasting, procurement and storage are carried out by the MoH at the central level or by the health facility itself. Procurement planning and forecasting is based on the estimations of yearly historic consumptions and adjusted with real supply and expirations of medicines as reported by the health unit per month (Granados-Cosme et al. 2011; López-Moreno et al. 2011).

For the supply of medicines, health facilities inform about their stock availability, their consumption and the monthly requirements to the procurement authorities. Procurement authorities communicate these requirements to the central warehouse and supply management area. The central warehouse distributes the medicines to the health facilities through periodic visits, often weekly (Granados-Cosme et al. 2011; López-Moreno et al. 2011).

Outsourced Model

Many state MoH and health facilities have adopted public-private partnerships for the supply of medicines (Moye-Holz 2019; López-Moreno et al. 2011). These partnerships have frequently led to the outsourcing of pharmacy services. The outsourced model also includes contracting compounding pharmacies for chemotherapeutic and parenteral treatment (Granados-Cosme et al. 2011; López-Moreno et al. 2011). The compounding pharmacy is a private provider that provides chemotherapy bags according to each patient's requirements.

Through this procurement mechanism, health facilities have transferred the pharmacy service to an outsourced (private) pharmacy provider. The contracted provider should guarantee the supply of medicines and satisfy all the medicines requirements of the population at all times. The contracted provider is responsible for stock management, storage and distribution of medicines and should implement a system to control information during all the stages of medicines supply. The medicines listed in the contract are supplied regularly. To mitigate shortages or stock-outs and guarantee access to treatment, the outsourced pharmacies supply medicines at different dosages and presentations (Moye-Holz 2019; López-Moreno et al. 2011; Granados Cosme and Garduño Andrade 2009). The contracts to outsource the pharmacy service can determine to pay only for medicines supplied to patients or by capitation independently of the final consumption. At health facilities, there could be pharmacies and warehouses managed by the outsourced company. Supply is registered in a system that collects daily information about supply and medicines in stock. In the contract, sanctions to providers are specified if medicines are not available and supply is not guaranteed (Granados-Cosme et al. 2011; López-Moreno et al. 2011).

Hybrid Model

Health facilities transitioning from the conventional model to the outsourced model develop a hybrid model. This model combines the advantages of the conventional and outsourced models: the organizational abilities of the former and the operational abilities of the latter, which include pooled procurement, more precision in the identification of real requirements and monitoring of medicines supply. Planning follows a combination of SP coverage and demand. However, there is a lack of involvement and participation of health facilities in procurement planning. Some states continue to manage the storage and warehouse activities where there is more experience with stock management while others outsource storage management to the company. Frequently, supply and distribution are carried out by dividing the volume of medicines among the delivery outlets. Facilities in the transition to the outsourced model face several obstacles including a limited control of the supply process and providers not supplying according to contract (Granados-Cosme et al. 2011; López-Moreno et al. 2011).

A survey conducted in 2017 (Moye-Holz 2019) on the availability and price of 31 cancer medicines covered by SP showed that cancer medicines were more available in facilities using the outsourced and hybrid models than the conventional model (Table 7.6). However, the values of the median price ratios (MPR)—when comparing procurement prices against SP reference prices—suggest that prices of medicines in facilities using the conventional model were lower than in facilities using the outsourced and hybrid models. The survey results also showed that more than half of the surveyed hospitals (n = 11) use at least one outsourced service (compounding pharmacy, outsourced pharmacy or both).

Direct Purchase

Direct purchases in the MoH facilities are made for unavailable medicines that are urgently needed and to complement the other procurement models (Granados-Cosme et al. 2011; López-Moreno et al. 2011). To carry out direct purchases, health facilities require three quotes from three different providers and the approval from a board or committee assessing the need of the medicine. The selection of the provider will depend on the price of the medicine and the delivery times (Granados-Cosme et al.

Table 7.6 Availability and prices of cancer medicines in public facilities according to their procurement model, 2017

Procurement system	% availability[a]	Median MPR[b]	25%ile MPR	75%ile MPR	Min MPR	Max MPR
Conventional model (n = 10)	66.1%	1.00	0.97	1.02	0.5	1.49
Outsourced model (n = 6)	83.3%	1.08	1.00	1.19	0.58	1.52
Hybrid model (n = 5)	74.2%	1.20	1.11	1.45	0.49	2.9

MoH, Ministry of Health; *MPR*, median price ratio; min, minimum; max, maximum
[a]%availability is the mean percentage of facilities with the medicines available
[b]Median MPR is the median of the median price ratios when comparing surveyed prices with the SPS reference prices 2017 survey (Moye-Holz 2019)

2011; López-Moreno et al. 2011). Making direct purchases can affect procurement planning at the facility level (Granados-Cosme et al. 2011), and the bureaucracy related to administrative procedures may limit the capacity of the institution to get treatments in a timely manner. In addition, direct purchases can jeopardize the budgets of health facilities when medicines without coverage are procured and because direct purchases are made at retail and at higher prices than those from tenders.

Discussion

In Mexico, the health reform that led to the implementation of SP has expanded access to healthcare to the Mexican population, getting closer to UHC (Chertorivski 2013). SP has developed policies to provide health coverage to prevalent diseases, including some of those catalogued as "causing catastrophic expenditure", like cancer, and has been able to address the components outlined by the WHO to promote equitable access to cancer medicines for those cancers with coverage. This chapter presents an overview of how SP has addressed the main components outlined by the WHO Access to Medicines Framework (World Health Organization 2004) to provide access to medicines with a focus on essential cancer medicines. We discuss how each component of the WHO Access Medicines Framework (selection, financing, pricing and procurement and supply) has been addressed by SP and how these components have influenced on the availability, pricing and final access to cancer medicines in Mexico. We also discuss the future challenges that SP should address to improve and increase access to cancer medicines and care in Mexico.

Influence of Medicines Selection and Standard Treatment Guidelines on the Availability of Cancer Medicines in the Public Sector of Mexico

SP provides coverage to a number of cancers for which treatment guidelines that include medicines have been developed. SP covers more than 90% of cancer medicines listed in the WHO-EML (World Health

Organization 2015; O'she Cuevas 2016). Over the last decade, coverage of medicines has increased. SP covers less than half of the cancer medicines listed in the national formulary because it strives to cover the most cost-effective treatments only (Consejo de Salubridad General 2017). It is necessary to explore if the treatment protocols developed and updated by SP truly provide the best level of care and if medicines outlined in such protocols are in fact covered by SP and available in health facilities.

A study conducted in 2017 (Moye-Holz 2019) reported that treatment guidelines are outdated and do not represent the best standard of care (Moye-Holz 2019; Reynoso-Noverón et al. 2016; Hess and Pohl 2013). This has forced clinicians to use other clinical guidelines (national and/or international guidelines) and prescribe medicines not covered by SP. We found treatment guidelines dated in 2011 and 2012 that were not updated until 2017 and 2018 (Consejo General de Salubridad 2018). Some clinicians believe that these guidelines should be updated or at least revised every two or three years to guarantee the best treatment available. Furthermore, according to health professionals (Moye-Holz 2019), SP does not cover treatment for advanced stages of cancer. This is worrisome since many patients in Mexico are diagnosed at advanced stages (Reynoso-Noverón et al. 2016; López-Carrillo et al. 2001).

SP's protocols should be regularly revised and updated using scientific and health-economic evidence in order to expand coverage with the most cost-effective interventions and "resource-appropriate strategies" (Knaul et al. 2011), to guarantee the best level of care. The update and revision of these protocols could also consider clinicians' and experts' opinions and experiences to prevent disagreement. Adequate implementation of these treatment guidelines should promote standard, equitable and quality treatment to all Mexican patients (Gutiérrez-Alba et al. 2015). Furthermore, the Mexican government should expand efforts to provide coverage to people with other prevalent types of cancers, such as lung and stomach cancer.

Influence of SP Financing and Reference Prices on the Prices and Affordability of Essential Cancer Medicines in the Public Sector of Mexico

Through SP reimbursement, health facilities can provide cancer treatment. FPGC has pooled funds to guarantee that patients receive cancer care. It finances validated cases—that is, patients actually diagnosed and treated—to guarantee the rational use of resources. This fund has financed and paid more than 80% of these validated cases, representing 30% of the funds covering FPGC interventions. A considerable proportion of these funds are allocated to cover pharmaceutical treatment, which, for some cancers, represent more than half of the treatment costs (Knaul et al. 2011; Comisión Nacional de Protección Social en Salud 2017).

One challenge that SP needs to address is the delayed reimbursement to health facilities causing supply problems and pushing these facilities to use resources allocated to other activities (Granados Cosme and Garduño Andrade 2009). Delays in the validation process have been reported (Orozco-Núñez et al. 2016). The validation procedures should be revised and inefficiencies should be addressed by the authorities to guarantee the timely availability of resources (Orozco-Núñez et al. 2016; Aracena-Genao et al. 2011).

Health facilities face resource challenges mostly to finance medicines (e.g. when patients do not respond to treatment covered by SP) or cancers not covered by SP. When this happens, health facilities try to cover all or most treatment costs so that patients do not incur in catastrophic expenditure or stop treatment. However, some hospitals charge patients without SP coverage for treatment. Some charge patients the procurement price of medicines, but others charge them prices that are 10 to 20% higher (Moye-Holz 2019). These patients make out-of-pocket payments and/or turn to charity organizations for support (Pérez-Cuevas et al. 2013; Dorantes-Acosta et al. 2012).

On the other hand, by setting reference prices and establishing tabulators, SP seeks to control the costs of cancer care while guaranteeing access. In general, SP medicine prices are comparable or lower than IRP, and health facilities have (mostly) procured medicines at the prices indicated by SP. Providing reference prices can influence procurement procedures, where procurement authorities seek to contract providers bidding at prices according to SP reference prices. However, previous research has reported high variability in procurement prices of medicines covered by SP. The survey conducted in 2017 reported that 21% of the cancer medicines were procured above the 20% allowed by SP (Moye-Holz 2019). Therefore, monitoring compliance is imperative in Mexico to guarantee that the SP resources are spent efficiently and according to regulation.

Influence of Procurement and Supply of Cancer Medicines on the Availability of Cancer Medicines in the Public Sector of Mexico

In order to provide healthcare for diseases covered by FPGC, including cancer medicines, an increasing number of health facilities have been accredited by SP (Sistema de Protección Social en Salud 2016, 2017). In most states, less than one facility per 100 thousand affiliated inhabitants are available for diseases covered by FPGC, and it is even less for facilities providing paediatric cancer care. Considering that traveling costs (Moye-Holz 2019) and distance to health facilities are barriers to access to cancer medicines and care, expanding accreditation will bring treatment closer to patients and will reduce out-of-pocket payments.

SP has improved the availability of medicines, including cancer medicines, in health facilities (Garrido-Latorre et al. 2008). However, a recent survey showed that, overall, the availability of cancer medicines is lower than the international recommendation of 80% availability and affordability of essential medicines (Moye-Holz 2019; World Health Assembly 2018). Differences in procurement and supply systems between hospitals had an influence in medicine availability. In facilities using the conventional model, distribution systems, warehouse maintenance and storage tend to be deficient with lower availability of medicines (Granados-Cosme et al. 2011; López-Moreno et al. 2011), while facilities using the outsourced model have reported timelier and better access to cancer medicines than hospitals supplied through the conventional model (López-Moreno et al. 2011; Contreras-Loya et al. 2013). The outsourced model, however, may not promote equity since it tends to be limited to easily accessible facilities only, reducing the possibility of increasing supply coverage in remote areas (Granados-Cosme et al. 2011; López-Moreno et al. 2011).

Health facilities still use direct purchases to complement their supply system for unavailable and urgently needed medicines, but more frequently for medicines not covered by SP (Moye-Holz 2019; Granados-Cosme et al. 2011). The persistent use of direct purchases to procure this type of medicines can harm the institution's budgets, procurement planning and forecasting and ultimately the effectiveness of the procurement model in place. WHO (World Health Organization 2002; Nguyen et al. 2015) does not recommend direct purchases, as these may interfere with procurement projections (López-Moreno et al. 2011), medicines could be overpriced (Granados-Cosme et al. 2011) and institutions may inefficiently use resources (Granados Cosme and Garduño Andrade 2009) to cover these medicines.

The heterogeneity between the supply and procurement models and the multiplicity of procedures in the supply stages have led to variations on the final availability and supply of medicines (Granados Cosme and Garduño Andrade 2009). The government, procurement agencies and health institutions should assess the supply and procurement models in place and strive to move towards the most cost-effective, efficient and reliable supply and procurement mechanisms that guarantee the timely supply and access to the required medicines.

Furthermore, the portability of SP and the accreditation of cancer facilities across the country seek to provide harmonized, high-quality and equitable access to cancer care. However, regional differences in the availability of medicines (Murayama-Rendón 2011; Moye-Holz et al. 2018) and access to cancer care persist. Mexico continues to concentrate resources in big cities (e.g. Mexico City, Monterrey and Guadalajara) generating an "overwhelming influx of patients" (Moye-Holz et al. 2018; Goss et al. 2013), and the overall cancer burden continues to grow across the country (Lazcano-Ponce et al. 2016; Gómez-Dantés et al. 2016a). Moreover, geographical barriers and traveling costs can contribute to late diagnosis and prevent patients from seeking healthcare and getting treatment (Dorantes-Acosta et al. 2012; Verastegui and Mohar 2010; Knaul et al. 2012), resulting in poor health outcomes (Knaul et al. 2011). Therefore, decentralization of healthcare is necessary and accreditation of health facilities needs to expand geographically to bring treatment closer to patients (Gómez-Dantés et al. 2016a, b). To achieve wider accreditation, the government needs to invest in infrastructure (e.g. roads and health facilities) and capacity building of existent and new health facilities, increase the participation of the private sector as health providers and improve budget allocation according to the health needs and priorities of each state.

Future Challenges

SP is considered a successful health reform experience. Regarding medicines, SP has in place mechanisms that address the WHO Access to Medicines Framework to promote equitable access to medicines, including medicines to treat cancers with coverage. However, the availability of cancer medicines in public facilities is not optimal, causing mistrust and dissatisfaction with public health services (Moye-Holz 2019; Contreras-Loya et al. 2013). Although out-of-pocket expenditure has been significantly reduced, it still represents 40% of total health expenditure (OECD 2019), despite strategies to strengthen supply systems and the strategic purchase of medicines by SP (González-Block 2017; Wirtz et al. 2012). Therefore, efforts and strategies implemented by SP to guarantee access to medicines should be aligned with a national pharmaceutical policy. Developing a national pharmaceutical policy as a guide for action for all relevant stakeholders to promote equitable access to medicines is a pending task in Mexico (Moye-Holz et al. 2017; Granados Cosme and Garduño Andrade 2009).

Furthermore, SP needs to address several challenges to strengthen its sustainability and operation. The actions to reinforce SP could include (Knaul et al. 2011) regular revisions of the clinical treatment guidelines; (Shulman et al. 2016) mobilizing additional financial resources to expand the number of covered interventions, including other prevalent adult cancers (e.g. stomach and lung cancer); (Strasser-Weippl et al. 2015) timely reimbursement procedures; (Gray et al. 2015) expanding care for advanced cancer stages and for patients not responding to covered treatment, coupled with disease prevention and early diagnosis strategies; and (Hogerzeil et al. 2013) increasing the accreditation of health facilities throughout the country, including second-level and private facilities (González-Block 2017), in order to bring healthcare closer to patients. These actions should aim at strengthening the overall healthcare system to guarantee access to cancer medicines and, furthermore, reduce the current reliance on out-of-pocket expenditure and charity (Moye-Holz 2019; Dorantes-Acosta et al. 2012; Sesma-Vázquez et al. 2011).

To guard the financial sustainability of SP, price and procurement monitoring systems are necessary. Currently, different systems have been implemented but are not widely used, probably due to health decentralization and the platforms being not user-friendly: CompraNet and CesMed (Moye-Holz et al. 2017). The wide use of these systems can provide relevant information to analyse trends, access, inefficiencies and use of medicines and other resources. These actions should be part of an integrated institutional effort to find the gaps and barriers that prevent effective access to medicines.

A new government came into power in late 2018. This government has proposed the re-centralization of the health system and the abolition of SP (Frenk et al. 2019; Rodríguez 2019), despite the increased public expenditure in health, the promoted cost-effective use of financial resources and the increased health coverage (Knaul et al. 2012; Frenk et al. 2009; Nigenda et al. 2015). If the government removes SP, it is worth keeping in place those mechanisms that have rendered positive results and made UHC a reachable goal.

Limitations

In this chapter, we discuss the SP components that address access to medicines aspects as described by the WHO framework (World Health Organization 2004). The MoH concentrates nearly half of all healthcare infrastructure in the country and covers approximately 40% of the total population. Therefore, this chapter does not represent the entire public sector in Mexico, and further research should explore how social security agencies (e.g. IMSS and ISSSTE) address all components of access to medicines.

Conclusions

SP has expanded healthcare coverage, including treatment for various types of cancer, to a large population (particularly the most vulnerable groups) and moved towards UHC. It has addressed the major components outlined by the WHO Access to Medicines Framework to provide access to cancer medicines through the selection of medicines and interventions to treat cancer and the development of treatment protocols to guide prescription and selection of cancer medicines in health facilities. SP functions as a financing mechanism to guarantee that resources to provide cancer care and medicines are available. It has also provided reference prices to guide the procurement of medicines and drive the efficient use of resources. Furthermore, its accreditation mechanisms seek to harmonize and provide equitable and quality access to treatment and care across the country.

However, SP needs to address a series of challenges such as ensuring equitable access to quality care, adequate financing of a cancer medicines benefit package, timely reimbursement of facilities and regular updates of standard treatment guidelines.

In Mexico and other LMICs, efforts to improve access to cancer medicines should be part of a strong national pharmaceutical policy coupled with a coherent national cancer control plan that considers better access to screening, prevention and treatment.

Annex 1. List of Cancer Medicines Covered by SP and its Characteristics

Medicine	Dose		Generic/ patented	Medicine in WHO-EML? (2015)	Reference price SP (USD) (2016)	Negotiated by CCNMPMIS in 2015?	Ratio survey price (2017)/SP ref. price	Ratio SP Ref$/ IRP	CCNPMIS$/ MRP
Amifostine	500 mg	Package with one vial	Generic	No	137.16				
Anastrozole	1 mg	Package with 28 tablets	Generic	Yes	38.41		0.95	2.57	
Aprepitant	125 mg - 80 mg	Package with one 125 mg capsule and two 80 mg capsules	Patented	No	39.19	Yes			0.03
Bleomycin	15 UI/5 ml	Package with vial and 5 ml thinner	Generic	Yes	12.25			1.00	
Buserelin	9.45 mg	Package with pre-filled syringe with implant	Patented	No	266.99	Yes			
Busulfan	2 mg	Package with 25 tablets	Patented	No	21.39	Yes		1.52	
Capecitabine	500 mg	Package with 120 tablets	Generic	Yes	101.70		1.39	0.50	
Carboplatin	150 mg	Package with vial	Generic	Yes	8.27		1.23	0.55	
Carmustine	100 mg/3 ml	Package with vial and 3 ml thinner	Generic	No	43.81				
Cyclophosphamide	50 mg	Package with 30 tablets	Generic	Yes	7.42			0.80	

(*continued*)

(continued)

Medicine	Dose		Generic/ patented	Medicine in WHO-EML? (2015)	Reference price SP (USD) (2016)	Negotiated by CCNMPMIS in 2015?	Ratio survey price (2017)/SP ref. price	Ratio SP Ref$/ IRP	CCNPMIS$/ MRP
Cyclophosphamide	50 mg	Package with 50 tablets	Generic	Yes	8.73			0.57	
Cyclophosphamide	200 mg	Package with five vials	Generic	Yes	7.03		1.14	0.33	
Cyclophosphamide	500 mg	Package with two vials	Generic	Yes	7.71		0.97	0.47	
Cisplatin	10 mg	Package with one vial	Generic	Yes	1.39			0.56	
Cytarabine	500 mg	Package with one vial	Generic	Yes	6.73		1.19	1.43	
Dacarbazine	200 mg	Package with one vial	Generic	Yes	6.37			0.92	
Dactinomycin	0.5 mg	Package with one vial	Generic	Yes	24.34			2.76	
Daunorubicin	20 mg	Package with one vial	Generic	Yes	6.22		1.01	0.32	
Dexrazoxane	500 mg	Package with one vial	Generic	No	141.31				
Docetaxel	80 mg/6 ml	Package with 80 mg vial and 6 ml thinner	Generic	Yes	223.98				
Docetaxel	20 mg/1.5 ml	Package with 20 mg vial and 1.5 ml thinner	Generic	Yes	64.82				

Docetaxel trihydrate	80 mg	Package with 80 mg and 4 ml vial	Generic	Yes	223.98	0.99	12.63
Docetaxel trihydrate	20 mg	Package with 20 mg and 1 ml vial	Generic	Yes	64.82	1.04	12.37
Doxorubicin	20 mg/10 ml	Package with 10 ml (2 mg/ml) vial	Generic	No	161.31		
Doxorubicin	10 mg	Package with one vial	Generic	Yes	7.57	0.53	3.52
Doxorubicin	50 mg	Package with one vial	Generic	Yes	7.68	1.36	1.04
Epirubicin	10 mg	Package with one vial	Generic	No	6.59	1.04	1.20
Etoposide	100 mg/5 ml	Package with ten vials of 5 ml	Generic	Yes	24.68	1.06	6.31
Exemestane	25 mg	Package with 15 tablets	Generic	No	57.49		1.81
Exemestane	25 mg	Package with 30 tablets	Generic	No	114.97	0.97	1.81
Exemestane	25 mg	Package with 90 tablets	Generic	No	344.92		1.81
Filgrastim	300 µg	Package with five vials or syringes	Generic	Yes	63.58		1.57
Finasteride	5 mg	Package with 30 tablets	Generic	No	1.43		
Fludarabine	10 mg	Package with 15 tablets	Patented	Yes	291.63		
Fluorouracil	250 mg	Package with ten vials of 10 ml	Generic	Yes	9.58	1.12	0.36
Flutamide	250 mg	Package with 90 tablets	Generic	No	19.43		1.92

(*continued*)

(continued)

Medicine	Dose		Generic/ patented	Medicine in WHO-EML? (2015)	Reference price SP (USD) (2016)	Negotiated by CCNMPMIS in 2015?	Ratio survey price (2017)/SP ref. price	Ratio SP Ref$/ IRP	CCNPMIS$/ MRP
Folinic acid	3 mg/ml	Package with six vials of 1 ml	Generic	Yes	4.13				
Folinic acid	15 mg/5 ml	Package with five vials of 5 ml	Generic	Yes	17.47				
Folinic acid	50 mg/4 ml	Package with 4 ml vial	Generic	Yes	9.99			4.22	
Folinic acid	15 mg	Package with 12 tablets	Generic	Yes	9.90			0.63	
Gemcitabine	1 g	Package with one vial	Generic	Yes	18.77		1.25	0.73	
Goserelin	3.6 mg	Package with syringe with implant	Patented	No	89.55	Yes			
Goserelin	10.8 mg	Package with syringe with implant	Patented	No	201.49	Yes			
Granisetron	20 mg/100 ml	Package with 30 ml and dispenser	Generic	No	2.20				
Granisetron	1 mg	Package with two tablets	Generic	No	8.56			31.70	
Granisetron	3 mg/3 ml	Package with 3 ml vial	Generic	No	5.72				
Hydroxycarbamide	500 mg	Package with 100 tablets	Patented	Yes	64.25			2.92	

Ifosfamide	1 g	Package with one vial	Generic	Yes	15.34		0.94	1.40	
Imatinib	400 mg	Package with 30 tablets	Patented	Yes	352.07	Yes	1.00	0.46	0.16
Imatinib	100 mg	Package with 60 tablets	Patented	Yes	183.93	Yes	1.00	4.37	0.20
Irinotecan	100 mg/5 ml	Package with 5 ml vial	Generic	Yes	30.04		1.24	1.03	
Lapatinib	250 mg	Package with 70 tablets	Patented	No	524.97	Yes			0.61
L-Asparaginase	10,000 UI	Package with one vial	Patented	Yes	43.64		1.35	0.81	
Letrozole	2.5 mg	Package with 30 tablets	Generic	No	3.12		1.35	0.25	
Leuprorelin	11.25 mg/2 ml	Package with vial, 2 ml thinner vial and dispenser equipment	Generic	No	171.12				
Melphalan	2 mg	Package with 25 tablets	Generic	No	39.66				
Mercaptopurine	50 mg	Package with 20 tablets	Patented	Yes	44.46	Yes	0.80	0.98	
Mesna	400 mg/4 ml	Package with five vials of 4 ml (100 mg/ml)	Generic	Yes	11.30			3.71	
Methotrexate	50 mg	Package with one vial	Generic	Yes	3.83		0.85	0.79	
Methotrexate	500 mg	Package with one vial	Generic	Yes	11.02		1.09	0.23	

(*continued*)

(continued)

Medicine	Dose		Generic/ patented	Medicine in WHO-EML? (2015)	Reference price SP (USD) (2016)	Negotiated by CCNMPMIS in 2015?	Ratio survey price (2017)/SP ref. price	Ratio SP Ref$/ IRP	CCNPMIS$/ MRP
Methotrexate	1 g	Package with one vial	Generic	Yes	22.05				
Methotrexate	2.5 mg	Package with 50 tablets	Generic	Yes	2.87		1.12	0.36	
Mitomycin	5 mg	Package with one vial	Generic	No	10.22			0.40	
Mitoxantrone	20 mg/10 ml	Package with 10 ml vial	Generic	No	49.10				
Nilutamide	150 mg	Package with 30 tablets	Patented	No	108.46	Yes			
Ondansetron	8 mg	Package with 10 tablets	Generic	Yes	1.31			0.51	
Ondansetron	8 mg/4 ml	Package with three vials of 4 ml	Generic	No	0.75			0.19	
Oxaliplatin	50 mg	Package with one vial	Generic	Yes	22.75		1.00	0.78	
Oxaliplatin	100 mg	Package with 20 ml vial	Generic	Yes	34.00		0.10	0.45	
Paclitaxel	300 mg/50 ml	Package with 50 ml vial, with equipment for free venoclysis of polyvinylchloride (PVC) and filter with membrane no greater than 0.22 μm	Generic	Yes	37.28		1.20	0.57	

Palonosetron	0.25 mg/5 ml	Package with 5 ml vial	Patented	No	24.36				
Pegfilgrastim	6 mg/0.60 ml	Package with vial with pre-filled syringe with 6 mg/0.60 ml	Patented	No	726.93				0.02
Rituximab	100 mg/10 ml	Package with 10 ml vial	Patented	Yes	69.99			0.51	
Rituximab	100 mg/10 ml	Package with two vials of 10 ml	Patented	Yes	139.99	Yes	1.00	0.51	
Rituximab	500 mg/50 ml	Package with 50 ml vial	Patented	No	289.30	Yes	1.00	0.32	
Rituximab	500 mg/50 ml	Package with two vials of 50 ml	Patented	No	578.61			0.32	
Tamoxifen	20 mg	Package with 14 tablets	Generic	Yes	1.09			0.68	
Temozolomide	100 mg	Package with five tablets	Generic	No	112.17			1.13	
Temozolomide	100 mg	Package with ten tablets	Generic	No	224.34			1.13	
Temozolomide	100 mg	Package with 20 tablets	Generic	No	448.67			1.15	
Temozolomide	20 mg	Package with five tablets	Generic	No	35.62				
Temozolomide	20 mg	Package with ten tablets	Generic	No	71.23				
Temozolomide	20 mg	Package with 20 tablets	Generic	No	142.46				

(*continued*)

(continued)

Medicine	Dose		Generic/ patented	Medicine in WHO-EML? (2015)	Reference price SP (USD) (2016)	Negotiated by CCNMPMIS in 2015?	Ratio survey price (2017)/SP ref. price	Ratio SP Ref$/ IRP	CCNPMIS$/ MRP
Trastuzumab	440 mg/20 ml	Package with vial with powder and 20 ml thinner vial	Patented	Yes	1159.88	Yes	1.00		
Tropisetron	5 mg	Package with vial	Generic	No	22.79			9.38	
Vinblastine	10 mg/10 ml	Package with vial and 10 ml thinner vial	Generic	Yes	6.52			2.53	
Vincristine	1 mg/10 ml	Package with vial and 10 ml thinner vial	Generic	Yes	2.71		1.06	0.82	
Vinorelbine	30 mg	Package with one tablet	Generic	No	101.17				
Vinorelbine	10 mg/ml	Package with 1 ml vial	Generic	Yes	10.24			0.46	
Zoledronic acid	4.0 mg/5 ml	Package with vial	Generic	No	3.48			0.15	

[a]Medicine prices converted from Mexican pesos to US dollars using the average exchange rate in 2017 as reported by the Bank of Mexico (Banco de México 2019) and adjusted for inflation (Inflation Calculator 2019)

Annex 2. Number of Healthcare Facilities with SP Accreditation to Treat FPGC Interventions

State	Number of SP beneficiaries (2017)	Number of accredited facilities for FPGC per 100,000 SP affiliates (2017)	Number of facilities with accreditation for cancer < 18 years per 100,000 SP affiliates (2017)
Aguascalientes	379,869	2.11	0.26
Baja California	997,251	1.00	0.30
Baja California Sur	207,118	2.41	0.00
Campeche	474,324	1.05	0.21
Coahuila	705,624	1.28	0.14
Colima	253,182	2.37	0.39
Chiapas	3,470,352	0.02	0.002
Chihuahua	1,220,272	1.31	0.33
Mexico City	2,749,580	1.53	0.29
Durango	736,442	0.01	0.00
Guanajuato	3,011,165	0.76	0.10
Guerrero	2,241,345	0.31	0.04
Hidalgo	1,666,161	0.36	0.06
Jalisco	3,014,388	0.56	0.10
Mexico State	7,077,137	0.57	0.01
Michoacan	2,309,934	0.26	0.04
Morelos	977,755	0.92	0.10
Nayarit	526,660	1.14	0.19
Nuevo Leon	1,174,818	0.77	0.17
Oaxaca	2,637,811	0.23	0.08
Puebla	3,349,337	0.33	0.03
Queretaro	881,601	1.02	0.11
Quintana Roo	600,393	1.17	0.17
San Luis Potosi	1,484,429	0.61	0.07
Sinaloa	1,068,594	1.12	0.09
Sonora	868,430	0.69	0.12
Tabasco	1,472,861	0.61	0.14
Tamaulipas	1,293,441	1.55	0.15
Tlaxcala	786,202	0.89	0.13
Veracruz	4,050,186	0.25	0.12
Yucatan	949,958	0.63	0.21
Zacatecas	868,567	0.69	0.12
Total	**53,505,187**	**0.25**	0.04

Source: Accredited health units (Secretaría de Salud 2019d), SPS affiliation (Seguro Popular 2017), SPS reports (Sistema de Protección Social en Salud 2017)

References

Knaul FM, Frenk J, Shulman L, for the Global Task Force on Expanded Access to Cancer Care and Control in Developing Countries. Closing the Cancer Divide: a Blueprint to Expand Access in Low and Middle Income Countries. Boston; 2011.

Shulman LN, Wagner CM, Barr R, Lopes G, Longo G, Robertson J, et al. Proposing essential medicines to treat cancer: Methodologies, processes, and outcomes. Journal of Clinical Oncology. 2016.

Strasser-Weippl K, Chavarri-Guerra Y, Villarreal-Garza C, Bychkovsky BL, Debiasi M, Liedke PER, et al. Progress and remaining challenges for cancer control in Latin America and the Caribbean. The Lancet Oncology. 2015.

Gray AL, Wirtz VJ, 'T Hoen EFM, Reich MR, Hogerzeil HV. Essential medicines are still essential. The Lancet. 2015.

Hogerzeil H V, Liberman J, Wirtz VJ, Kishore SP, Selvaraj S, Kiddell-Monroe R, et al. Promotion of access to essential medicines for non-communicable diseases: Practical implications of the UN political declaration. Lancet. 2013;

Robertson J, Barr R, Shulman LN, Forte GB, Magrini N. Essential medicines for cancer: WHO recommendations and national priorities. Bull World Heal Organ [Internet]. 2016;94:735–42. Available from: https://doi.org/10.2471/BLT.15.163998

WHO. Programas nacionales de control del cáncer [Internet]. Geneva; 2004. Available from: https://www.paho.org/hq/dmdocuments/2012/OPS-Programas-Nacionales-Cancer-2004-Esp.pdf

World Health Organization. Cancer [Internet]. 2018 [cited 2019 Mar 15]. Available from: https://www.who.int/news-room/fact-sheets/detail/cancer

Wirtz VJ, Hogerzeil H V, Gray AL, Bigdeli M, de Joncheere CP, Ewen MA, et al. Essential medicines for universal health coverage. Lancet. 2017;389:403–76.

Secretaría de Salud. Decreto por el que se reforma y adicional la Ley General de Salud [Internet]. Diario Oficial de la Federación; 2003. Available from: http://dof.gob.mx/website/nota_to_imagen_fs.php?codnota=695626&fecha=15/05/2003&cod_diario=28260

World Health Organization. Equitable access to essential medicines: a framework for collective action. WHO Policy Perspect Med. 2004;6.

Moye-Holz D. Access to Innovative Medicines in a Middle-Income Country. The Case of Mexico and Cancer Medicines. University of Groningen; 2019.

Gómez Dantés O, Sesma S, Becerril V, Knaul FM, Arreola H, Frenk J. Sistema de salud de México [The health system of Mexico]. Salud Publica Mex. 2011;53(Suppl 2):S220–32.

González-Block MÁ. ¿Qué compra, cómo y de quién el Seguro Popular de México? Experiencia con la compra estratégica nacional y en una entidad pionera [What is purchased, how and from whom by Seguro Popular in Mexico? Experience with strategic purchasing at national level and. Salud Publica Mex [Internet]. 2017;59(1):59–67. Available from: https://doi.org/10.21149/7768

Reynoso-Noverón N, Mohar A. El cáncer en México: Propuestas para su control. Salud Publica Mex. 2014;56(5):418–20.

Reynoso-Noverón N, Alejandro J. Epidemiología del cáncer en México: carga global y proyecciones 2000-2020 [Epidemiology of cancer in México: global burden and projections 2000–2020]. Rev Latinoam Med Conduct. 2000;8(1):9–15.

Shalkow J. Cáncer infantil en México. Situación actual y retos [Internet]. Washington, D.C.: PAHO, UICC, SSa; 2017 [cited 2018 Dec 27]. Available from: https://www.paho.org/hq/dmdocuments/2017/Cancer-infantil-en-MEXICO.pdf

Secretaría de Salud. Cáncer Infantil en México [Internet]. 2015 [cited 2018 Dec 27]. Available from: https://www.gob.mx/salud/articulos/cancer-infantil-en-mexico

International Agency for Research on Cancer. Global Cancer Observatory [Internet]. [cited 2019 Apr 5]. Available from: https://gco.iarc.fr/

Hernández-Peña P, Lazcano-Ponce EC, Ruiz PA De, Cruz-Valdez A, Meneses-González F, Hernández-Avila M. Analisis costo beneficio del programa de deteccion oportuna del cancer cervicouterino. Salud Publica Mex. 1997.

Secretaria de Salud. Programa de Acción Específico Prevención y Control del Cáncer de la Mujer 2013–2018. México, D.F.; 2013.

Secretaría de Salud. Programa de Acción Específico. Cáncer en la Infancia y la Adolescencia 2013–2018 [Internet]. Programa Sectorial de Salud. Mexico City; 2014. Available from: http://www.censia.salud.gob.mx/contenidos/descargas/transparencia/especiales/PAE_Cancer.pdf

Secretaría de Salud. Programa de Acción: Cáncer de Próstata [Internet]. 2001 [cited 2019a May 21]. Available from: http://www.salud.gob.mx/unidades/cdi/documentos/cancer_prostata.pdf

Torres-Mejía G, Ortega-Olvera C, Ángeles-Llerenas A, Villalobos-Hernández AL, Salmerón-Castro J, Lazcano-Ponce E, et al. Utilization patterns of prevention and early diagnosis for cancer in women. Salud Publica Mex. 2013;

Bright K, Barghash M, Donach M, de la Barrera MG, Schneider RJ, Formenti SC. The role of health system factors in delaying final diagnosis and treatment of breast cancer in Mexico City, Mexico. Breast. 2011;20 (Suppl 2):S54–9.

Pérez-Cuevas R, Doubova S V., Zapata-Tarres M, Flores-Hernández S, Frazier L, Rodríguez-Galindo C, et al. Scaling up cancer care for children without medical insurance in developing countries: The case of Mexico. Pediatr Blood Cancer. 2013;60:196–203.

Reynoso-Noverón N, Meneses-García A, Erazo-Valle A, Escudero-de los Ríos P, Antonio Kuri-Morales P, Mohar-Betancourt A, et al. Challenges in the development and implementation of the National Comprehensive Cancer Control Program in Mexico. Salud Publica Mex. 2016;58(2):325–33.

Mohar A, Reynoso N, Villarreal-Garza C, Bargalló-Rocha JE, Arce-Salinas C, Lara-Medina F. Cáncer de mama en el Instituto Nacional de Cancerología. Experiencia del Seguro Popular 2007–2013. Rev Mex Mastología. 2015;

Moye-Holz D, van Dijk JP, Reijneveld SA, Hogerzeil H V. Policy approaches to improve availability and affordability of medicines in Mexico - an example of a middle income country. Global Health. 2017;13(53).

Rivas R, Rico Alba I. n.d. Efecto de la solicitud de evaliaciones económicas en la integración del Cuadro Básico Mexicano. In: ISPOR 1st Latin America Conference. GuiaMark.

Consejo de Salubridad General. REGLAMENTO Interior de la Comisión Interinstitucional del Cuadro Básico y Catálogo de Insumos del Sector Salud, publicado en el Diario Oficial de la Federación el 22 de junio de 2011 [Internet]. Diario Oficial de la Federación; 2011 p. 15. Available from: http://www.csg.gob.mx/descargas/pdf/priorizacion/cuadro-basico/normatividad/Reglamento_CI_CByCISS_05092011.pdf

Ríos PR, Rivera AG, Oropeza IR, Rivas Bocanegra RE. Análisis del Proceso de Actualización de Medicamentos en el Cuadro Básico y Catálogo de Insumos del Sector Salud. Value Heal Reg Issues. 2013;2:387–91.

Barraza-Lloréns M, Campos-Hernández Á. Elementos para mejorar la regulación farmacéutica en México: la experiencia del Reino Unido. México, D.F.; 2007.

Moïse P, Docteur E. Las políticas de precios y reembolsos farmacéuticos en México, OCDE, 2007 [Pharmaceutical pricing and reimbursement policies in Mexico, OECD, 2007]. Salud Publica Mex. 2008;50(Suppl 4):S504–510.

Centro Nacional de Excelencia Tecnológica en Salud. Guías de Práctica Clínica [Internet]. 2018 [cited 2018 Dec 27]. Available from: https://cenetec-difusion.com/gpc-sns/

Centro Nacional de Excelencia Tecnológica en Salud. Atribuciones de CENETEC [Internet]. 2017 [cited 2018 Dec 27]. Available from: https://www.gob.mx/salud/cenetec/documentos/atribuciones-de-cenetec?

Gómez-Dantés O, Wirtz VJ, Reich MR, Terrazas P, Ortiz M. A new entity for the negotiation of public procurement prices for patented medicines in Mexico. Bull World Health Organ. 2012;90:788–92.

Secretaria de Salud. Cátalogo Universal de Servicios de Salud - CAUSES. Seguro Popiular Mexico: Comición Nacional de Protección Social en Salud; 2018 p. 950.

Comisión Nacional de Protección Social en Salud. Catálogo Universal de Servicios de Salud CAUSES 2016.Seguro Popiular Mexico: Comición Nacional de Protección Social en Salud; 2016.

Consejo de Salubridad General. REGLAMENTO Interior de la Comisión para Definir Tratamientos y Medicamentos Asociados a Enfermedades que Ocasionan Gastos Catastróficos. Mexico: Diario Oficial de la Federación; 2017.

World Health Organization. WHO Model List of Essential Medicines. 19th List [Internet]. World Health Organization; 2015. p. 51. Available from: http://www.who.int/medicines/publications/essentialmedicines/en/

González-Block MÁ, Figueroa A, García-Téllez I, Alarcón J. Asignación financiera en el Sistema de Protección Social en Salud de México: Retos para la compra estratégica [Financial allocations in the System for Social Protection in Health in Mexico: challenges for strategic purchasing]. Salud Publica Mex. 2016;58(5):522–32.

Chemor Ruiz A, Ratsch AEO, Alamilla Martínez GA. Mexico's *Seguro Popular*: Achievements and Challenges. Health Syst Reform. 2018;

Servan-Mori E, Heredia-Pi I, Montañez-Hernandez J, Avila-Burgos L, Wirtz VJ. Access to medicines by Seguro Popular beneficiaries: Pending tasks towards universal health coverage. PLoS One. 2015;

Lozano R, Garrido F. Improving Health Systems Efficiency. Mexico: Catastrophic Health Expenditure Fund. 2015.

Sistema de Protección Social en Salud. Informe de Resultados. Enero – Diciembre 2016. México; 2016.

Sistema de Protección Social en Salud. Informe de resultados Enero - Diciembre 2017 [Internet]. Mexico; 2017. Available from: http://www.transparencia.seguro-popular.gob.mx/contenidos/archivos/transparencia/planesprogramaseinformes/informes/2017/InformedeResultadosdelSPSSenero-diciembre2017.pdf

Orozco-Núñez E, Alcalde-Rabanal J, Navarro J, Lozano R. Eficiencia de los procesos administrativos para la gestión del fondo de protección contra gastos catastróficos en México. Salud Publica Mex. 2016.

Seguro Popular. Tabuladores del Fondo de Protección contra Gastos Catastróficos [Internet]. [cited 2019 Mar 15]. Available from: http://www.transparencia.seguro-popular.gob.mx/index.php/transparencia-focalizada/24-gestion-de-servicios-de-salud/50-tabuladores-del-fondo-de-proteccion-contra-gastos-catastroficos

Comisión Nacional de Protección Social en Salud. Tabulador Cáncer de Mama (Clave CIE-10: C50) [Internet]. 2017 [cited 2019 Mar 15]. Available from: http://www.transparencia.seguro-popular.gob.mx/contenidos/archivos/transparencia/gestioserviciossalud/fpgc/Tabuladores2015-2018/2017/5Cánceres en adultos/5.3Cáncerdemama.pdf

O'she Cuevas GJ. LINEAMIENTOS para la adquisición de medicamentos asociados al Catálogo Universal de Servicios de Salud y al Fondo de Protección contra Gastos Catastróficos, por las entidades federativas con recursos transferidos por concepto de cuota social y de la aport. Mexico: Diario Oficial de la Federación; 2016 p. 38.

OECD Reviews of Health Systems: Mexico 2016. 2016; Available from: http://www.oecd-ilibrary.org/social-issues-migration-health/oecd-reviews-of-health-systems-mexico-2016_9789264230491-en

Secretaría de Salud. Comisión Coordinadora para la Negociación de Precios de Medicamentos e Insumos para la Salud.[Internet]. 2018 [cited 2019b Mar 15]. Available from: https://www.gob.mx/salud/es/acciones-y-programas/comision-coordinadora-para-la-negociacion-de-precios-de-medicamentos-e-insumos-para-la-salud-91422

Moye-Holz D, Dijk JP Van, Reijneveld SA, Hogerzeil HV. The Impact of Price Negotiations on Public Procurement Prices and Access to 8 Innovative Cancer Medicines in a Middle-Income Country – The Case of Mexico. Value Heal Reg Issues [Internet]. 2019;20:129–35. Available from: https://doi.org/10.1016/j.vhri.2019.04.006

Comisión Interinstitucional del Cuadro Básico y Catálogo de Insumos del Sector Salud. Cuadro Básico y Catálogo de Medicamentos [Internet]. Mexico: Consejo de Salubridad General; 2016 p. 1–113. Available from: http://www.csg.gob.mx/descargas/pdf/priorizacion/cuadro-basico/med/catalogo/2016/EDICION_2016_MEDICAMENTOS.pdf

García Saisó S. Manual para la acreditación de establecimientos y servicios de atención médica. Diario Oficial de la Federación; 2016.

Secretaría de Salud. Reportes de Acreditación de Establecimientos [Internet]. [cited 2019c Jun 5]. Available from: http://www.dgis.salud.gob.mx/contenidos/sinais/ReportesClues.html

Congreso de la Unión, Cámara de Diputados. Reglamento de la ley de adquisiciones, arrendamientos y servicios del sector público. 2010.

Granados-Cosme JA, Tetelboin-Henrion C, Garduño-Andrade M de los A, Rivera-Márquez JA, Martínez-Ojeda RH. Análisis cualitativo del abasto de medicamentos en México. Evaluación en los servicios a población no asegurada [A qualitative approach to drug supply in Mexico. Evaluation in the services for population with no medical insurance]. Salud Publica Mex. 2011;53(Suppl 4):S458–69.

López-Moreno S, Martínez-Ojeda RH, López-Arellano O, Jarillo-Soto E, Castro-Albarrán JM. Organización del abasto de medicamentos en los servicios estatales de salud. Potenciales consecuencias de la mezcla público-privada [Organization of the drug supply chain in state health services. Potential consequences of the public-private mix]. Salud Publica Mex. 2011;53(Suppl 4):S445–57.

Granados Cosme JA, Garduño Andrade M de los A, Jarillo Soto EC, Garrido Latorre F. Cadena de Abasto de Medicamentos en México: Evaluación cualitativa. XXVII Congr la Asoc Latinoam Sociol VIII Jornadas Sociol la Univ Buenos Aires Asoc Latinoam Sociol. 2009;

Chertorivski S. Planning cancer control-a Mexican perspective. Lancet Oncol. 2013;14.

Hess LM, Pohl G. Perspectives of quality care in cancer treatment: a review of the literature. Am Heal Drug Benefits 2013;6(6):321–9.

Consejo General de Salubridad. Protocolos Técnicos de Gastos Catastróficos [Internet]. [cited 2018 Dec 26]. Available from: http://www.csg.gob.mx/contenidos/priorizacion/gastos-catastroficos/protocolos.html

López-Carrillo L, Torres-Sánchez L, López-Cervantes M, Rueda-Neria C. Identificación de lesiones mamarias malignas en México. Salud Publica Mex. 2001.

Gutiérrez-Alba G, González-Block MÁ, Reyes-Morales H. Desafíos en la implantación de guías de práctica clínica en instituciones públicas de México: estudio de casos múltiple [Challenges in the implementation of clinical practice guidelines in major public health institutions in Mexico: A multiple case study]. Salud Publica Mex. 2015.

Aracena-Genao B, González-Robledo MC, González-Robledo LM, Palacio-Mejía LS, Nigenda-López G. El Fondo de Protección contra Gastos Catastróficos: tendencia, evolución y operación [Fund for Protection against Catastrophic Expenses]. Salud Publica Mex. 2011;53(Suppl 4):S407–15.

Dorantes-Acosta E, Zapata-Tarrés M, Liliana Miranda-Lora A, Reyes-López A, Muñoz Hernández O, Cortés-Gallo G, et al. Apoyo de organizaciones no gubernamentales a pacientes pediátricos con leucemia linfoblástica aguda afiliados al Seguro Popular en México [Support from nongovernmental organizations to pediatric patients with acute lymphoblastic leukemia affiliated with the Seguro Popular in Mexico]. Bol Med Hosp Infant Mex. 2012;69(3):212–7.

Garrido-Latorre F, Hernández-Llamas H, Gómez-Dantés O. Surtimiento de recetas a los afiliados al Seguro Popular de Salud de México [Dispensing prescriptions to persons affiliated with Popular Health Insurance in Mexico]. Salud Publica Mex. 2008;50(Suppl 4):S429–36.

World Health Assembly. Follow-up to the Political Declaration of the High-level Meeting of the General Assembly on the Prevention and Control of Non-communicable Diseases [Internet]. Sixty-Sixth World Health Assembly. 2013 [cited 2018 Apr 17]. Available from: http://apps.who.int/gb/ebwha/pdf_files/WHA66/A66_R10-en.pdf?ua=1

Contreras-Loya D, Reding-Bernal A, Gómez-Dantés O, Puentes-Rosas E, Pineda-Pérez D, Castro-Tinoco M, et al. Abasto y surtimiento de medicamentos en unidades especializadas en la atención de enfermedades crónicas en méxico en 2012 [Supply of essential drugs in units specialized in the treatment of chronic diseases in Mexico in 2012]. Salud Publica Mex. 2013;55(6):618–26.

World Health Organization. Practical Guidelines on Pharmaceutical Procurement for Countries with Small Procurement Agencies. World Health Organizational Regional Office For The Western Pacific. 2002.

Nguyen TA, Knight R, Roughead EE, Brooks G, Mant A. Policy options for pharmaceutical pricing and purchasing: Issues for low- and middle-income countries. Health Policy and Planning. 2015.

Murayama-Rendón C. Adquisición de medicamentos en el seguro popular: Ineficiencia e inequidad. Gac Med Mex. 2011;

Moye-Holz D, Soria Saucedo R, Van Dijk JP, Reijneveld SA, Hogerzeil H V. Access to innovative cancer medicines in a middle-income country - The case of Mexico. J Pharm Policy Pract. 2018;11(25):1–8.

Goss PE, Lee BL, Badovinac-Crnjevic T, Strasser-Weippl K, Chavarri-Guerra Y, Louis JS, et al. Planning cancer control in Latin America and the Caribbean. The Lancet Oncology. 2013.

Lazcano-Ponce E, Mohar-Betancourt A, Meneses-García A, Hernández-Ávila M. Cancer burden in Mexico: Urgent challenges to be met. Salud Publica de Mexico. 2016;

Gómez-Dantés H, Lamadrid-Figueroa H, Cahuana-Hurtado L, Silverman-Retana O, Montero P, González-Robledo MC, et al. The burden of cancer in Mexico, 1990–2013. Salud Publica Mex. 2016a;

Verastegui E, Mohar A. Colorectal cancer in Mexico: Should a middle income country invest in screening or in treatment? Eur J Heal Econ. 2010;10(Suppl 1):S107–14.

Knaul FM, González-Pier E, Gómez-Dantés O, García-Junco D, Arreola-Ornelas H, Barraza-Lloréns M, et al. The quest for universal health coverage: Achieving social protection for all in Mexico. Lancet. 2012;

Gómez-Dantés H, Fullman N, Lamadrid-Figueroa H, Cahuana-Hurtado L, Darney B, Avila-Burgos L, et al. Dissonant health transition in the states of Mexico, 1990–2013: a systematic analysis for the Global Burden of Disease Study 2013. Lancet. 2016b;

OECD. Health Spending (indicator) [Internet]. 2019 [cited 2019 Feb 28]. Available from: https://data.oecd.org/healthres/health-spending.htm

Wirtz VJ, Santa-Ana-Tellez Y, Servan-Mori E, Avila-Burgos L. Heterogeneous effects of health insurance on out-of-pocket expenditure on medicines in Mexico. Value Heal. 2012;

Sesma-Vázquez S, Gómez-Dantés O, Wirtz VJ, Castro-Tinoco M. Abasto, surtimiento y gasto de bolsillo en medicamentos en hospitales públicos de México en 2009 [Supply prescription filling and out-of-pocket expenditures on medicines in public hospitals in Mexico in 2009]. Salud Publica Mex. 2011;

Frenk J, Gã O, Marie Knaul F. A dark day for universal health coverage. 2019; Available from: https://doi.org/10.1016/S0140-

Rodríguez R. AMLO sustituirá el Seguro Popular en México por un nuevo sistema de salud.CNN [Internet]. CNN. 2018 [cited 2019 Jun 12]. Available from: https://cnnespanol.cnn.com/video/desaparicion-seguro-popular-mexico-amlo-nuevo-plan-nacional-salud-pkg-rey-rodriguez/

Frenk J, Gómez-Dantés O, Knaul FM. The democratization of health in Mexico: Financial innovations for universal coverage. Bulletin of the World Health Organization. 2009.

Nigenda G, Wirtz VJ, González-Robledo LM, Reich MR. Evaluating the Implementation of Mexico's Health Reform: The Case of *Seguro Popular*. Health Syst Reform. 2015.

Banco de México. Mercado cambiario (tipos de cambio) [Internet]. [cited 2019 Jan 20]. Available from: http://www.anterior.banxico.org.mx/portal-mercado-cambiario/

Inflation Calculator. US Dollar's Value from 1913–2019 [Internet]. [cited 2019 Jan 20]. Available from: https://www.usinflationcalculator.com/

Secretaría de Salud. Directorio de Unidades Médicas Acreditadas [Internet]. [cited 2019d Mar 15]. Available from: https://www.gob.mx/cms/uploads/attachment/file/16323/Directorio_UMA.pdf

Seguro Popular. Beneficiarios de Protección Social en Salud de Seguro Popular [Internet]. 2017 [cited 2019 Mar 15]. Available from: https://datos.gob.mx/busca/dataset/beneficiarios-de-proteccion-social-en-salud-de-seguro-popular

8

Access to Medicines: Case Studies from Russia and Kyrgyzstan

Liliya Eugenevna Ziganshina, Chinara M. Razzakova, Syed Shahzad Hasan, and Zaheer-Ud-Din Babar

Brief Historical Background

According to the World Bank, Russia is an upper middle-income economy and Kyrgyzstan is a lower middle-income economy.[1] Both post-Soviet countries face the same problems of transition to market economies, and their pharmaceutical markets reflect all the challenges of the transition, depriving the most in need of access to medicines.

[1] World Bank Country and Lending Groups https://datahelpdesk.worldbank.org/knowledgebase/articles/906519-world-bank-country-and-lending-groups. Accessed June 2019.

L. E. Ziganshina (✉) • C. M. Razzakova
Cochrane Russia, Kazan Federal University, Kazan, Russia

Department of Pharmacology, Kazan State Medical University, Kazan, Russia

S. S. Hasan
Centre for Pharmaceutical Policy and Practice Research, Department of Pharmacy, University of Huddersfield, Huddersfield, UK

Z. Babar (ed.), *Global Pharmaceutical Policy*,
https://doi.org/10.1007/978-981-15-2724-1_8

These challenges have historic routes. While they were still within the Soviet Union, all republics depended on the centrally managed medicine supply system. The central government allocated the amounts of medicine supply and maintained uniform medicine prices all over the country and a health regulatory environment. After the collapse of the Soviet Union, the centralized medicine provision stopped. Pharmaceutical markets developed in severe economic, social and political crisis. This abrupt transition resulted in total reliance of countries on market forces.[2]

Over the years of transition, governments of post-Soviet countries started working on their pharmaceutical policies to develop measures for price containment. These measures and the implementation success vary substantially across these countries.[3]

Russia and Kyrgyzstan present diverse examples of legislative and regulatory approaches to medicine pricing, while the same pharmaceutical and biotechnology companies operate in the two countries. The Russian government introduced price control measures in 2010: setting the maximum wholesale and retail mark-ups, the maximum selling prices for essential medicines[4,5,6] and protection of domestic pharmaceutical market by supporting the domestic pharmaceutical industry development.[7]

---

[2] Shakhovskaya L.S., Evstratov A.V., Peskova O.S. The formation of regional pharmaceutical clusters in modern Russia. RUDN Journal of Economics 2011. № 2. 49–56.

[3] Martinenko G.I., Martinenko I.P. Legal protection of competition. Ltd. "Yustitsinform", 2016. 380–385. (In Russ.) ISBN: 9785720513023.

[4] The resolution of the Russian Federation government № 654 issued at 08.08.2009 (ed. on 03.02.2016) "About the improvement of government regulation of prices for medications included into the panel of vital and most important medications". (In Russ.). Available at: http://pravo.gov.ru/proxy/ips/?docbody=&nd=102131938. Access date: June 2019.

[5] State Committee on Tariffs in the Republic of Tatarstan. List of pharmaceutical organizations engaged in the retail sale of VED in the Republic of Tatarstan by type and form of ownership. Available at: http://kt.tatarstan.ru/rus/file/pub/pub_918685.pdf. Access date: 25.06.2019.

[6] State Committee on Tariffs in the Republic of Tatarstan. List of pharmaceutical organizations engaged in the wholesale sale of VED in the Republic of Tatarstan by type and form of ownership. Available at: http://kt.tatarstan.ru/rus/file/pub/pub_489550.pdf. Access date: 25.06.2019.

[7] The resolution of the Russian Federation government № 91 issued at 17.02.2011 (In Russ.) "About the federal targeted program 'Development of pharmaceutical and medical industry in the

---

Z. Babar
Centre for Pharmaceutical Policy and Practice Research,
University of Huddersfield, Huddersfield, UK
e-mail: z.babar@hud.ac.uk

The Kyrgyzstan situation is different. The pharmaceutical market is in private hands with no public pharmacies. Prices are formed by competitive pricing. Government does not regulate medicine prices: pharmaceutical distributors and retailers set price mark-ups.[8]

Reliable and trustworthy information on medicine prices and availability forms the evidence base for interventions towards fairer access to medicines. The Lancet Commission on Essential Medicines for Universal Health Coverage reiterates that "Data on prices need to be analysed and understood to design interventions to improve affordability. However, substantial gaps in the availability and quality of systematically gathered and analysed data on price and affordability of medicines exist at a global level."[9,10]

To help countries, in 2001, Health Action International (HAI, Amsterdam) in collaboration with the World Health Organization (WHO) Team on Pharmaceutical Policies, Access to Medicines and Rational Use of Medicine, established a joint project and developed a comprehensive methodology to measure medicine prices, availability and affordability. This allowed cross-country and time-series comparisons. This methodology remains the unique international instrument for obtaining reliable information on medicine prices. The results of HAI surveys are in the public domain at the HAI website in the form of a database. It serves as an evidence base for governments. It is also a starting point for developing and changing governmental policies to improve public access to information about medicine pricing and to foster access to medicines.

This chapter reports the medicine prices, availability and affordability in Russia and Kyrgyzstan by using the WHO/HAI methodology. The first pricing survey results (2010) were published on the HAI website, supplementing a Russian governmental price monitoring system.

Russian Federation for the period till 2020 and further perspectives'". Available at: http://pravo.gov.ru/proxy/ips/?docbody=&nd=102145869. Access date: 25.06.2019.

8 World Health Organization. Essential Medicines and Health Products Information Portal. Program of the Government of the Kyrgyz Republic on Development of the area of drugs circulation in the Kyrgyz Republic for 2014–2020. (Approved By the Resolution of the Government of the Kyrgyz Republic № 376 as of "8" July 2014). 2014. 1–22 Available at: http://apps.who.int/medicinedocs/en/m/abstract/Js23022en/. Access date: 25.06.2019.

9 Wirz V.J., Hogerzeil H.V., Gray A.L. et al. (the Lancet Commission on Essential Medicines) Essential medicines for universal health coverage. Lancet. 2017. 389(10067): 403–76. doi:https://doi.org/10.1016/S0140-6736(16)31599-9.

10 Wirz V.J., H.H.V., Gray A.L. et al. Essential medicines for universal health coverage. Kazan Medical Journal. 2019. 1 (C), 1–111. DOI: https://doi.org/10.17816/KMJ2019-4.

Comparison of Access to Cardiovascular Medicines in Russia and Kyrgyzstan, 2015

The cardiovascular diseases (CVDs) are a significant problem in low- and middle-income countries.[11] Alongside lifestyle measures, medicines play an important role in CVD treatment. Therefore, access to CVD medicines is important for Russia and Kyrgyzstan, where patients pay for their medicines out-of-pocket, except for limited categories, where they are entitled for state benefit schemes especially in Russia.

We carried out a comparative analysis of cardiovascular medicine prices, availability and affordability in the private sector of Russia (Tatarstan) and Kyrgyzstan (2015), using the WHO/HAI methodology.[12] We collected patient prices in private pharmacies of the capitals and five other survey areas. The study included 30 retail pharmacies in each country; five pharmacies were randomly selected in the capital and the same number in each survey area. In Tatarstan, the survey areas included the capital Kazan and Nizhnekamsky, Chistopolsky, Almetyevsky and Tukayevsky areas. In Kyrgyzstan the survey areas were the capital Bishkek and Chuy, Osh, Jalalabad, Issyk-Kul and Talas.

Selection of Medicines

We included 14 international and 16 national (Russian) medicines and 65 CVD medicines on the survey list; in total, there were 95 medicines. For each medicine in specific predetermined dosage forms, we recorded availability and price of the lowest-priced generic (LPG) and originator brand (OB). After excluding non-CVD medicines, we had 71 cardiovascular medicines.

To ensure comparability of medicine prices between the two countries, we selected medicines, which were available in both countries. We

[11] World Health Organization: Cardiovascular diseases (CVDs). Available at: https://www.who.int/cardiovascular_diseases/en/. Access date: 25.06.2019.

[12] Health Action International; World Health Organization. Measuring medicine prices, availability, affordability and price components 2nd edition. Available at: http://www.haiweb.org/medicineprices/manual/documents.html. Access date: 25.06.2019.

removed medicines, for which international reference prices (IRPs) were not available (Management Sciences for Health Price Indicator Guide, 2015[13]). Finally, for Russia-Kyrgyzstan comparisons, we had the complete price data for 23 LPGs and 7 OBs of cardiovascular medicines (Table 8.4).

Calculations and Statistical Analyses

We calculated the unit prices in local currency. We entered the data into the automated MS Excel WHO/HAI Workbook software. The Workbook automatically verified imputed values for accuracy after double-entry.

The Workbook calculated the median price ratio (MPR) by dividing the local price to IRP (converted into rubles or soms) for each medicine. At the time of the survey (August 2015), the ruble and some exchange rates were equal: 1 ruble equaled 1007 soms; 1 US dollar was 61 rubles or soms.[14] We used median prices (direct comparisons) and MPRs for comparisons.

Statistics: The final 30 medicines were included in the two-way ANOVA analysis. We calculated "median unit price" for each medicine. Then the "median-median" for matched sets of medicines among the two countries was compared using estimated marginal means. P-values and 95% CI were adjusted for multiple comparisons using Bonferroni method. Entry method: Two-way ANOVA was used (country and medicines category as fixed factors and MPs and MPRs as dependent variables).

For availability indicators, we calculated the percentage of pharmacies where the drugs were found. We also calculated the mean availability. The availability data reflects availability on the day of data collection at each site and may not represent the average monthly or annual availability of medicines in the country.

We calculated the affordability of a 30-day standard treatment course of hypertension using daily wages of the lowest-paid unskilled government

---

[13] MSH. The Management Sciences for Health Price Indicator Guide. 2015. Available at: https://www.msh.org. Access date: 25.06.2019.

[14] XE Currency Converter. Available at: https://www.xe.com/currencyconverter//. Access date: 25.06.2019.

worker and expressed the results as the number of paid working days necessary to cover the costs of treatment. The daily wages of the lowest-paid unskilled government worker in 2015 were 199 rubles/day (USD 3.3) in Russia[15]and 32.3 soms/day (USD 0.53) in Kyrgyzstan.[16]

Results

Availability of Cardiovascular Medicines

The availability of individual medicines varied from 0 to 100% in both countries. In Russia, the mean availability was 61% for LPGs and 35% for OBs (Table 8.1). On survey days we did not find generics of:

- Captopril 50 mg+hydrochlorothiazide 25 mg
- Felodipine 5 mg+metoprolol 47.5 mg
- Fluvastatin 20 mg
- Fosinopril 20 mg+hydrochlorothiazide 12.5 mg
- Reserpine 0.25 mg

Table 8.1 Differences in mean availability of CVD medicines by country and category

Country	Category	Mean availability, %	SD	Number of included medicines
Russia	OBs	35	36	38
	LPGs	61	35.5	59
Kyrgyzstan	OBs	10	22	12
	LPGs	58	42.5	42

[15]The minimum wage established simultaneously throughout the territory of the Russian Federation by federal law. Available at: http://publication.pravo.gov.ru/Document/View/0001201412020012. Access date: 25.06.2019.

[16]National Statistical Committee of the Kyrgyz Republic. Standard of living of the population of the Kyrgyz Republic 2013–2017. (In Russ.) Available at: http://www.stat.kg/media/publicationarchive/9f79e4d0-eb39-4013-8544-1784dc6bacd4.pdf. Access date: 25.06.2019.

We found two of them (captopril 50 mg+hydrochlorothiazide 25 mg, felodipine 5 mg+metoprolol 47.5 mg) as OBs.

We did not find any of these medicines in Kyrgyzstan pharmacies either generic or OBs.

We found the highest availability of medicines in Kazan, the capital of Tatarstan, 71% for LPGs and 42% for OBs, and the lowest availability in Chistopolsky, 56% for LPGs and 28% for OBs. In other surveyed areas, availability of generics was about 1.5–2 times higher than that of OBs:

- Almetyevsky (LPGs at 63%, OBs at 31%),
- Nizhnekamsky (LPGs at 60%, OBs at 40%),
- Tukayevsky (LPGs at 58%, OBs at 37%).

In Kyrgyzstan, medicine availability was lower than in Russia: LPGs at 57% and OBs at 10%. Among 71 studied medicines, 19 LPGs and 46 OBs were unavailable. Among the missing generics were medicines included on the Kyrgyzstan National EML[17]:

- Amiodarone 200 mg
- Amiodarone 50 mg/ml (OB available)
- Epinephrine 1 mg/ml
- Isosorbide dinitrate 10 mg

In the capital Bishkek, Chuy and Osh, availability of LPGs (62%, 60%, 60%) and OBs (16%, 12%, 13%) was higher than in other regions:

- Jalalabad, (LPGs at 54%, OBs at 7%)
- Issyk-Kul, (LPGs at 56%, OBs at 10%)
- Talas (LPGs at 55%, OBs at 5%)

[17] Ministry of Justice of the Kyrgyz Republic. Resolution «On Approval of the List of Essential Medicines in the Kyrgyz Republic» issued at 9 October 2012 № 693. (In Russ.). Available at: http://cbd.minjust.gov.kg/act/view/ru-ru/93116. Access date: 25.06.2019.

Medicine Prices

Of the included 23 LPGs and 7 OBs, all belonged to the National EMLs of Russia[18] and Kyrgyzstan, except for perindopril 4 mg, which is not included in Kyrgyzstan.[19]

Prices were higher than IRPs in both countries (Table 8.2). Mean MPRs in Russia were consistently lower than in Kyrgyzstan (OBs and LPGs). In Russia, OB prices were on average 20 times higher than IRPs. In Kyrgyzstan OBs were priced on average 33 times higher than IRPs. LPG prices exceeded IRPs by 3 times (Russia) and 4.5 times (Kyrgyzstan). In Kyrgyzstan, compared to Russian median prices, MPRs of OBs were 1.6 times higher; those of LPGs were 1.5 times higher. In both countries, OB prices were five times (compared by median prices) and seven times (compared by MPRs) higher than LPG prices.

Median prices and MPRs of six **OBs** were up to four times higher in Kyrgyzstan than in Russia. The only exception was the OB of indapamide (Arifon, Servier). Its median price and the MPR were approximately two

Table 8.2 Differences in median prices and MRPs of CVD medicines by country and category

Country	Category	Mean	Std. deviation	Std. error
Median prices in local currency (rubles and soms)				
Russia	OBs	16.73	9.75	3.69
	LPGs	3.48	2.93	0.61
Kyrgyzstan	OBs	26.96	15.15	5.73
	LPGs	5.29	5.52	1.15
Median MPRs				
Russia	OBs	20.76	24.27	9.17
	LPGs	3.09	2.99	0.62
Kyrgyzstan	OBs	33.20	36.00	13.61
	LPGs	4.49	4.39	0.92

[18] List of vital and essential drugs for medical use in 2019. The order of the Government of the Russian Federation from December 30, 2014. № 2782–173. Available at: https://www.rosminzdrav.ru/documents/8159. Access date: 25.06.2019.

[19] Ministry of Justice of the Kyrgyz Republic. Resolution "On Approval of the List of Essential Medicines in the Kyrgyz Republic" issued at 9 October 2012. № 693. (In Russ.). Available at: http://cbd.minjust.gov.kg/act/view/ru-ru/93116. Access date: 25.06.2019.

times higher in Russia. However, LPG of indapamide was up to four times more expensive in Kyrgyzstan than in Russia.

The MPRs of eight **LPGs** in Russia were two times higher than in Kyrgyzstan; the MPRs of the remaining 15 LPGs were four times higher in Kyrgyzstan (Table 8.3).

Price Variation in Russia

According to the State Committee on Tariffs, the density of pharmacies in Kazan was the highest in Tatarstan.[20] Pharmaceutical organizations engaged with wholesale delivery were also mainly located in Kazan (74%),[21] the main distribution hub for pharmaceuticals in Tatarstan.

The prices of OBs and LPGs in Kazan and Nizhnekamsky were lower than in other Tatarstan areas (Tables 8.4 and 8.5). Medicines were the most expensive in Chistopolsky and Almetyevsky areas.

In all surveyed pharmacies, there were 5–10% discounts for the entire range of surveyed medicines for the elderly.

Price Variation in Kyrgyzstan

The capital Bishkek hosts the highest number of retail and wholesale pharmaceutical organizations. Medicines are supplied to other regions from the capital.

Medicine prices varied across the surveyed areas. In Bishkek medicine prices were lower than in other areas (Tables 8.4 and 8.5). MPRs of OBs and LPGs were 38.5 and 3.5 times the IRPs, respectively. In Osh, the prices of OBs were lower than in other areas except for Bishkek, but the prices for generics were higher than in Issyk-Kul and Talas. The highest prices of LPGs and OBs were in Jalalabad, with MPRs ranging from 5.9 to 64.7, respectively.

We did not find any discounts for medicines in Kyrgyzstan.

---

[20] State Committee on Tariffs in the Republic of Tatarstan. List of pharmaceutical organizations engaged in the retail sale of VED in the Republic of Tatarstan by type and form of ownership. Available at: http://kt.tatarstan.ru/rus/file/pub/pub_918685.pdf. Access date: 25.06.2019.

[21] State Committee on Tariffs in the Republic of Tatarstan. List of pharmaceutical organizations engaged in the wholesale sale of VED in the Republic of Tatarstan by type and form of ownership. Available at: http://kt.tatarstan.ru/rus/file/pub/pub_489550.pdf. Access date: 25.06.2019.

Table 8.3 Comparison of median prices and MPRs of 30 CVD medicines between Kyrgyzstan (K) and Russia (R)

Medicine name	Category	Difference in median prices	Difference in median price ratios
1. Amlodipine 5 mg (Norvasc)	OB	1.41 times ↑ in K	1.61 times ↑ in K
2. Amlodipine 10 mg (Norvasc)	OB	1.26 times ↑ in K	1.45 times ↑ in K
3. Carvedilol 6.25 mg (Dilatrend)	OB	1.64 times ↑ in K	1.87 times ↑ in K
4. Enalapril 10 mg (Renitec)	OB	1.15 times ↑ in K	1.15 times ↑ in K
5. Furosemide 10 mg/ml (Lasix)	OB	3.26 times ↑ in K	3.73 times ↑ in K
6. Indapamide 2.5 mg (Arifon)	**OB**	**2.09 times ↑ in R**	**1.82 times ↑ in R**
7. Nimodipine 30 mg (Nimotop)	OB	3.16 times ↑ in K	3.62 times ↑ in K
1. Amlodipine 5 mg	**LPG**	**1.62 times ↑ in R**	**1.42 times ↑ in R**
2. Amlodipine 10 mg	**LPG**	**1.95 times ↑ in R**	**1.70 times ↑ in R**
3. Atenolol 50 mg	**LPG**	**1.29 times ↑ in R**	**1.23 times ↑ in R**
4. Atenolol 100 mg	**LPG**	**1.38 times ↑ in R**	**1.21 times ↑ in R**
5. Bisoprolol 5 mg	LPG	2.71 times ↑ in K	3.11 times ↑ in K
6. Captopril 25 mg	LPG	1.25 times ↑ in K	1.44 times ↑ in K
7. Captopril 50 mg	LPG	1.97 times ↑ in K	2.26 times ↑ in K
8. Carvedilol 6.25 mg	LPG	1.88 times ↑ in K	2.15 times ↑ in K
9. Enalapril 10 mg	LPG	2.12 times ↑ in K	2.43 times ↑ in K
10. Enalapril 20 mg	LPG	1.50 times ↑ in K	1.72 times ↑ in K
11. Enalapril 5 mg	**LPG**	**2.28 times ↑ in R**	**1.99 times ↑ in R**
12. Furosemide 40 mg	LPG	1.03 times ↑ in K	1.18 times ↑ in K
13. Furosemide 10 mg/ml	LPG	1.29 times ↑ in K	1.48 times ↑ in K
14. Hydrochlorothiazide 25 mg	**LPG**	**1.00 same**	**1.30 times ↑ in R**
15. Indapamide 2.5 mg	LPG	3.28 times ↑ in K	3.76 times ↑ in K
16. Lisinopril 10 mg	LPG	1.49 times ↑ in K	1.70 times ↑ in K
17. Lisinopril 20 mg	LPG	2.18 times ↑ in K	2.50 times ↑ in K
18. Losartan 50 mg	LPG	1.90 times ↑ in K	2.17 times ↑ in K
19. Nifedipine 10 mg	**LPG**	**2.55 times ↑ in R**	**2.23 times ↑ in R**
20. Nifedipine 20 mg	LPG	2.18 times ↑ in K	2.50 times ↑ in K
21. Perindopril 4 mg	LPG	1.04 times ↑ in K	1.20 times ↑ in K
22. Propranolol 40 mg	**LPG**	**1.55 times ↑ in R**	**1.36 times ↑ in R**
23. Verapamil 40 mg	LPG	1.06 times ↑ in K	1.21 times ↑ in K

Table 8.4 MPRs of 30 CVD medicines in private sector retail pharmacies by country and surveyed areas

Country	Surveyed areas	Category	Mean	Std. deviation	Std. error
Russia	Kazan	OBs	21.64	24.12	9.85
		LPGs	2.66	2.12	0.44
	Tukayevsky	OBs	23.07	25.73	10.51
		LPGs	3.15	2.95	0.62
	Nizhnekamsky	OBs	22.15	24.47	9.99
		LPGs	2.77	2.99	0.64
	Chistopolsky	OBs	26.31	27.97	12.51
		LPGs	3.23	3.24	0.69
	Almetyevsky	OBs	26.03	27.68	12.38
		LPGs	3.26	3.21	0.68
Kyrgyzstan	Bishkek	OBs	38.47	37.56	15.33
		LPGs	3.48	3.71	0.79
	Chuy	OBs	52.50	42.90	21.45
		LPGs	5.34	5.32	1.13
	Osh	OBs	41.80	40.59	18.15
		LPGs	5.59	5.74	1.22
	Jalalabad	OBs	64.67	35.18	20.31
		LPGs	5.88	6.83	1.46
	Issyk-Kul	OBs	51.84	42.42	21.21
		LPGs	4.89	5.00	1.06
	Talas	OBs	61.49	31.88	18.41
		LPGs	4.32	4.52	0.94

In Kyrgyzstan median prices were six times higher than in Russia. In both countries OB prices were 23 times (by MPRs) and 17 times (by median prices) higher than LPG prices (Table 8.6).

Affordability

The cost of a one-month hypertension treatment with OBs in Russia ranged from 0.9 to 8 days' wages. In Kyrgyzstan it ranged from 6.6 to 156.5 days' wages. The OBs were less affordable than their LPG equivalents in both countries. For example, to afford a one-month treatment with OB of amlodipine 5 mg in Kyrgyzstan, a patient had to pay 27 days' wages, while it is 1.6 days' wages in the case of its LPG.

Table 8.5 Mean prices of 30 CVD medicines in private sector retail pharmacies by country and surveyed areas

Country	Surveyed areas	Category	Mean	Std. deviation	Std. error
Russia	Kazan	OBs	16.02	9.81	4.00
		LPGs	2.96	2.09	0.44
	Tukayevsky	OBs	17.36	10.52	4.30
		LPGs	3.61	3.06	0.64
	Nizhnekamsky	OBs	16.84	9.92	4.05
		LPGs	3.17	2.60	0.57
	Chistopolsky	OBs	17.50	11.94	5.34
		LPGs	3.58	3.49	0.74
	Almetyevsky	OBs	17.30	11.80	5.28
		LPGs	3.69	3.57	0.76
Kyrgyzstan	Bishkek	OBs	30.23	13.80	5.63
		LPGs	4.54	5.36	1.14
	Chuy	OBs	37.73	9.83	4.92
		LPGs	5.66	5.41	1.15
	Osh	OBs	31.34	15.15	6.77
		LPGs	5.79	5.54	1.18
	Jalalabad	OBs	38.29	8.45	4.88
		LPGs	5.98	5.83	1.24
	Issyk-Kul	OBs	36.78	9.31	4.65
		LPGs	5.41	5.79	1.23
	Talas	OBs	37.47	9.66	5.58
		LPGs	5.27	5.77	1.20

Table 8.6 Pairwise comparison of MRPs of 30 CVD medicines by country and medicine category

			95% confidence interval for difference	
Item	Mean difference	Sig.	Lower bound	Upper bound
Median prices				
Kyrgyzstan-Russia	6.013	0.007	1.683	10.342
OBs-LPGs	17.463	0.001	13.133	21.792
MPRs				
Kyrgyzstan-Russia	6.912	0.126	−2.014	15.838
OBs-LPGs	23.188	0.001	14.262	32.114

The majority of LPGs in Russia were affordable (with standard hypertension treatment costing one day's wages or less). Only the following four LPGs required more than one day's wages to afford a one-month hypertension treatment:

- Carvedilol 6.25 mg (2.1 days' wages)
- Lisinopril 10 mg (2.8 days' wages)
- Lisinopril 20 mg (1.4 days' wages)
- Perindopril 4 mg (1.3 days' wages)

In Kyrgyzstan the one-month hypertension treatment was affordable only with five LPGs:

- Atenolol 50 mg
- Atenolol 100 mg
- Enalapril 5 mg
- Propranolol 40 mg
- Captopril 25 mg

The affordability of the remaining LPGs ranged from 1.5 days' wages to 25.2 days' wages to pay for a one-month treatment. On average, the affordability of antihypertensives in Kyrgyzstan was lower than in Russia by 11 times for OBs and 9 times for LPGs (Table 8.7).

Considering governmental efforts on price containment, we see the fundamental differences in approaches taken by the countries and the impact on medicine prices and affordability.

In Russia, the legislation establishes the limits of wholesale and retail mark-ups for all medicines included on the National EML: 11–15% for wholesale and 23.4–30% for retail outlets.[22] However, the high OB prices adversely impact on generic prices by creating an opportunity to raise generic prices and to use the maximum allowed mark-ups. This problem was addressed by the Federal Antimonopoly Service of the Department of Social Control and Trade in its report in 2013.[23]

[22] Decree of the Russian Federation government № 654 issued at 08.08.2009 (ed. on 03.02.2016) "About the improvement of government regulation of prices for medications included into the panel of vital and most important medications". (In Russ.). Available at: http://pravo.gov.ru/proxy/ips/?docbody=&nd=102131938. Access date: 25.06.2019.

[23] Federal antimonopoly service, Department of Social Control and Trade. Results of the evaluation of affordability of medications on the basis of retail prices analysis and medicines price setting in the Russian Federation (Federal subjects included) and on comparable markets of other countries, including member-countries of the European Union and BRICS. 2013. p. 30–95. (In Russ.) Available at: https://fas.gov.ru/attachment/138241/download?1504613550 Access date: 25.06.2019.

Table 8.7 Affordability: the number of days' wages of the lowest-paid unskilled worker required to purchase a standard one-month hypertension/CVD treatment

Medicines name	Total of units per treatment	Category	Russia	Kyrgyzstan	KR/RF
1. Amlodipine 5 mg	30	OB	3.1	26.9	9
2. Amlodipine 10 mg	30	OB	5.4	42.5	8
3. Carvedilol 6.25 mg	60	OB	5.2	53.3	10
4. Enalapril 10 mg	30	OB	0.9	6.6	7
5. Furosemide 10 mg	60	OB	2.7	56.5	21
6. Indapamide 2.5 mg	60	OB	4.4	13	3
7. Nimodipine 30 mg	120	OB	8	156.5	20
					M 11 [3–21]
1. Amlodipine 5 mg	30	LPG	0.8	1.6	2
2. Amlodipine 10 mg	30	LPG	0.6	1.8	3
3. Atenolol 50 mg	30	LPG	0.1	*0.6*	6
4. Atenolol 100 mg	30	LPG	0.2	*0.7*	4
5. Bisoprolol 5 mg	30	LPG	0.6	9.3	16
6. Captopril 25 mg	60	LPG	0.1	1.1	11
7. Captopril 50 mg	60	LPG	0.3	3.5	12
8. Carvedilol 6.25 mg	60	LPG	*2.1*	18.6	9
9. Enalapril 10 mg	30	LPG	0.4	5.0	13
10. Enalapril 20 mg	30	LPG	0.8	6.8	9
11. Enalapril 5 mg	30	LPG	0.3	*1.0*	3
12. Furosemide 40 mg	60	LPG	0.2	1.1	6
13. Furosemide 10 mg/ml	60	LPG	0.8	6.7	9
14. Hydrochlorothiazide 25 mg	30	LPG	0.5	2.0	4
15. Indapamide 2.5 mg	60	LPG	0.4	11.6	29
16. Lisinopril 10 mg	60	LPG	*2.8*	25.2	9
17. Lisinopril 20 mg	30	LPG	*1.4*	19.4	14
18. Losartan 50 mg	30	LPG	*1.1*	12.9	12
19. Nifedipine 10 mg	120	LPG	0.6	1.5	2.5
20. Nifedipine 20 mg	60	LPG	1.0	13.6	14
21. Perindopril 4 mg	30	LPG	*1.3*	8.0	6
22. Propranolol 40 mg	60	LPG	0.2	*0.9*	5
23. Verapamil 40 mg	90	LPG	0.4	2.5	6
					M 9 [2–29]

Another problem is that patients may not know about the availability of cheaper generic alternatives. When a patient asks for a medicine, pharmacists offer the most expensive OBs.[24] Currently the Federal Government is taking measures to raise public awareness of LPGs. At the end of 2018, the Federal Antimonopoly Service prepared draft legislation, binding pharmacy organizations by law to inform patients about availability of the cheapest generic and its price.[25]

In Kyrgyzstan, LPGs and OBs were overpriced exceeding IRPs by 4.5 and 33 times and exceeding corresponding Russian prices by 6 times. Kyrgyz medicine prices were high regardless of whether the medicines were on the National EML or not.

Despite the above-described problems in Russia, the central price reduction efforts bring positive results.[26,27] The governmentally regulated public sector drug procurement system and the private sector retail pharmacies present the model for Kyrgyzstan. Other studies showed that the free market economy and the increase in the number and variety of generics on the market are not an effective tool for reducing prices.[28] Kyrgyz pharmaceutical market consists of imported medicines (97%), which contributes to high prices. Meanwhile in Russia the government planned for domestic production of 50% of all medicines and of 90% of essential medicines by 2020 according to the Strategy of Pharmaceutical Industry Development 2020.[29]

---

[24] Lvov V. Drug discrimination as a state problem. Rossiyskaya Gazeta - Federal issue № 7769 (11). (In Russ.) Available at: https://rg.ru/2019/01/18/lekarstvennaia-diskriminaciia-kak-gosudarstvennaia-problema.html. Access date: 25.06.2019.

[25] Order of the Government of the Russian Federation on approval of the action plan "Development of competition in health care" issued at 12 January 2018. N. 9-p. (In Russ.) Available at: http://static.government.ru/media/files/vyoWQD6EZYQkBaqKfKFKAPZqqgtmcHDH.pdf. Access date: 25.06.2019.

[26] Razzakova Ch.M., Ziganshina L.E., Change in affordability of medication in Kazan in 2011 and 2015 as a reflection of state initiatives to regulate medicines prices. Kazan Medical Journal. 2017. 5822–826. doi: https://doi.org/10.17750/KMJ2017-822.

[27] Razzakova C.M., Ziganshina L.E. Cardiovascular medicine prices as an indicator of access to medicines and their rational use. Rational Pharmacotherapy in Cardiology. 2019.15(2):215–223. (In Russ.) doi: https://doi.org/10.20996/1819-6446-2019-15-2-215-223.

[28] Babar Z.U.D., Ibrahim M.I., Singh H. et al., Evaluating Medicines Prices, Availability, Affordability, and Price Components: Implications for Access to Medicines in Malaysia. PLoS Med 2007. 4(3):e82. doi: https://doi.org/10.1371/journal.pmed.0040082.

[29] Decree of the Russian Federation government № 91 issued at 17.02.2011 (In Russ.) "About the federal targeted program 'Development of pharmaceutical and medical industry in the Russian

Summing-Up

1. Availability of cardiovascular medicines in private sector retail pharmacies was higher for LPGs than for OBs: in Russia by two times (LPGs at 61%, OBs at 35%) and in Kyrgyzstan by six times (LPGs at 57%, OBs at 10%) with three essential medicines not available in any of the surveyed Kyrgyz pharmacies. The availability was higher in the capitals with no association between availability and remoteness from the capital.
2. In both countries OB CVD prices were higher than LPG prices. OB MPRs were 21 and 33 times higher than IRPs in Russia and Kyrgyzstan, respectively.
3. Median CVD prices in Kyrgyzstan were six times higher than in Russia.
4. LPG CVD prices in Russia were 3 times higher than IRPs, while in Kyrgyzstan it is 4.5 times higher than IRPs.
5. Prices varied across surveyed areas of the two countries and were lower in the capitals with no clear association with remoteness from the capitals.
6. The affordability of CVD medicines in Kyrgyzstan on average was lower than in Russia by 11 times for OBs and by 9 times for LPGs.
7. Antihypertensive pharmacotherapy was affordable in Russia but not in Kyrgyzstan.

Medicine Price Monitoring in Fostering Government Interventions for Price Containment and Access to Medicines in Russia: 2010–2015–2017 Time Series

We evaluated the progress in access to medicines and the viability of Russian pharmaceutical policies using the WHO/HAI methodology. We present results using lists of global and regional essential and cardiovascular medicines (Tables 8.8, 8.9, 8.10, and 8.11), following the methodology for CVD medicine selection as described above.

Federation for the period till 2020 and further perspectives'". Available at: http://fcp.economy.gov.ru/cgi-bin/cis/fcp.cgi/Fcp/File/FcpPass/350. Access date: 25.06.2019.

Table 8.8 Median price ratios for the global and regional essential medicines: patient prices in the **public sector** as compared to IRPs

	2010		2015		2017	
Government sector	OB	LPG	OB	LPG	OB	LPG
Mean MPR	8.96	2.28	2.79	1.43	4.52	1.3
[25%–75%]	[3.1–11.38]	[1.59–3.32]	[1.88–6.58]	[0.93–2.43]	[2.6–9.9]	[0.99–1.86]
Min MPR	2.08	0.56	1.36	0.49	1.53	0.31
Max MPR	12.2	11.31	26.26	4	20.43	4.72
Number of medicines included	7	27	8	26	14	27

Table 8.9 Median price ratios for the global and regional essential medicines: patient prices in the **private sector** as compared to IRPs

	2010		2015		2017	
Private sector	OB	LPG	OB	LPG	OB	LPG
Mean MPR	9.12	3.39	2.83	2.06	11.1	3.25
[25%–75%]	[3.62–11.8]	[2.04–5.26]	[1.99–8.49]	[1.48–2.91]	[2.6–18.98]	[1.65–5.09]
Min MPR	2.64	0.99	1.4	0.57	1.4	0.67
Max MPR	114.64	17.17	13.93	6.11	56	30.97
Number of medicines included	9	25	8	26	14	29

Table 8.10 Median price ratios for cardiovascular medicines: patient prices in the **public sector** as compared to IRPs

Government	2011	2015		2017		
sector	OB	LPG	OB	LPG	OB	LPG
Mean MPR	13.28	2.17	12.57	1.38	6.88	1.14 [0.43–1.82]
[25%–75%]	[11.23–17.36]	[1.09–4.37]	[10.52–31.43]	[0.82–2.63]	[4.57–10.04]	
Min MPR	6.00	0.11	5.59	0.22	1.71	0.03
Max MPR	66.88	57.47	62.84	5.11	54.22	12.77
Number of medicines included	10	38	8	34	15	39

Table 8.11 Median price ratios for cardiovascular medicines: patient prices in the **private sector** as compared to IRPs

	2011		2015		2017	
Private sector	OB	LPG	OB	LPG	OB	LPM
Mean MPR	12.4	2.79	10.98	2.40	12.38	2.23
[25%–75%]	[9.47–17.58]	[1.36–5.35]	[8.14–13.39]	[0.82–3.9]	[7.75–16.59]	[1.13–11.03]
Min MPR	3.95	0.16	1.97	0.21	2.33	0.4
Max MPR	27.35	28.5	14.91	7.27	66.61	11.06
Number of medicines included	12	30	10	32	19	43

Patient Prices of Russian Essential Medicines

Prices for essential medicines in 2015 tended to decrease compared to the baseline pricing survey results of 2010–2011 (Tables 8.10 and 8.11). The OB MPRs decreased in 2015 by about three times, but still exceeding IRPs by three times. The LPG prices were over two times higher than IRPs in 2010–2011, but they came closer to IRPs in 2015 and became acceptable. However, there was no further progress in price reductions in 2017 in the public sector: LPG prices remained at the 2015 level, while OB prices became higher than in 2015.

In private sector, essential medicine prices were higher than in the public sector, with price reduction from 2010–2011 to 2015, which was not sustained and reverted by 2017 (Table 8.11).

Patient Prices of Cardiovascular Medicines

MPRs of OBs and LPGs of cardiovascular medicines in public and private sectors decreased from 2010 to 2015, with some further decrease in 2017 in the public sector, but not in the private sector (Tables 8.10 and 8.11).

Over the studied time periods, the lowest and highest MPRs were found for the same CVD medicines. Among the medicines with the lowest MPRs in the private sector was furosemide 10 mg/ml, prices of which exceeded international reference prices (IRPs) by two to four times. Amlodipine had the highest MPRs (60+) over the years even in the public sector.

In the public sector LPG prices in 2015 and 2017 were close to IRPs and became acceptable (WHO/HAI recommendations, Table 8.10).

The most successful price reductions were for:

- Acetylsalicylic acid 100 mg
- Digoxin 0.25 mg
- Hydrochlorothiazide 25 mg
- Isosorbide mononitrate 20 mg
- Nifedipine 10 mg
- Simvastatin 40 mg

Procurement Prices of Russian National Essential and Cardiovascular Medicines

Not all medicines selected for the study were purchased by the surveyed public hospitals. We collected data on state procurement of 61 medicines in 2010 and 29 medicines in 2015.

In 2010, 48 medicines were procured as generics (11, global; 12, regional; 25, CVD list) and 13 as OBs (2, global; 2, regional; 9, CVD list). MPRs for generics were 2.9 [1.8–5.5] and for OBs 12.3 [4.4–14.9]. Of 71 CVD medicines, 42 were procured for public hospitals: 31 as generics and 11 as OBs. MPRs amounted to 3.08 [1.16–5.66] for generics and to 12.4 [5.71–15.96] for OBs.

In 2015 public hospitals procured 28 medicines as generics (6, global; 3, regional; 19, CVD list) and only 1 medicine as an OB (amiodarone 50 mg/ml). MPR for generics was 1.1 [0.2–2.6] and for OB –2.0. We see reduction of state procurement prices from 2010 to 2015, by two times for generics and six times for OBs. Of 71 CVD medicines, 22 were procured for public hospitals: only one (amiodarone 50 mg/ml) as OB. MPR of 21 generics was 0.77 [0.22–2.39].

Procurement prices for CVD generics reduced by four times and by six-plus times for OB of amiodarone 50 mg/ml.

These price reductions were due to the 2013 Decree of the Russian government, which restricted procurement of OBs, by means of creating a special list of medicines allowed for procurement as OBs.

Summing-Up

Government interventions on price regulation contributed to a 1.5–3 times reduction of patient retail prices from 2010 to 2015 both for LPGs and OBs in public and private sectors.

Generic price reductions in the public sector achieved the recommended MPRs of 1.

Not all positive changes were sustained up to 2017.

These findings confirm that government interventions on price containment are effective for reduction of public procurement of OBs and preferential procurement of LPGs, with the overall reduction of procurement prices by at least two times for generics and six times for OBs.

Summing-Up and Looking Forward

We used the WHO/HAI methodology to compare access to cardiovascular medicines in Russia and Kyrgyzstan. We confirmed that central government regulation and targeted interventions for price containment provide advantages over market forces in the two post-Soviet countries, Russia and Kyrgyzstan:

- Three of essential CVD medicines were not available in any of the surveyed Kyrgyz pharmacies on the date of the survey.
- In Kyrgyzstan, the median prices of CVD medicines in the private sector were six times higher than in Russia. Affordability of CVD medicines was lower than in Russia by 9 times for LPGs and by 11 times for OBs.
- Antihypertensive pharmacotherapy was affordable in Russia, but not in Kyrgyzstan.
- We did not manage to obtain information on price components in both countries.

We used the WHO/HAI methodology for monitoring patient and procurement prices in public hospitals over the years 2010–2017 in Russia.

- We documented reduction of essential and CVD medicine prices from 2010 onwards, achieving the recommended MPRs of 1 for generics in the public sector.
- Price containment government interventions were successful in achieving preferential procurement of LPGs with overall reduction of procurement prices by two times for LPGs and six times for OBs.
- Continued price monitoring in 2017–2018 proved the need for more interventions to sustain all achievements.

Acknowledgements We would like to thank Dr. Margaret A. Ewen (HAI) for the support and expert advice at all levels of the Russian/Tatarstan pricing project, Ms. Ekaterina Ivacheva for providing data on drug prices for 2010 and Professor Hans V. Hogerzeil for all the support and inspiration through many happy years with essential medicines.

9

Access and Use of Medicines in Ukraine

Grintsova Olga and Zaheer-Ud-Din Babar

Introduction

Ukraine is a country in the east of Europe, a former republic of the Soviet Union that gained independence in 1991. According to the World Bank classification, Ukraine belongs to lower middle-income countries with GNI per capita of 2660 USD (World Bank Data 2019). The total population of Ukraine is around 44,439,000 (World Health Organization 2019). The life expectancy is 68 years (males) and 77 years (females), and this is significantly below the average in the countries in WHO European region. The main mortality indicators are ischemic heart disease, stroke, Alzheimer's disease, cirrhosis, cardiomyopathy and cancer (lung, colorectal and stomach). The frequency of cardiovascular mortality decreased

G. Olga (✉)
Apotheke am Meilenstein, Bielefeld, Germany

Z. Babar
Centre for Pharmaceutical Policy and Practice Research,
University of Huddersfield, Huddersfield, UK
e-mail: z.babar@hud.ac.uk

Z. Babar (ed.), *Global Pharmaceutical Policy*,
https://doi.org/10.1007/978-981-15-2724-1_9

during the past decade (2007–2017), in contrary to Alzheimer's disease (+30%, 2007–2017) (Institute for Health Metrics and Evaluation 2019).

The birth and mortality rates are showing a dramatic tendency—in November 2018 state statistic centre reported an average of 59 births per 100 deaths, showing that the population of Ukraine is decreasing very fast. It can be partially explained by bias in the data collection, as well as by the military losses in eastern regions of Ukraine (UNIAN Information Agency 2018).

During the past decade, the public health spending was consistently low in Ukraine, 3.9% in 2005 and 4.4% in 2010, and this is below the average of the WHO European region (5%) and of the European Union (6%). Starting from 2014, the political instability and military conflict in the east part of Ukraine, as well as annexation of the Crimean Peninsula, contributed to economic recession. The public health spending in 2014 decreased to 3.8% of GDP and to 2.9% of GPD in 2015. As a consequence, the out-of-pocket payments were consistently high over time, reaching 48% of total household budget in 2015 (Goroshko A. 2018).

The recent WHO review suggests that majority of Ukrainian citizens experienced the financial hardship by the use of the health services, including medicines (Goroshko A. 2018). To improve the access and use of healthcare services and medicines in Ukraine, a range of healthcare reforms has been implemented since 2017.

Healthcare System Before 2017

The **universal health coverage** is guaranteed by the Constitution of Ukraine (Article 29) (Parliament of Ukraine 2019): It states that "Each citizen has right for health care, medical help and medical insurance". Healthcare is provided by state financing for the relevant socio-economic, medical and preventive programmes. In the state healthcare establishments, the healthcare is provided free-of-charge.

Unfortunately, the Constitution right for the universal access and free-of-charge services is not practically implemented for the Ukrainian citizens due to a range of reasons: the insufficient management, lack of state financing, ineffective allocation of available resources as well as non-transparency in public procurement practices. Till 2017, **the healthcare system organization and financing** in Ukraine was based on the integrated Semashko model—a hierarchical, nationally controlled system, where medical staff is state-employed (Lekhan V. 2015).

The majority of healthcare institutions are owned, managed and financed by state. The outpatient primary care was provided in polyclinics as well as in primary care units in rural areas. The inpatient care was provided in city and regional hospitals.

The financing model for healthcare institutions was based on the statistical indicators—size of the area served, patient number and level of healthcare. Despite the use of statistic and demographic indicators, according to Article 49 of the Constitution of Ukraine (Parliament of Ukraine 2019), the existing number of public healthcare facilities (hospitals, polyclinics, etc.) must remain unchanged. This restriction was a serious burden for the effective use of the existing resources and has been abolished in the new regulation.

The **distribution and dispensing of medicines** are granted via public and private pharmacies in Ukraine. The pharmacy business is regulated and controlled from the regulatory perspective; the pharmacy license is provided by the State Service of Ukraine on Medications and Drugs Control (SSUMDC) (State Service of Ukraine on Medications and Drugs Control 2019). The pharmacy licenses register is publicly available via the online platform (SSUMDC 2018). The re-licensing of pharmacies is done every five years by regional departments of SSUMDC. Over 80% of pharmacies in Ukraine are located in urban areas, and in many rural areas the number of pharmacies is not sufficient. Special regulations on the access to medicines in remote rural areas allow pharmacy specialists with college degree (pharmacy technicians) or even nurses to manage the small pharmacy branches and dispense medicines.

Healthcare Reform 2017

In 2015, the Government of Ukraine initiated the transformative reforms and new financial mechanisms for the health system with the goal to improve health outcomes and to ensure the financial protection from excessive out-of-pocket payment through increasing efficiency, modernizing the obsolete service delivery systems and improving access for better quality of care (WHO & World Bank 2019).

As a first step, in 2017 Ukrainian parliament approved a new Law on State Finance Guarantees of Health Care Services to the Population (Law of Ukraine 2168-VIII) (Parliament of Ukraine 2018).

The programme of State Finance Guarantees of Health Care Services to the Population is a programme that defines the **catalogue and extent of healthcare services** (including medical devices) and medicines that will be completely covered by the state. The catalogue of services includes all levels of healthcare, from the emergency and primary care to specialized treatment, medical rehabilitation and maternity.

In Ukraine Law 2168-VIII, it is also stated that the state budget for the programme of the State Finance Guarantees of Health Care Services to the Population must be yearly assigned and it should not be less than 5% of gross domestic product (GDP). The financing of the programme is a fixed and protected position in the state budget (Parliament of Ukraine 2018).

The major principle of the financing of the healthcare is "money follows the patient". Ukrainian citizens received the right to choose the primary care physician and are not forced to use the local healthcare establishments according to their residence. In less than a year, 27 million or 65% of Ukrainians made a choice and signed declarations with primary care physicians (WHO & World Bank 2019).

For the purchasing of healthcare services, a single national healthcare purchaser is being established, the National Health Service of Ukraine (National Health Service of Ukraine 2019).

Access to Medicines

Medicines have not been officially excluded from the free-of-charge healthcare, but in reality, 99% of all spending on medicines in 2015 and 96% in 2017 were covered by the patients. The expenses for medicines by Ukrainian patients cover both in- and outpatient use. From the perspective of patients, out-of-pocket spending on medicines makes about a half of total spending of households on health, continuously growing from 51.7% in 2010 to 56.5% in 2017 (Goroshko A. 2018).

A new national essential medicines list (EML) was adopted by the Government of Ukraine in March 2017 (Cabinet of Ministers of Ukraine 2017). It includes medicines eligible for public procurement and reimbursement, such as Affordable Medicines Programme (Програма Доступні Ліки). Currently there are 427 INN medicines on the list (Cabinet of Ministers of Ukraine 2017).

The services and medicines that are not included into the programme might be covered from other special targeted programmes from the state budget of Ukraine (oncology, insulins, orphan drugs, etc.). New opportunities opened also for regional governments that according to local needs can design and finance healthcare services, which are not included into the programme of finance guarantees. To improve access to medicines, the government covers public procurement of vaccines and medicines for HIV, tuberculosis, cancer, transplants, diabetes, hepatitis B, hepatitis C and rare diseases, as well as the treatment for acute neonatal and obstetric conditions.

Use of Medicines

The total pharmaceutical expenditure in Ukraine is about 70 billion hryvna (ca 2 billion euros) in 2017, represented by 1.2 billion packages. The market is strongly dominated by local pharmaceutical producers that represent around 70% in volume and 40% in value. In general, over 90% medicines are generics (World Health Organization 2019).

Despite the existing clinical treatment guidelines, the evaluation of medicines use is not actively monitored and controlled in Ukrainian healthcare system. One of the factors supporting these practices is the high proportion of out-of-pocket spending for the medicines. The prescription habits of medical doctors according to current studies show that there is a tendency for overprescribing as well as irrational prescribing (e.g. use of brand names when generics are available).

The survey data from 2018 indicate that 94% of people using outpatient services received a prescription for medicines and, on average, four different medicines were prescribed per patient, and 97% of the patients paid for medicines out-of-pocket (KIIS & NaUKMA 2018).

Affordable Medicines Programme

A key component of the reform of the healthcare system is the design and implementation of the Affordable Medicines Programme (AMP) since April 2017 (World Health Organization 2019).

According to the prevalence and burden of diseases and in terms of medicines effectiveness in Ukraine, the State Expert Committee identified three key areas for the reimbursement of medication: cardiovascular diseases, type 2 diabetes and asthma.

The Ministry of Health granted 100% reimbursement for the cheapest products. In this programme, manufacturers and pharmacies are participating voluntarily.

As of September 2018, a total of 23 international nonproprietary name (INN) medicines are part of the scheme. These medicines are listed below (Table 9.1).

Figure 9.1 (World Health Organization 2019) represents how this system is working in practice

Medical doctors that are registered by the National Health Service of Ukraine are able to prescribe the medicines from the Affordable Medicines Programme list to the patients. Patient receives a paper-based or electronic prescription and goes to one of the 8000 pharmacies that participate in the programme. Pharmacy staff dispenses the medicines according to the prescription and reports to the regional government twice per month for the reimbursement. Regional governments in this case provide financing. The Ministry of Health allocates the responsible budget based on the population size by the regional government and is its responsibility to reimburse the prescriptions.

After the introduction of AMP in April 2017, the patients' access to medicines increased significantly. On average, 2 million prescriptions have been dispensed each month in the framework of the AMP programme. Altogether, up to September 2018, more than 28 million prescriptions have been reimbursed through the AMP. In 2017 more than 8 million Ukrainians benefited, of whom 7.2 million suffered from cardiovascular diseases, 700,000 from type 2 diabetes and about 160,000 from bronchial asthma. They account for half of the patients registered for these diseases (46%, 65% and 85% respectively).

Table 9.1 List of international nonproprietary name (INN) medicines that are currently reimbursed by the Affordable Medicines Programme in Ukraine (September 2018)

Cardiovascular diseases	Type 2 diabetes	Asthma
Amiodarone	Glibenclamide	Beclomethasone
Amlodipine	Gliclazide	Budesonide
Atenolol	Metformin	Salbutamol
Bisoprolol		
Verapamil		
Hydrochlorothiazide		
Digoxin		
Isosorbide dinitrate		
Carvedilol		
Clopidogrel		
Losartan		
Metoprolol		
Nitroglycerin		
Simvastatin		
Spironolactone		
Furosemide		
Enalapril		

The participation in the AMP seemed to be attractive for the pharmaceutical manufacturers' point of view as well. From April 2017 till June 2018, the use of a number of brand-name generics in the AMP programme increased from 6 to 15 for bronchial asthma medicines, from 24 to 43 for diabetes medicines and from 127 to 203 for cardiovascular medicines.

Between January 2016 and June 2018, the diabetes drugs consumption increased to 139%, antithrombotic agents to 441%, cardiovascular drugs to 117% and asthma drugs up to 50%. These growth rates exceed by far the dynamic of the rest of the market in the corresponding groups, and this also concludes that the increase in consumption is linked directly to implementation of the programme.

The AMP also had a significant impact on the prices of the medicines included. In all but one of the therapeutic areas covered (bronchial asthma), prices decreased after initiation, and this remained consistent over time. Such reductions were particularly significant for cardiovascular diseases—notably for lipid-modifying agents, diuretics and calcium

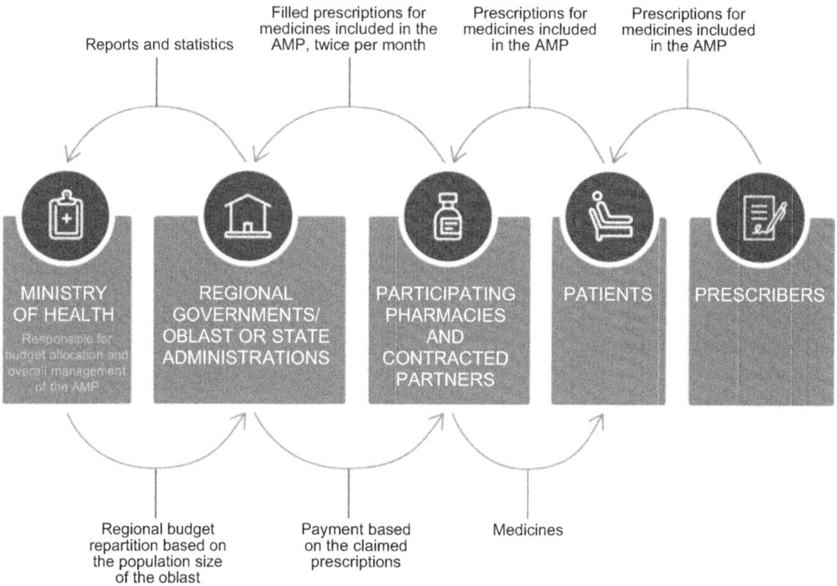

Fig. 9.1 The roadmap of the practical implementation of the Affordable Medicines Programme in Ukraine. (Source: Evaluation of the Affordable Medicines Programme in Ukraine. WHO 2019)

channel blockers (with reductions ranging from 30% to 40%). The programme led to an 85% average reduction in patient copayments, which is equivalent to a saving of 1020 hryvna annually, as is shown in Fig. 9.2 (World Health Organization 2019).

The programme received good feedback from the prescribers. They state that AMP provides increased access to medicines. For many of the patients, the programme was their only chance to receive treatment, especially in the case of vulnerable patients.

Access to Insulin

Diabetes is a significant public health issue in Ukraine. The official number of the diabetes prevalence is between 7 and 9%. According to WHO data, in 2016 about 9.1% of Ukrainian population had diabetes (8.3% of

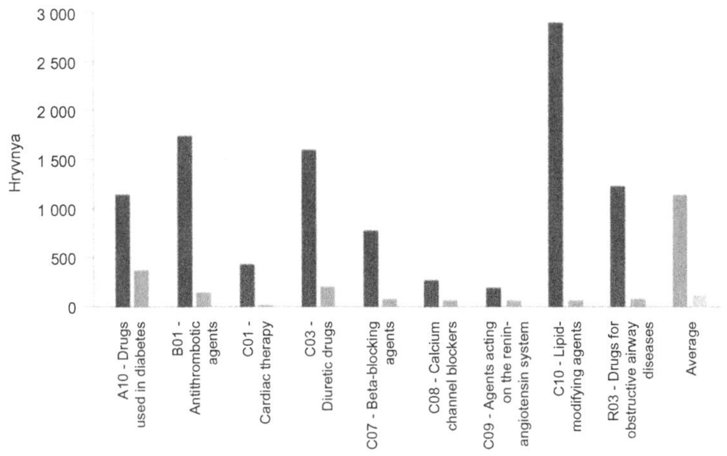

	A10	B01	C01	C03	C07	C08	C09	C10	R03	Average
Average annual co-payments before the initiation of the AMP (in hryvnya, for one patient)	1 144	1 738	434	1 596	776	272	195	2 893	1 228	1 142
Average annual co-payments after the initiation of the AMP (in hryvnya, for one patient)	372	146	18	205	79	67	64	65	81	122

Fig. 9.2 Annual copayments before and after implementation of the Affordable Medicines Programme in Ukraine (absolute values). (Source: Evaluation of the Affordable Medicines Programme in Ukraine. WHO 2019)

males and 9.7% of females, based on population of 44,824,000 people) (World Health Organization 2016). The World Bank defines the diabetes prevalence of 7.11% of population at the age between 20 and 79 years old (World Bank 2017). The International Diabetes Federation stated that in Ukraine the diabetes prevalence in adults is 8.4% of population (based on total number of 33,860,000 citizens). The real figures including undiagnosed diabetes might be even higher, because the prevalence of diabetes risk factors indicates that over 57% of Ukrainians are overweight, every fourth person has obesity (21.7%) and about 14.4% of the population is physically inactive.

The supply of insulin to patients with diabetes is one of the key functions of the national healthcare. The decentralization of the healthcare financing after Ukrainian independence in 1991 influenced the structure for insulin supply.

Formerly, before 2016, the public procurement of insulins was done by local governments using tender procedure. The funding was provided partly by the Ministry of Healthcare and by the local governments. However, this process had shown problems and was not efficient. In 2017, to overcome the challenges with the insulin supply, the state government made a decision for the introduction of the National Registry of patients with insulin-treated diabetes and implementation of the programme for insulin reimbursement (Ministry of Health Care of Ukraine 2017).

The "Bylaw № 239 of the Cabinet of Ministers of Ukraine from 23.03.2016" defines the key issues of the insulin reimbursement programme: groups of patients, as well as the type and dosage form of insulin they may receive, and reference prices. In the bylaw they also define the categories of patients that have the right to receive insulins free-of-charge or with the copayments (Table 9.2) (Cabinet of Ministers of Ukraine 2016).

The 40–50% financing of the insulin reimbursement was planned to be covered from the state budget, and the rest was supposed to be financed from the regional budgets. But this structure was not working properly in all regions, contributing to delays and complete stop of the dispensing of insulins due to insufficient reimbursement to pharmacies from the regional budgets.

However, starting from 2019, the state government guaranteed to reimburse 100% of insulins in all regions of the country. The total budget allocation for insulin programme was 925 million hryvna (about 31 million euros) (Segodnya.ua 2018).

Since 2016 the government and Ministry of Health Care introduced a range of new regulatory and financial mechanisms to improve access to insulins for diabetes patients in Ukraine. The National Registry enables the new precise data aggregation and evaluation to define the current number and need of patients for the insulin supply. The reimbursement procedures enable the access to insulin for patients free-of-charge or with copayment in all regions of Ukraine.

Table 9.2 List of diabetes patient categories for the reimbursement of insulins in Ukraine according to the Bylaw № 239 of the Cabinet of Ministers of Ukraine from 23.03.2016

	Category of patients with diabetes that receive defined art and form of insulin	Art of insulin	Reimbursement
1.	Adults that were diagnosed with diabetes after 18 years old	Human insulin (flacon)	Full reimbursement
2.	Adults that have diabetes since childhood	Human insulin (cartridge, insulin pen)	
3.	Pupils of schools or students of higher educational establishments	Human insulin (cartridge, insulin pen)	
4.	Diabetes patients with a condition, when vision with correction makes less than 0.4 for an eye that sees better	Human insulin (cartridge, insulin pen)	
5.	Diabetes patients with allergy on insulin (documented in specialized endocrinologic inpatient facility)	Human insulin (flacon, cartridge) or insulin analogue (flacon, cartridge, insulin pen)	
6.	Children younger than 18 years old and pregnant women	Human insulin or insulin analogue (cartridge, insulin pen)	
7.	Diabetes patients that received insulin analogues in the age younger than 18 years with a satisfactory disease compensation (HbA1c<7.5%)[a]	Insulin analogue (flacon, cartridge, insulin pen)	
8.	Adults that formerly received continuous treatment with insulin analogues. By the treatment duration not less than 1 year, HbA1c<7.5%[a]	Insulin analogue (flacon, cartridge, insulin pen)	
	Adults that received insulin analogues and have HbA1c>7.5%, but had often acute diabetic complications (severe hypoglycaemic conditions)[a]	Insulin analogue (flacon, cartridge, insulin pen)	
9.	Adults that formerly received continuous treatment with human insulin in cartridges. By the treatment duration not less than 1 year, HbA1c<7.5%[a]	Human insulin (cartridge, insulin pen)	

(continued)

Table 9.2 (continued)

	Category of patients with diabetes that receive defined art and form of insulin	Art of insulin	Reimbursement
10.	Adult patients, diagnosed with diabetes after 18 years, that receive human insulin in flacons for the first time. By willingness to co-finance the human insulin in cartridge form, insulin pen	Human insulin (cartridge, insulin pen)	Partial reimbursement
11.	Adults that receive human insulin and don't have contraindication for the use of insulin analogues and are willing to co-finance the price for insulin analogues	Insulin analogue (cartridge, insulin pen)	

[a]During the first year after the introduction of the bylaw, in following diabetes patient's category, the HbA1c level must not be higher than 8%. In patients older than 65 years with two or more macrovascular events in the anamneses (myocardial infarction and/or stroke) that are proven by ECG and/or MRT/CT of the brain, the HbA1c level must not be higher than 8.5%

Conclusions

Since 2017, the Ukrainian government has increased its efforts to improve the efficiency and quality of the healthcare services, as well as to increase the financial protection for its citizens. It has also instituted mechanisms to enable the access to essential medicines including insulins. The healthcare reform and new financing mechanisms in Ukraine received a positive feedback from the international organizations such as WHO and World Bank. Based on the analysis of current situation, it is concluded that the efforts of the Ukrainian government in the health financing reform and Affordable Medicines Programme were successful and these programmes should be continued. In the future, more attention is needed to evaluate reform results, restructure the hospitals and further extend the Affordable Medicines Programme.

References

Cabinet of Ministers of Ukraine. (2016, 03 23). Bylaw 239 "Some questions of the insulin reimbursement". Kyiv. Retrieved from https://zakon.rada.gov.ua/laws/show/239-2016-п

Cabinet of Ministers of Ukraine. (2017, 12 13). National List of Essential Medicines. Bylaw 1081. Kyiv, Kyiv, Ukraine.

Goroshko A. S. N. (2018). *Can people afford to pay for health care? New evidence on financial protection in Ukraine.* Copenhagen: WHO Regional Office for Europe.

Institute for Health Metrics and Evaluation, U. P. (2019, 12 02). Retrieved from http://www.healthdata.org/ukraine

KIIS&NaUKMA. (2018). *Health Index Ukraine 2019. Results of the National Household Survey.* Kyiv: Kyiv International Institute of Sociology (KIIS). National University of Kyiv-Mohyla Academy (NaUKMA). Retrieved from http://health-index.com.ua/zvit_index_2018_eng.pdf

Lekhan V. R. V. (2015, 01 01). Ukraine. Health System Review. *Health Systems in Transition, 17*(2), pp. 1–153.

Ministry of Health Care of Ukraine. (2017, 10 23). *Cabinet of Ministers of Ukraine – News.* Retrieved from https://www.kmu.gov.ua/news/250365837

National Health Service of Ukraine. (2019, 12 02). Retrieved from https://nszu.gov.ua/en

Parliament of Ukraine. (2018, 10 19). Law of Ukraine About state financial guarantees of health service for population 2168-VIII. *Відомості Верховної Ради*(5), p. 31.

Parliament of Ukraine. (2019, 02 07). Constitution of Ukraine, Article 49. *Відомості Верховної Ради України*(9), p. 50.

Segodnya.ua. (2018, 10 19). Insulin 2019 will be fully paid by state-Ministry of Health. Retrieved from https://ukr.segodnya.ua/economics/enews/insulin-v-2019-godu-polnostyu-oplatit-gosudarstvo-minzdrav-1181211.html

SSUMDC. (2018, 11 23). *Licence registry for production of medicines (in the pharmacy), wholesale and retail of medicines.* Retrieved from http://dls.gov.ua/державні-реєстри/ліцензійний-реєстр-з-виробництва-лік/

State Service of Ukraine on Medicines and Drugs Control. (2019, 03 13). Retrieved from http://dls.gov.ua/en/state-service-of-ukraine-on-medicines-and-drugs-control/

UNIAN Information Agency. (2018, 11 20). Retrieved from unian.info: https://www.unian.info/society/10344180-deaths-in-ukraine-almost-twice-birth-rate-in-nine-months-document.html

WHO&World Bank. (2019). *Ukraine: Review of Health Financing Reforms 2016–2019. WHO-World Bank Joint Report.* Copenhagen: World Health Organization.

World Bank. (2017). *The World Bank Data. Diabetes Prevalence.* Retrieved from https://data.worldbank.org/indicator/SH.STA.DIAB.ZS?view=map

World Bank Data, C. P. (2019, 12 02). Retrieved from https://data.worldbank.org/country/ukraine

World Health Organization. (2016). *Diabetes Country Profiles-Ukraine.* Retrieved from https://www.who.int/diabetes/country-profiles/ukr_en.pdf?ua=1

World Health Organization. (2019). *Evaluation of Affordable Medicines Programme in Ukraine.* Copenhagen: World Health Organization.

World Health Organization, C. P. (2019, 12 02). Retrieved from https://www.who.int/countries/ukr/en/

10

Public Participation in Access to Medicines

Sofia Crisóstomo and Filipa Alves da Costa

Context

Citizens have the right to participate in health decision-making (Declaration of Alma-Ata 1978; Council of Europe 2000), with participation at political and institutional levels commonly taking place through representative organizations—usually organizations of people living with disease or health service users and in some cases consumer organizations. Public involvement, either individually or through representative

S. Crisóstomo (✉)
The Centre for Research and Studies in Sociology (CIES-IUL), University Institute of Lisbon (ISCTE-IUL), Lisbon, Portugal

Treatment Activists Group (GAT), Lisbon, Portugal

F. A. da Costa
Centre for Interdisciplinary Research Egas Moniz (CiiEM), University Institute Egas Moniz, Caparica, Portugal

Research Institute for Medicines (iMED.ULisboa), Faculty of Pharmacy, University of Lisbon, Lisbon, Portugal

Z. Babar (ed.), *Global Pharmaceutical Policy*,
https://doi.org/10.1007/978-981-15-2724-1_10

organizations, in collective decision-making in health, i.e. decisions about health policy and services, is usually referred to as public participation, to differentiate from individual involvement in decisions about one's own health, together with health professionals—also known as shared decision-making (Florin 2004; Mitton et al. 2009).

By contributing with citizens' perspective to inform collective decision-making, representative organizations play a key role not only in defending the rights and interests of their constituency (Council of Europe 2000; European Patients' Forum 2015) but also in strengthening health governance (European Patients' Forum 2015; Kickbusch and Gleicher 2012) and pushing for people-centred health systems (World Health Organization 2016). Citizens' experiential knowledge about the health system and healthcare delivery and, where applicable, of living with disease is crucial to align health policy with people's unmet needs and societal preferences and make services more responsive to the individuals and communities (World Health Organization 2016; Ives et al. 2013; International Alliance of Patients' Organizations 2005; Frankish et al. 2002) and thus improve the quality of decision-making and facilitate its implementation (Tallon et al. 2000; Barnes et al. 2008; Van De Bovenkamp et al. 2010). Together with citizens' empowerment, health outcomes will improve (Florin 2004; Van De Bovenkamp et al. 2010). Public involvement in health decision-making leads to democratic decision-making and, in turn, to increased legitimacy and better accountability (Council of Europe 2000; Kickbusch and Gleicher 2012; Tritter and McCallum 2006; Cooper et al. 1995).

Civil society organizations, in particular, advocacy organizations for people living with disease, have been at the forefront calling for greater and meaningful public participation at all levels (national, regional and local) and areas of health decision-making, including policy making, service organization and delivery (European Patients' Forum 2015; International Alliance of Patients' Organizations 2005; Terzi 2013). Other health stakeholders, like the World Health Organization (Declaration of Alma-Ata 1978; World Health Organization 2016), the Organisation for Economic Co-operation and Development (2001), the European Council and the European Commission (2007), also joined the movement by calling for and supporting increased public participation in health systems.

Consequently, various initiatives to promote public participation in health decision-making have been implemented across the world. Formal spaces are currently in place to involve citizens in medicines research, regulatory procedures or health technology assessment, to name a few. National advocacy organizations, which are increasingly organized under global or regional umbrella organizations, have thus an increasing outreach and influence, by informing medicines development and other decision-making and advocating for early and equal access to medicines.

Public Participation in Medicines Use and Access Research

The demand from organizations of people living with disease for involvement in research–initiated in the 1980s by the HIV/AIDS movement—has grown with increasing support from other stakeholders. These resulted from advocacy efforts to put public participation in the health agenda, the arising evidence of differences between beliefs and perceptions of researchers, health professionals and other decision-makers from the needs and preferences directly expressed by individuals or the community (Montgomery and Fahey 2001; Sewitch et al. 2003; Harrison 2008; da Silva et al. 2010; Miravitlles et al. 2013). The value of public participation in medicines research and development, particularly when it comes to the involvement of people living with disease and their representative organizations, is now widely recognized by other health stakeholders, especially among those most directly involved in research and development—scientists, pharmaceutical companies and research funding agencies. Despite the prevalence of public engagement in research still being poor (Fergusson et al. 2018), this scenario is expected to change dramatically in the coming years given the increasing trend towards a people-centred approach.

Organizations of people living with disease may contribute to optimize pharmaceutical research and better meet the needs and preferences of medicine users and trial participants, by being involved in trial design (Sacristan et al. 2016; Geissler et al. 2017; Cook et al. 2019) and ethical or safety reviews (Regulation (EU) 2014; AVAC 2011), in improving access to clinical trials (Sacristan et al. 2016; Huang et al. 2018) or in co-developing materials for trial participants or lay summaries of trial results (Sacristan et al. 2016; Summaries of Clinical Trial Results for Laypersons 2018). Furthermore, they may be involved in the identification of daily challenges of medicines use and strategies to address those challenges (Sacristan et al. 2016; Garfield et al. 2016), thus contributing to better use across the medicines lifecycle. Advocacy organizations are also increasingly engaged in setting the research agenda and raising funds for research (Sacristan et al. 2016; Oliver 2006), most commonly for rare or neglected diseases (Mavris and Le Cam 2012).

In an attempt to establish a structured approach and standards for public engagement in health research, various organizations in different countries have set their guidance on public participation—e.g. the US Patient-Centered Outcomes Research Institute (PCORI) (2016), the Canadian Institutes of Health Research (2014) and the INVOLVE advisory group from the UK National Institute for Health Research (NIHR) (2018). Current existing guidance establishes public involvement from early stages of pharmaceutical research throughout the whole duration of medicines lifecycle, in a process of co-production, where research is made with and by individuals and communities, in order to deliver medicines and outcomes that are relevant to them and better address their needs and preferences. The European Patients' Academy (EUPATI), a pan-European consortium, which includes organizations of people living with disease, academic groups, non-governmental organizations (NGOs) and pharmaceutical companies, besides issuing specific guidance on patient involvement in medicines research and development (Warner et al. 2018), also addressed patient involvement in ethical review of clinical trials (Klingmann et al. 2018) and rolled-out a comprehensive training programme for patient experts in pharmaceutical development.

As part of the discussions on patient and people-centricity in research, several organizations have emphasized the importance of patient-reported outcome measures (PROMs). Quality of life (QoL) conceptualization started in the 1990s, and not long after that, clinical trials started to include it as an endpoint. However, QoL has sometimes been confused with experienced symptoms. A breast cancer trial comparing tamoxifen with placebo showed similar results in physical and psychological functioning, although higher frequency of various symptoms was reported by patients on tamoxifen (Ganz 2001). These findings highlight the need to consider PROs and patient-reported experiences (PREs), which according to the illness, severity and phase of disease may be valued differently by people living with illness, in research and in clinical practice. Subsequent trials comparing tamoxifen with anastrozole opened the door to shared decision-making, using results to inform women about drug-induced symptoms associated with each drug (Ganz et al. 2016). PROs are valued by regulators [although the European Medicines Agency (EMA) seems to be more likely to accept PRO data compared to the US Food and Drugs Administration (FDA)], pharmaceutical industry and the public, but to date debate continues as to which are the most suitable outcomes to be measured (Kluetz et al. 2016). Public engagement in this debate is also important because consensus may only be reached once all stakeholders are involved. Another recent trend in research has been the development of core outcomes sets (COS) that could be recommended for use in any study so that, in the future, indirect comparisons and meta-analysis are more common and easier to perform. Evidence showing that outcomes prioritized by patients do not always coincide with those prioritized by health professionals and disease experts (Milman et al. 2019) has also pushed for patient engagement in COS development, progressively extending into various disease areas.

More recently, patient and public involvement extended to medical research journals. The *British Medical Journal* is leading this effort, through a structured strategy (Richards et al. 2015) introducing several editorial changes: requesting authors of research papers to document patient and public involvement in the research question; requesting authors of other articles to co-produce their papers with patients and carers; subjecting all relevant research papers to patient review; publishing a monthly patient-led, patient (and carer) written series called "What Your Patient Is Thinking"; publishing examples of initiatives where patients and health professionals are working together to co-produce change; and appointing patient and carer editors as members of the editorial team.

Patient advocacy organizations aiming to raise awareness about the use of patient data and building confidence on their use to improve outcomes have also emerged. "Use My Data" is one such organization that created a patient data citation "This work uses data provided by patients and collected by the NHS as part of their care and support" to acknowledge the use of their data.

Another important development is the consideration of patient and public participation in research funding calls. The US PCORI has an engagement award in place where patients participate as reviewers of research funding applications, and patient engagement is a merit review criterion (PCORI 2019). In research programmes funded through the UK NIHR, research applicants have to describe patient and public involvement in the development of their research proposal and in the research study itself (National Institute for Health Research 2017). Public engagement has also been integrated in the European Union research and innovation programme (European Commission 2020) through the establishment of participatory multi-actor dialogues, co-creation of research and innovation and input to policy agendas.

Finally, public participation and involvement is the basis for people-centred research and evidence, and in the upcoming future, it will become increasingly relevant for the subsequent dialogue with regulators, health technology assessment (HTA) bodies and payers. Therefore, public participation may and should take place in all research phases and activities, including in the identification of research gaps and priorities, definition of research strategies, development of research protocols or PROMs, training of researchers and community experts, publication of results and funding calls.

Public Participation in Regulatory Agencies: FDA and EMA

Both leading agencies in pharmaceutical regulation—FDA and EMA—have a long history of public and patient engagement, though with greater focus on the latter. Patient and public involvement is now well-established and acknowledged as a positive and added-value experience, providing a crucial and unique "real-life" perspective in scientific discussions on medicines and, therefore, contributing to better outcomes of the regulatory process (e.g. increased transparency and trust, or enriched quality of the opinion given by the scientific committees).

In the US, the HIV/AIDS movement pushed for changes in regulatory approval processes at FDA, marking the beginning of patient engagement in FDA activities (Food and Drug Administration n.d.). In 1988, FDA founded an HIV/AIDS patient group and, three years later, this group expanded to include cancer and other conditions. The same year (1991) a patient representative sat for the first time at an FDA Advisory Committee, and in 1996, patient representatives received voting rights. In 2001, as part of the FDA Patient Representative Program, patients became consultants for the regulatory medical product review process. Today, under this programme, over 200 FDA patient representatives—patients or primary caregivers—share their knowledge and experience of living with one or more conditions and participate in FDA Advisory Committees and panels, providing direct input to the decision-making process associated with medical products for drugs, biologics and medical devices. Training is provided by the FDA to patient representatives, through webinars, workshops, mentoring by senior representatives and one-on-one support as needed.

Over the last decade, several other institutional mechanisms have been put in place by the FDA to expand and evolve patient engagement. In 2012, the FDA Patient Network web page was launched. The same year, FDA launched the Patient-Focused Drug Development initiative to systematically gather patients' perspectives on conditions and treatments. Under this initiative, a glossary was developed to provide standardized nomenclature and terminologies and 24 disease-specific meetings were conducted, with summaries of patients and patient representatives' input provided at these public meetings published through a series of reports called "The Voice of the Patient". In 2013, FDA established a discussion group that later evolved to become the FDA Patient Council, which brings together all FDA centres and offices to better coordinate and integrate the role of patient perspectives in regulatory decision-making over the product lifecycle. In 2015, FDA released the Patient Preference Information framework and guidance and held the first Patient Engagement Advisory Committee to provide advice on complex issues relating to medical devices, the regulation of devices and their use by patients. In 2017, FDA together with the Clinical Trials Transformation Initiative created the Patient Engagement Collaborative, a working group with patient advocacy organizations to discuss how to achieve more meaningful patient engagement at FDA, including in product development and other regulatory discussions. The Patient Engagement Collaborative is led by the FDA's Patient Affairs Staff, which was also launched the same year and is responsible for the coordination of agency-wide and cross-centre projects related to patient engagement.

More recently, FDA signed a Memorandum of Understanding (MOU) with the National Organization for Rare Disorders (NORD) to promote early and iterative patient engagement into clinical and regulatory discussions, through rare disease listening sessions aimed at providing a common understanding of the most urgent needs and informing drug development programmes. FDA is also developing a series of four methodological patient-focused drug development guidance documents on (i) collecting comprehensive and representative input; (ii) methods to identify what is important to patients; (iii) selecting, developing or modifying fit-for-purpose clinical outcomes assessments (COA); and (iv) COA-related endpoint development and interpretation. These guidance documents are intended "to facilitate the advancement and use of systematic approaches to collect and use robust and meaningful patient and caregiver input that can better inform product development and regulatory decision making". The latest development has been the launch of the online portal "Request to Connect", where patients and caregivers can ask questions to the FDA or request meetings to share disease experiences or better understand the FDA's work.

In Europe, EMA and patients have been actively interacting since the creation of the agency in 1995 to "bring a 'real-life' experience as well as specific knowledge and expertise to scientific discussions on medicines and on the impact of regulatory decisions" (European Medicines Agency n.d.). In 1996 the first dialogue with patients was established, and in 2000, patients became committee members. In 2003, this engagement extended to consumer groups, but it was only in 2005 that a framework for interaction with patients' and consumers' organizations was endorsed by EMA's Management Board. This framework describes the scope, objectives and working methodology for involving patients and consumers in the agency's activities and aims at supporting EMA to assess disease experiences, their management and information on current use of medicines, contributing to more efficient and targeted communication to patients and consumers and enhancing understanding of the role of the EU medicines regulatory network. In 2006, EMA put in place the Patients' and Consumers' Working Party, a platform for information exchange and discussion of common interest issues between EMA, patients and consumers, also providing recommendations to EMA and its human scientific committees on all matters of interest in relation to medicines. In 2014, EMA's Public Engagement Department was established, and since 2017, EMA has been conducting public hearings and involving young people too.

Currently, patients and consumers are involved in a wide range of activities at EMA. They are members of the Management Board and scientific committees, where they have equal voting capacity as formal members. They are also consulted on disease-specific requests by the scientific committees and working parties and take part in discussions on the development and authorization of medicines. Other activities where patients and consumers are involved include the review of written information on medicines prepared by EMA, preparation of guidelines and involvement in EMA's conferences. EMA provides training sessions to patient and consumer representatives invited to participate in its activities plus a collection of training videos and documents for anyone interested in learning more about EMA's activities.

The work done by both FDA and EMA on public and patient involvement has led these agencies to join efforts and create a working group called the FDA/EMA Patient Engagement Cluster, to share best practices involving patients along drug and biologic regulatory lifecycles. Other regulatory authorities around the world have then started to engage patients and members of the public, but such initiatives are mostly still in the planning or pilot stage. Those that have not yet begun will surely follow soon. With this context in mind, EUPATI published in 2018 a dedicated guidance for patient involvement in regulatory processes, at national and European level (Haerry et al. 2018).

Public Participation in HTA

Involving patients and the public in HTA is not about advocating for a particular health technology but rather about better reflecting public needs and preferences in HTA and increasing the relevance of decision-making. In addition, it responds to the quest from patients and public for increased transparency and knowledge about HTA decision-making (Knox 2009). Although patient and public involvement in HTA varies across agencies and countries and in many cases improvement is needed to achieve meaningful involvement in HTA, there is growing interest for patients' experiences and preferences (Boutin et al. 2017; Scott and Wale 2017; Hunter et al. 2018).

Probably the widest experience of patient and public involvement in HTA has been gained with the UK National Institute for Health and Care Excellence (NICE). NICE involves patients, service users, carers and the public, including voluntary, charitable and community organizations, in its work, since 1999. As part of NICE patient and public involvement policy (National Institute for Health and Care Excellence 2019), patients, service users, carers and the public can be involved directly, as formal members of committees and working groups, in producing or promoting guidance documents and quality standards among others. They can also be involved in commenting draft guidance scopes and recommendations and by submitting evidence. Patient, service user, carer and public involvement is developed and supported by a NICE dedicated team—the Public Involvement Programme (PIP). Working alongside the PIP, there is an independent coalition of over 80 patient organizations—Patients Involved in NICE (PIN)—that provides patient organizations with a system of mutual support and information sharing enabling them to engage productively with NICE and to act as equal partners in developing and shaping aspects of NICE work. NICE also has a Citizens Council—a panel of 30 citizens—that addresses challenging questions, including fairness of resource allocation and needs prioritization to be considered when producing guidance.

The Canadian Agency for Drugs and Technologies in Health (CADTH) was one of the first HTA agencies to follow NICE's approach to patient and public involvement early in 2010 (Boutin et al. 2017). In 2013,

CADTH launched the Patient Community Liaison Forum which for five years contributed to develop a formal approach to incorporating patients' perspectives within CADTH. In 2019, the CADTH Framework for Patient Engagement in HTA was published, setting out "why CADTH engages with patients, families, and communities, with a focus on how CADTH engages, and with who, across different programs and processes". CADTH also has put in place a Patient and Community Advisory Committee, to provide CADTH with "advice on issues relevant to its mandate, from the perspective of those using the Canadian healthcare system". Input from patient groups is also considered by the Canadian Drug Expert Committee (CDEC) in the CADTH Scientific Advice Program and when making formulary listing recommendations, as part of the Common Drug Review.

In Germany, patient perspective is also taken into consideration in benefit assessment performed by the Institute for Quality and Efficiency in Health Care (IQWiG) (n.d.). This can be done through the spokesperson of the coordination committee of patient representatives at the Federal Joint Committee (G-BA). Patients may also directly approach IQWiG at different stages of the benefit assessment process, for example, by submitting comments on preliminary reports and report plans, participating in discussions of patient-relevant outcomes, providing patients' perspectives and proposing topics for HTA reports. Patient and the public are also represented in the IQWiG Board of Trustees, which includes five representatives of patient organizations and one patient representative commissioned by the Federal government—the Federal Commissioner for Patients' Affairs—among its 30 members.

More recently, subsequently to some pressure from a patient and consumer group initiative to advance public participation in health decision-making (Crisóstomo and Santos 2018), the Portuguese National Authority of Medicines and Health Product (INFARMED) launched an initiative to include patient input in HTA of new medicines (INFARMED 2019). After public consultation, the framework document for patient involvement at the agency was published in 2018. This sought the involvement of patient organizations, in particular within the PICO (population, intervention, comparator and outcomes) framework to inform HTA.

Given the varying extent and quality of patient involvement in HTA across countries and in order to improve patient involvement in HTA, EUPATI has issued guidance on the interaction between HTA bodies and patients and their representatives in medicines assessment. The guidance provides recommendations for supporting patient involvement in HTA and specific guidance for individual HTA processes (Hunter et al. 2018).

Case Studies

Selected case studies, illustrating how public and patient involvement played a key role in securing access to medicines, are presented in this section.

HIV Infection

Back in the 1980s when the HIV/AIDS epidemics arose, people were struggling with a lack of an effective treatment that could prevent infected people from dying shortly after diagnosis. Fear and stigma led to generalized discrimination of people with HIV/AIDS. Simultaneously, governments and social and health services lacked appropriate answers to the growing epidemics. Such context boosted the genesis of the HIV/AIDS social movement, where people with HIV/AIDS and members of the affected communities joined together to pledge for societal support and non-discrimination, involvement at every level of decision-making, access to experimental treatments and information about treatment risks and benefits to be able to engage in informed decisions (Advisory Committee 1983).

The first promising treatment identified was zidovudine (AZT). However, the regulations clearly stated that for this drug to be approved and available to all, research trials had first to demonstrate its efficacy and safety. Such trials normally had a minimum duration of eight years, during which access to AZT was restricted to those enrolled in the clinical trial. In addition, as in every trial, participants would have a 50% chance of taking the active drug (AZT) and another 50% of receiving a placebo (as there was no alternative treatment by then). People infected with HIV could not afford waiting that long to be treated or take the chance of not getting a "real treatment". As a result, many individuals organized in informal buyers' clubs started to import drugs not yet approved by the FDA that they thought might be useful in treating HIV and opportunistic infections, including cheaper counterfeit versions of AZT. Under a huge pressure from HIV/AIDS advocates, the AZT trial was stopped prematurely, because patients on the placebo group were dying faster. As a result, AZT was approved in 1987 by the FDA, in a record time and including only the results of one single and unfinished trial in humans. In fact, the plan was to involve 282 patients for 24 weeks, but when the trial was interrupted, data was available for 179 patients, of which 27 had completed the 24 weeks, 152 had completed 16 weeks and the remainder had completed between 8 and 16 weeks (Fischl et al. 1987). It was considered that the need to meet an unmet medical need outweighed the demand for additional efficacy and safety data. This decision was strongly based on one of the fundamental ethical pillars, the principle of benevolence, i.e. it would be unethical to deprive patients from a potentially life-saving treatment.

After AZT's approval, concerns arose about the high cost of treatment, the lack of political will and funding for research and how such factors would jeopardize equitable access to safe and effective treatment for HIV/AIDS and opportunistic infections. Such concerns led HIV/AIDS activists to continue advocating for changes to secure a faster access to safe and effective medicines and equal access for everyone in need, including an accelerated approval process. This implied fighting against double-blind placebo trials and in favour of including all affected population in clinical trials, alongside meaningful involvement in decision-making—a claim institutionalized under the motto "nothing about us, without us" (Crimp 2011; Lessem 2019). Following huge protests like the "Seize Control of the FDA" (1988) and the "Storm the NIH" (1990) demonstrations, the investment in HIV/AIDS research dramatically increased and major changes took place on the conduction of clinical trials and medicines approval process. Advocacy groups were involved in redesigning clinical trial protocols and influencing FDA and NIH discussions, paving the way for accelerated development and access to highly effective combination antiretroviral therapy (1996) and ultimately for the range of prevention and treatment options available today.

During the 2000s, HIV advocacy groups played a key role in calling for policy and organizational changes needed to reduce the barriers to testing and treatment and achieving earlier diagnosis, linkage to care and sustained treatment and viral suppression. More recently, they have also pushed for research, approval and public financing of HIV pre-exposure prophylaxis (PrEP), while informal buyers' clubs resurged, this time to procure generic PrEP internationally, ramping the pressure on decision-makers. Today as before, equitable access to prevention and treatment continues on the top priorities of the HIV activists, who keep asking for a reduction in medicines prices, challenging patent rights and advocating for the importance of community engagement and research on HIV prevention, diagnostics, treatment of co-infections and cure.

Hepatitis C

Hepatitis C virus (HCV) has for long been on top of the most prevalent HIV co-infections. HCV infection was particularly worrisome, both in clinical and epidemiological terms, as effective treatments were inexistent. Direct-acting antivirals (DAAs) marked a shift in the treatment paradigm of HCV infection, from a disease representing a major public health threat to a disease where all infected people can be expected to achieve cure. DAAs are safer, better tolerated and more efficacious than interferon-based therapies, offering over 95% sustained viral response, including in patients with HIV infection and injectable drug users and independently of prior treatment experience and presence of cirrhosis. DAAs offer for the first time the possibility to eliminate HCV epidemics (Heffernan et al. 2019).

Notwithstanding, the extremely high price but outstanding comparative efficacy of DAA-containing regimens, combined with a 1% global prevalence of HCV infection (World Health Organization 2017), has put huge pressure on governments and payers that were not prepared to deal with the challenges of this new "cost-effective but unaffordable" paradox (Lomas et al. 2018). Restrictive policies on access to DAA treatment were then imposed in an attempt to contain the impact on healthcare budgets. In the US, the high prices of DAAs prompted health plans and payers to institute restrictions based on the liver fibrosis stage, the documented alcohol and drug abstinence and the practitioner's clinical specialty and complex preauthorization procedures for treatment (Millman et al. 2017). In the UK, NICE deemed DAAs as cost-effective for treating many patients with HCV, but the implementation period of NICE guidance was extended beyond the usual timeframe (Lomas et al. 2018). In Australia, the Pharmaceutical Benefits Advisory Committee (PBAC) judged DAAs by more stringent criteria (a lower cost per QALY "threshold") than the usually considered, given the significance of the estimated budget impact (Lomas et al. 2018). In Portugal, treatment with DAAs was initially restricted to patients with severe cirrhosis who required a liver transplant (Douglass et al. 2018). In Brazil, the National Committee for Technology Incorporation in the National Health System (CONITEC) recommended the inclusion of DAAs for HCV treatment, but excluding patients at F1 and F2 fibrosis stages (Kieslich et al. 2016).

Such policies posed a substantial barrier to treating people with HCV. As a result, learnings and tactics from the HIV/AIDS social movement have been taken over by HCV advocacy groups to force pharmaceutical companies to lower DAA prices and governments and payers to secure equitable access and to scale-up HCV testing and treatment, including to the most vulnerable and affected populations (e.g. people co-infected with HIV and/or injectable drug users). These included meeting directly with representatives from governments and pharmaceutical companies to discuss prices; challenging intellectual property rights through patent oppositions and advocacy for the use of compulsory licenses; collaborating with researchers, healthcare professionals and policy makers to build the case for unrestricted HCV treatment access; and establishing buyers' clubs (Kaplan 2015; Grillon et al. 2018).

In the US, some states and insurers have relaxed their rules and begun to lift restrictions in response to pressure and lawsuits filled by individuals with HCV and advocacy groups (Chapman and Buckley 2017).

Pharmaceutical companies have also come under pressure to disclose information about the development costs and profits of these drugs and to explain the pricing rationale (Chapman and Buckley 2017).

In countries where buyers' clubs operated effectively (including in Australia, New Zealand, Italy and Switzerland), advantageous price reductions and risk-sharing agreements for DAAs were finalized rapidly (Grillon et al. 2018). For example, in Australia, a volume-based risk-sharing deal capped treatment costs at a fixed total amount annually, regardless of the number of people treated, with excess costs covered by pharmaceutical companies (Douglass et al. 2018). In Portugal, a risk-sharing and volume-based agreement was also signed (Douglass et al. 2018), but only after a fierce advocacy campaign in the media and at the parliament that put an end to a negotiation process lasting over two years. Access to treatment with DAAs regardless of fibrosis stage was granted, and only treatment leading to cure was paid.

Voluntary licenses also improved access to affordable generic medicines in low- and some middle-income countries, excluding from the latter those with high hepatitis C burdens (Douglass et al. 2018; Grillon et al. 2018). Malaysia issued a compulsory license. DAA patent applications were rejected by the Egyptian patent office. DAA patents were also opposed by civil society organizations in Argentina, Brazil, China, India, Russia, Ukraine and the US, while HCV treatment rationing in high-income countries led a coalition of civil society organizations and patient groups to oppose patents on HCV medicines before the European patent office. These initiatives led to the rejection or substantial weakening of key patents in several countries. Mercosur countries (Argentina, Brazil, Paraguay, Uruguay and Venezuela) and other associated countries (Chile, Colombia, Peru and Ecuador) completed, in 2015, the first joint procurement of DAAs. In Europe, concerns from the public and politicians over the availability and affordability of DAAs also opened the door to intergovernmental initiatives involving joint price negotiations and sharing of information on medicines prices and contractual agreements such as the Benelux Initiative on Pharmaceutical Policy (created in 2015 and involving Belgium, Netherlands, Luxemburg, Austria and Ireland) or the Valletta Declaration (created in 2017 and signed by Spain, Italy, Portugal, Greece, Malta, Cyprus, Ireland, Romania,

Slovenia and Croatia). Nevertheless, DAAs have not yet been addressed by these initiatives. Other alternative approaches proposed by HCV activists to increase access include new research and development paradigms and compassionate use, named-patient and early access programmes (Grillon et al. 2018).

Cancer

Public participation in cancer research, as well as in regulatory and funding decisions, has grown widely in the last decade (Pii et al. 2019), building upon many years of previous work on raising awareness on cancer prevention and early diagnosis. Most involvement experiences originate in the US or the UK, and breast cancer, as the most prevalent cancer type, has the longest history of public involvement. Unlike the experience in viral infections, where activism was, in many cases, in confront with pharmaceutical industry's interests, the major challenge in cancer has been the recognition of the added value of patients' involvement—given their unique perspective about living with a chronic condition and taking life-saving or life-prolonging treatments, which often seriously impair quality of life—in the face of decision-makers' perception of co-optation of patient organizations by pharmaceutical industry.

Various studies highlight the discrepancies between patients' and physicians' preferences about treatment and, consequently, the importance of adequately and clearly conveying risks and benefits associated with treatments. The time trade-offs for marginal benefits of chemotherapy were shown to vary significantly between patients and physicians. For example, Vaz-Luis et al. showed that 34% of patients, compared to 5% of physicians, would be willing to accept 6-month chemotherapy regimens leading to 2 months of additional survival (Vaz-Luis et al. 2017). Conversely, patients seem to value adverse events according to their impact on psychological, social and holistic well-being. Hair and nail loss is an example of a common adverse event in chemotherapy treatment, highly rated by women and undervalued by clinicians (Dika et al. 2016). Patients' willingness to accept or tolerate toxic effects is also related to the cancer type and particularly with the associated chance of cure and expected survival gain. Not surprisingly, lung cancer patients were shown to better accept dermatological toxicities of targeted therapies than breast cancer patients (Castellanos et al. 2015). Although cancer treatments are progressively becoming safer, even with the development of the so-called targeted therapies, the proportion of patients experiencing at least one type of toxicity is often above 75% (Macdonald et al. 2015). Recognizing the need to involve patients in reporting adverse events, adaptions of the Common Terminology Criteria for Adverse Events have been developed for citizens (Trask et al. 2018).

Another important issue is the patient's perspective on treatments' impact on quality of life (QoL), which should be taken into consideration in clinical trials and in real-world studies. Nonetheless, QoL as an endpoint is still only included in around half of phase III trials and, of these, a minority consider it a primary endpoint (Marandino et al. 2018). Furthermore, the impact of treatments on important aspects of patients' life is still poorly and inconsistently captured (Catt et al. 2017). PROs seem to be more a "back-up" measure (in case other endpoints traditionally seen as more robust like overall survival fail to demonstrate clear benefits), rather than a true effort to assess the patient's perspective.

One of the main goals of cancer advocacy groups has been to communicate the patients' perspective on cancer treatment benefits and risks and to put civil society, healthcare providers and decision-makers at the same table to make decisions about access to treatment. Particularly in high-cost pharmaceuticals, society and third-party payers may value more a life-saving treatment, irrespective of its quality of life impact, while people with cancer may have unique views on the impact of side effects on one's life. Bevacizumab was first approved by the FDA in 2004 for metastatic colorectal cancer, indication later expanded to non-small cell lung cancer, renal cell carcinoma and glioblastoma (Vitry et al. 2015). In 2008, it was granted conditional market access for advanced breast cancer and, in 2011, re-evaluation led to market withdrawal for this indication, as there was new evidence of risks outweighing benefits aside from various flaws identified in the trial supporting conditional approval. This decision led to strong manifestations both from women with advanced breast cancer and oncologists, who argued toxicity was manageable and, therefore, considered acceptable. In fact, patients and physicians are generally more willing to accept toxicities in the face of a life-threatening disease (as metastatic disease) and limited treatment options. Currently bevacizumab is still used for metastatic breast cancer, although in association and under specific situations where risks are considered justified. Situations like this, in particular when they are leveraged by media coverage, have been described as fitting the countervailing powers theory, as they tend to reinforce pharmaceutical industry interests and quest against regulators' or payers' decisions (Gabe et al. 2012).

Advocacy groups, like the European Cancer Patient Coalition (2019) or the UK Macmillan Cancer Support (2019), have also contributed to raise awareness for inequalities in cancer prevention, diagnosis and treatment and to mobilize politicians to take action, at European (Banks 2019) and national (The All Party Parliamentary Group on Cancer 2009) level, while actively involving patients and advocacy groups. Access to new oncology medicines is another area where cancer advocacy organizations have played a major role in disseminating information about ongoing clinical trials (like eligibility criteria, phase or centres) and, as such, in facilitating access to treatments otherwise unavailable.

Rare Diseases

From the cases studied in this chapter, public participation in the rare disease space is the most recent. Taking advantage of the learnings and tactics from other disease movements, new approaches were essayed to address the challenge of meeting the needs and preferences of people affected by rare diseases.

In the face of limited attention, information and treatment options, rare disease advocacy groups, mostly formed by child's parents, have taken a leading role in advancing research, raising awareness for the specificities of rare diseases and orphan medicines, shaping policies and services and advocating for adequate funding for rare diseases and orphan drugs. This movement has been strongly driven during the last two decades by the widespread use of the internet and social networks, which facilitated outreach to people affected by rare diseases, education and empowerment of rare disease advocates, public awareness raising and, ultimately, mobilization of a vast network of supporters which includes patients and their families, activists, researchers, health professionals, academics, pharmaceutical companies and the general public.

Probably the most distinctive feature of public participation in the field of rare diseases has been its strong and direct involvement in rare disease research, including in the discovery of new treatments and drug repurposing. Organizations like the Progeria Research Foundation (Gordon and Gordon 2014), the Amyotrophic Lateral Sclerosis (ALS) Association (2019), the Alkaptonuria (AKU) Society (2019) and the Parent Project Muscular Dystrophy (2019) or Findacure (2019), just to name a few, have engaged in extensive fundraising campaigns to support research. Millions raised have been used by these organizations not only to fund independent research grants but also to set up their own research programmes, including patient-led clinical trials. As a result, significant advancements have been made on the aetiology of many rare diseases, the diagnosis of people with a rare disease, the initiation of new clinical trials and the creation of rare disease registries.

Umbrella organizations like the US National Organization for Rare Disorders (NORD) or EURORDIS in Europe have also led the way in voicing the needs of the rare disease community, driving supportive policies and advancing research (NORD 2019). NORD was instrumental in the Orphan Drug Act of 1983, which created financial incentives for the development of treatments for rare diseases. Since then, NORD has worked to ensure that national- and state-level policy decisions are informed by the needs and perspective of people with rare diseases. Since 1989, NORD has also in place a research programme which provides grants that have resulted in at least two FDA-approved therapies. NORD is also working with rare disease organizations to launch disease-specific registries to support research. At the policy level, NORD works with policy makers on Capitol Hill, in the White House, in government agencies and at the local level to help inform policies that are reflective of the needs of people with rare diseases. Key to this advocacy work is Rare Action Network—NORD's advocacy network from a broad spectrum of stakeholders, ranging from patients to their families, caregivers and friends and from researchers to industry, physicians and academia. While working predominantly at the state level, the network informs NORD's national federal policy team to help address issues of national concern.

EURORDIS represents over 800 rare disease patient organizations in 70 countries. EURORDIS advocacy within the European Commission and other European institutions has contributed, among others, to the adoption of the EU Regulation on Orphan Medicinal Products, in 1999, and to the designation of over 1100 orphan drugs. Besides playing a pivotal role in obtaining EU-level legislation that encourages the development of medicinal products for rare diseases, EURORDIS is also a member of relevant scientific committees at EMA and has established the EURORDIS Round Table of Companies, bringing together pharmaceutical companies to discuss issues related to the development of treatments for rare diseases. Other EURORDIS initiatives focus on improving access to rare disease treatments throughout Europe. EURORDIS actively advocated for the European Committee of Experts on Rare Diseases (EUCERD) Recommendation on Improving Informed Decisions Based on the Clinical Added Value of Orphan Medicinal Products (CAVOMP) and for a value-based pricing approach for orphan medicines as elaborated in the Mechanism of Coordinated Access to Orphan Medicinal Products (MoCA) process launched in 2010.

In 2010, EURORDIS and NORD sealed a strategic partnership agreement to promote rare diseases as an international public health priority, and since then they have been working together on several initiatives, like the Rare Disease Day campaign and common positions on key advocacy priorities.

Future Perspectives on Public Participation in Access to Medicines

The trend towards patient-centred healthcare and increased public participation in activities related with access to medicines, illustrated in this chapter, will certainly spread across countries and soon become routine in medicines development and healthcare decision-making, starting in early development phases and spanning throughout the entire medicines' lifecycle. Furthermore, organizations of people living with disease, researchers, regulators and HTA agencies will be joined by other healthcare stakeholders—including health professionals and services' managers—in this quest for fully embracing the user's perspective. This is expected to contribute not only to further align on best practices for public involvement in the pharmaceutical space but also to promote the debate on individual participation in decisions about one's own health and medicines use.

References

Declaration of Alma-Ata. In: International Conference on Primary Health Care, 6–12 September [Internet]. Alma-ata, USSR: World Health Organization; 1978. Available from: www.who.int/publications/almaata_declaration_en.pdf?ua=1

Council of Europe. Recommendation No. R (2000) 5 of the Committee of Ministers to member states on the development of structures for citizen and patient participation in the decision-making process affecting health care [Internet]. Strasbourg, France: Council of Europe; 2000. Available from: http://wcd.coe.int/ViewDoc.jsp?id=340437&Site=CM

Florin D. Public involvement in health care. BMJ [Internet]. 2004 Jan 17;328(7432):159–61. Available from: http://www.bmj.com/cgi/doi/10.1136/bmj.328.7432.159

Mitton C, Smith N, Peacock S, Evoy B, Abelson J. Public participation in health care priority setting: A scoping review. Health Policy. 2009;91(3):219–28.

European Patients' Forum. Patient Empowerment Campaign [Internet]. 2015 [cited 2016 Oct 28]. Available from: www.eu-patient.eu/campaign/PatientsprescribE

Kickbusch I, Gleicher D. Governance for Health in the 21st Century [Internet]. Copenhagen: WHO Regional Office for Europe; 2012. Available from: www.euro.who.int/__data/assets/pdf_file/0019/171334/RC62BD01-Governance-for-Health-Web.pdf

World Health Organization. Framework on integrated people-centred health services. Report by the Secretariat. [Internet]. 2016. Available from: http://apps.who.int/gb/ebwha/pdf_files/WHA69/A69_39-en.pdf?ua=1&ua=1

Ives J, Damery S, Redwod S. PPI, paradoxes and Plato: who's sailing the ship?: Table 1. J Med Ethics [Internet]. 2013 Mar;39(3):181–5. Available from: http://jme.bmj.com/lookup/doi/10.1136/medethics-2011-100150

International Alliance of Patients' Organizations. Policy statement. Patient Involvement [Internet]. London; 2005. Available from: http://iapo.org.uk/sites/default/files/files/IAPOPolicyStatementonPatientInvolvement.pdftInvolvement.pdf

Frankish C, Kwan B, Ratner P, Wharf-Higgins J, Larsen C. Challenges of citizen participation in regional health authorities. Soc Sci Med. 2002;54:1471–80.

Tallon D, Chard J, Dieppe P. Relation between agendas of the research community and the research consumer. Lancet. 2000;355(9220):2037–40.

Barnes M, Skelcher C, Beirens H, Dalziel R, Jeffares S, Wilson L. Designing citizen-centered governance. Birmingham: Joseph Rowntree Foundation; 2008.

Van De Bovenkamp HM, Trappenburg MJ, Grit KJ. Patient participation in collective healthcare decision making: the Dutch model. Heal Expect [Internet]. 2010 Feb 17;13(1):73–85. Available from: http://doi.wiley.com/10.1111/j.1369-7625.2009.00567.x

Tritter JQ, McCallum, A. The snakes and ladders of user involvement: Moving beyond Arnstein. Health Policy (New York) [Internet]. 2006 Apr;76(2):156–68. Available from: http://linkinghub.elsevier.com/retrieve/pii/S0168851005001314

Cooper L, Coote A, Davies A, Jackson C. Voices off: tackling the democratic deficit in health. London: Institute for Public Policy Research; 1995.

Terzi A. The patients' involvement in health policies in Europe. [Internet]. Roma: Active Citizenship Network; 2013. Available from: http://www.activecitizenship.net/files/patients_rights/7th_EPRD/Patientsrights_acn_report_2013.pdf

OECD. Citizens as Partners [Internet]. Paris: OECD Publishing; 2001. Available from: http://www.oecd-ilibrary.org/governance/citizens-as-partners_9789264195561-en

European Commission. White Paper. Together for Health: A Strategic Approach for the EU 2008–2013 [Internet]. Brussels; 2007. Available from: http://ec.europa.eu/health/ph_overview/Documents/strategy_wp_en.pdf

Montgomery AA, Fahey, T. How do patients' treatment preferences compare with those of clinicians? Qual Saf Heal Care [Internet]. 2001 Sep 1;10(Supplement 1):i39–43. Available from: http://qualitysafety.bmj.com/lookup/doi/10.1136/qhc.0100039

Sewitch MJ, Abrahamowicz M, Dobkin PL, Tamblyn R. Measuring differences between patients' and physicians' health perceptions: the patient-physician discordance scale. J Behav Med [Internet]. 2003 Jun;26(3):245–64. Available from: http://www.ncbi.nlm.nih.gov/pubmed/12845937

Harrison JD. Patient and Physician Preferences for Surgical and Adjuvant Treatment Options for Rectal Cancer. Arch Surg [Internet]. 2008 Apr 1;143(4):389. Available from: http://archsurg.jamanetwork.com/article.aspx?doi=10.1001/archsurg.143.4.389

da Silva JAP, Ramiro S, Pedro S, Rodrigues A, Vasconcelos JC, Benito-Garcia E. Patients- and physicians- priorities for improvement. The case of rheumatic diseases. Acta Reumatol Port [Internet]. 2010;35(2):192–9. Available from: http://www.ncbi.nlm.nih.gov/pubmed/20734542

Miravitlles M, Ferrer J, Baró E, Lleonart M, Galera J. Differences between physician and patient in the perception of symptoms and their severity in COPD. Respir Med [Internet]. 2013 Dec;107(12):1977–85. Available from: http://linkinghub.elsevier.com/retrieve/pii/S095461111300231X

Fergusson D, Monfaredi Z, Pussegoda K, Garritty C, Lyddiatt A, Shea B, et al. The prevalence of patient engagement in published trials: a systematic review. Res Involv Engagem [Internet]. 2018 Dec 22;4(1):17. Available from: http://researchinvolvement.biomedcentral.com/articles/10.1186/s40900-018-0099-x

Sacristan JA, Aguaron A, Avendaño C, Garrido P, Carrion J, Gutierrez A, et al. Patient involvement in clinical research: why, when, and how. Patient Prefer Adherence [Internet]. 2016 Apr;631. Available from: www.dovepress.com/patient-involvement-in-clinical-research-why-when-and-how-peer-reviewed-article-PPA

Geissler J, Ryll B, di Priolo SL, Uhlenhopp M. Improving Patient Involvement in Medicines Research and Development: Ther Innov Regul Sci [Internet]. 2017 Sep 8;51(5):612–9. Available from: http://journals.sagepub.com/doi/10.1177/2168479017706405

Cook NS, Cave J, Holtorf A-P. Patient Preference Studies During Early Drug Development: Aligning Stakeholders to Ensure Development Plans Meet Patient Needs. Front Med [Internet]. 2019 Apr 24;6. Available from: www.frontiersin.org/article/10.3389/fmed.2019.00082/full

Regulation (EU) No 536/2014 of the European Parliament and of the Council of 16 April 2014 on clinical trials on medicinal products for human use, and repealing Directive 2001/20/EC [Internet]. 2014. Available from: http://ec.europa.eu/health/files/eudralex/vol-1/reg_2014_536/reg_2014_536_en.pdf

AVAC. Fact Sheet: Data Safety Monitoring Boards (DSMBs) [Internet]. 2011. Available from: www.avac.org/sites/default/files/resource-files/DataSafetyMonitoringBoards2011.pdf

Huang GD, Bull J, Johnston McKee K, Mahon E, Harper B, Roberts JN. Clinical trials recruitment planning: A proposed framework from the Clinical Trials Transformation Initiative. Contemp Clin Trials [Internet]. 2018 Mar;66:74–9. Available from: http://linkinghub.elsevier.com/retrieve/pii/S155171441730753X

Summaries of Clinical Trial Results for Laypersons. Recommendations of the expert group on clinical trials for the implementation of Regulation (EU) No 536/2014 on clinical trials on medicinal products for human use. Version 2 [Internet]. 2018. Available from: http://ec.europa.eu/health/sites/health/files/files/eudralex/vol-10/2017_01_26_summaries_of_ct_results_for_laypersons.pdf

Garfield S, Jheeta S, Husson F, Lloyd J, Taylor A, Boucher C, et al. The Role of Hospital Inpatients in Supporting Medication Safety: A Qualitative Study. Li D, editor. PLoS One [Internet]. 2016 Apr 19;11(4):e0153721. Available from: http://dx.plos.org/10.1371/journal.pone.0153721

Oliver S. Patient involvement in setting research agendas. Eur J Gastroenterol Hepatol [Internet]. 2006 Sep;18(9):935–8. Available from: http://insights.ovid.com/crossref?an=00042737-200609000-00001

Mavris M, Le Cam Y. Involvement of Patient Organisations in Research and Development of Orphan Drugs for Rare Diseases in Europe. Mol Syndromol [Internet]. 2012; Available from: www.karger.com/Article/FullText/342758

PCORI. Engagement Rubric for Applicants [Internet]. 2016. Available from: www.pcori.org/sites/default/files/Engagement-Rubric.pdf

Canadian Institutes of Health Research. Strategy for Patient-Oriented Research - Patient Engagement Framework [Internet]. 2014. Available from: http://www.cihr-irsc.gc.ca/e/documents/spor_framework-en.pdf

NIHR | INVOLVE. Guidance on co-producing a research project [Internet]. 2018. Available from: www.invo.org.uk/wp-content/uploads/2019/04/Copro_Guidance_Feb19front.jpg

Warner K, See W, Haerry D, Klingmann I, Hunter A, May M. EUPATI Guidance for Patient Involvement in Medicines Research and Development (R&D); Guidance for Pharmaceutical Industry-Led Medicines R&D. Front Med [Internet]. 2018 Oct 9;5. Available from: www.frontiersin.org/article/10.3389/fmed.2018.00270/full

Klingmann I, Heckenberg A, Warner K, Haerry D, Hunter A, May M, et al. EUPATI and Patients in Medicines Research and Development: Guidance for Patient Involvement in Ethical Review of Clinical Trials. Front Med [Internet]. 2018 Sep 7;5. Available from: www.frontiersin.org/article/10.3389/fmed.2018.00251/full

Ganz PA. Impact of Tamoxifen Adjuvant Therapy on Symptoms, Functioning, and Quality of Life. JNCI Monogr [Internet]. 2001 Dec 1;2001(30):130–4. Available from: http://academic.oup.com/jncimono/article-lookup/doi/10.1093/oxfordjournals.jncimonographs.a003450

Ganz PA, Cecchini RS, Julian TB, Margolese RG, Costantino JP, Vallow LA, et al. Patient-reported outcomes with anastrozole versus tamoxifen for postmenopausal patients with ductal carcinoma in situ treated with lumpectomy plus radiotherapy (NSABP B-35): a randomised, double-blind, phase 3 clinical trial. Lancet [Internet]. 2016 Feb;387(10021):857–65. Available from: http://linkinghub.elsevier.com/retrieve/pii/S0140673615011691

Kluetz PG, Slagle A, Papadopoulos EJ, Johnson LL, Donoghue M, Kwitkowski VE, et al. Focusing on Core Patient-Reported Outcomes in Cancer Clinical Trials: Symptomatic Adverse Events, Physical Function, and Disease-Related Symptoms. Clin Cancer Res [Internet]. 2016 Apr 1;22(7):1553–8. Available from: http://clincancerres.aacrjournals.org/cgi/doi/10.1158/1078-0432.CCR-15-2035

Milman N, McConville E, Robson JC, Boonen A, Tugwell P, Wells GA, et al. Updating OMERACT Core Set of Domains for ANCA-associated Vasculitis: Patient Perspective Using the International Classification of Function, Disability, and Health. J Rheumatol [Internet]. 2019 Feb 1;jrheum.181073. Available from: http://www.jrheum.org/lookup/doi/10.3899/jrheum.181073

Richards T, Snow R, Schroter S. Logging The BMJ's "patient journey." BMJ [Internet]. 2015 Aug 17;h4396. Available from: www.bmj.com/lookup/doi/10.1136/bmj.h4396

PCORI. Research Funding [Internet]. 2019. Available from: www.pcori.org/sites/default/files/PCORI-Research-Funding.pdf

National Institute for Health Research. Funding opportunities for research and career development [Internet]. 2017. Available from: www.nihr.ac.uk/funding-and-support/documents/NIHRFundingOpportunitiesBooklet2017.pdf

European Commission. Horizon 2020. Public Engagement in Responsible Research and Innovation [Internet]. Available from: http://ec.europa.eu/programmes/horizon2020/en/h2020-section/public-engagement-responsible-research-and-innovation

Food and Drug Administration. Learn About FDA Patient Engagement [Internet]. Available from: www.fda.gov/patients/learn-about-fda-patient-engagement

European Medicines Agency. Patients and consumers [Internet]. Available from: www.ema.europa.eu/en/partners-networks/patients-consumers

Haerry D, Landgraf C, Warner K, Hunter A, Klingmann I, May M, et al. EUPATI and Patients in Medicines Research and Development: Guidance for Patient Involvement in Regulatory Processes. Front Med [Internet]. 2018 Aug 17;5. Available from: www.frontiersin.org/article/10.3389/fmed.2018.00230/full

Knox S. Health economic decision making in Europe – a new priority for breast cancer advocacy. The Breast [Internet]. 2009 Apr;18(2):71–2. Available from: https://linkinghub.elsevier.com/retrieve/pii/S0960977609000356

Boutin M, Dewulf L, Hoos A, Geissler J, Todaro V, Schneider RF, et al. Culture and Process Change as a Priority for Patient Engagement in Medicines Development. Ther Innov Regul Sci [Internet]. 2017 Jan 20;51(1):29–38. Available from: http://journals.sagepub.com/doi/10.1177/2168479016659104

Scott AM, Wale JL. Patient advocate perspectives on involvement in HTA: an international snapshot. Res Involv Engagem [Internet]. 2017 Dec 10;3(1):2. Available from: http://researchinvolvement.biomedcentral.com/articles/10.1186/s40900-016-0052-9

Hunter A, Facey K, Thomas V, Haerry D, Warner K, Klingmann I, et al. EUPATI Guidance for Patient Involvement in Medicines Research and Development: Health Technology Assessment. Front Med [Internet]. 2018 Sep 6;5. Available from: www.frontiersin.org/article/10.3389/fmed.2018.00231/full

National Institute for Health and Care Excellence. Patient and public involvement policy [Internet]. [cited 2019 Jul 22]. Available from: www.nice.org.uk/about/nice-communities/nice-and-the-public/public-involvement/public-involvement-programme/patient-public-involvement-policy

IQWiG. Contributing the patients' perspective [Internet]. Available from: https://www.iqwig.de/en/participation/contributing-the-patients-perspective.3070.html

Crisóstomo S, Santos M. Participação pública na saúde: das ideias à ação em Portugal. Rev Crit Cienc Sociais [Internet]. 2018 Dec 1;(117):167–86. Available from: http://journals.openedition.org/rccs/8325

INFARMED. Doentes e associações de doentes: Incluir [Internet]. [cited 2019 Jul 22]. Available from: http://www.infarmed.pt/web/infarmed/cidadaos/doentes-e-associacoes-de-doentes

Advisory Committee of the People with AIDS. The Denver Principles [Internet]. 1983. p. Available from: www.actupny.org/documents/Denver.html

Fischl MA, Richman DD, Grieco MH, Gottlieb MS, Volberding PA, Laskin OL, et al. The Efficacy of Azidothymidine (AZT) in the Treatment of Patients with AIDS and AIDS-Related Complex. N Engl J Med [Internet]. 1987 Jul 23;317(4):185–91. Available from: http://www.nejm.org/doi/abs/10.1056/NEJM198707233170401

Crimp D. Before Occupy: How AIDS Activists Seized Control of the FDA in 1988. The Atlantic [Internet]. 2011 Dec 6; Available from: www.theatlantic.com/health/archive/2011/12/before-occupy-how-aids-activists-seized-control-of-the-fda-in-1988/249302

Lessem E. Nothing About Us Without Us: Community Engagement in Research to End the Epidemics. TAGline [Internet]. 2019;26(1). Available from: www.treatmentactiongroup.org/sites/default/files/tagline_may_2019_lessem_intro.pdf

Heffernan A, Cooke GS, Nayagam S, Thursz M, Hallett TB. Scaling up prevention and treatment towards the elimination of hepatitis C: a global mathematical model. Lancet [Internet]. 2019 Mar;393(10178):1319–29. Available from: https://linkinghub.elsevier.com/retrieve/pii/S0140673618322773

World Health Organization. Global Hepatitis Report 2017 [Internet]. Geneva: World Health Organization; 2017. Available from: http://apps.who.int/iris/bitstream/handle/10665/255016/9789241565455-eng.pdf?sequence=1

Lomas J, Claxton K, Martin S, Soares M. Resolving the "Cost-Effective but Unaffordable" Paradox: Estimating the Health Opportunity Costs of Nonmarginal Budget Impacts. Value Heal [Internet]. 2018 Mar;21(3):266–75. Available from: https://linkinghub.elsevier.com/retrieve/pii/S1098301517336136

Millman AJ, Ntiri-Reid B, Irvin R, Kaufmann MH, Aronsohn A, Duchin JS, et al. Barriers to Treatment Access for Chronic Hepatitis C Virus Infection: A Case Series. Top Antivir Med [Internet]. 2017;25(3):110–3. Available from: http://www.ncbi.nlm.nih.gov/pubmed/28820726

Douglass CH, Pedrana A, Lazarus J V., 't Hoen EFM, Hammad R, Leite RB, et al. Pathways to ensure universal and affordable access to hepatitis C treatment. BMC Med [Internet]. 2018 Dec 9;16(1):175. Available from: http://bmcmedicine.biomedcentral.com/articles/10.1186/s12916-018-1162-z

Kieslich K, Ahn J, Badano G, Chalkidou K, Cubillos L, Hauegen RC, et al. Public participation in decision-making on the coverage of new antivirals for hepatitis C. Kieslich, Peter Littlejohns and Alb K, editor. J Health Organ Manag [Internet]. 2016 Aug 15;30(5):769–85. Available from: http://www.emeraldinsight.com/doi/10.1108/JHOM-03-2016-0035

Kaplan K. Activist Satregies for Increasing Access to HCV Treatment in Low- and Middle-Income Countries [Internet]. TAG – Treatment Action Group; 2015. Available from: http://www.treatmentactiongroup.org/sites/default/files/201502/ActivistStrategiesforHCVTx.pdf

Grillon C, Krishtel PR, Mellouk O, Basenko A, Freeman J, Mendão L, et al. Treatment advocate tactics to expand access to antiviral therapy for HIV and viral hepatitis C in low- to high-income settings: making sure no one is left behind. J Int AIDS Soc [Internet]. 2018 Apr;21:e25060. Available from: http://doi.wiley.com/10.1002/jia2.25060

Chapman AR, Buckley T. Lowering the High Cost of Hepatitis C Drugs. J Pharm Care Heal Syst [Internet]. 2017;04(05). Available from: www.omicsonline.org/open-access/lowering-the-high-cost-of-hepatitis-c-drugs-2376-0419-1000187-95305.html

Pii KH, Schou LH, Piil K, Jarden M. Current trends in patient and public involvement in cancer research: A systematic review. Heal Expect [Internet]. 2019 Feb;22(1):3–20. Available from: http://doi.wiley.com/10.1111/hex.12841

Vaz-Luis I, O'Neill A, Sepucha K, Miller KD, Baker E, Dang CT, et al. Survival benefit needed to undergo chemotherapy: Patient and physician preferences. Cancer [Internet]. 2017 Aug 1;123(15):2821–8. Available from: http://doi.wiley.com/10.1002/cncr.30671

Dika E, Patrizi A, Ribero S, Fanti PA, Starace M, Melotti B, et al. Hair and nail adverse events during treatment with targeted therapies for metastatic melanoma. Eur J Dermatology. 2016;26(3):232–9.

Castellanos EH, Chen S, Drexler H, Horn L. Making the Grade: The Impact of Low-Grade Toxicities on Patient Preference for Treatment With Novel Agents. J Natl Compr Canc Netw [Internet]. 2015 Dec;13(12):1490–5. Available from: http://www.ncbi.nlm.nih.gov/pubmed/26656518

Macdonald JB, Macdonald B, Golitz LE, LoRusso P, Sekulic A. Cutaneous adverse effects of targeted therapies. J Am Acad Dermatol [Internet]. 2015 Feb;72(2):203–18. Available from: https://linkinghub.elsevier.com/retrieve/pii/S0190962214017630

Trask PC, Dueck AC, Piault E, Campbell A. Patient-Reported Outcomes version of the Common Terminology Criteria for Adverse Events: Methods for item selection in industry-sponsored oncology clinical trials. Clin Trials [Internet]. 2018 Dec 19;15(6):616–23. Available from: http://journals.sagepub.com/doi/10.1177/1740774518799985

Marandino L, La Salvia A, Sonetto C, De Luca E, Pignataro D, Zichi C, et al. Deficiencies in health-related quality-of-life assessment and reporting: a systematic review of oncology randomized phase III trials published between 2012

and 2016. Ann Oncol [Internet]. 2018 Dec 1;29(12):2288–95. Available from: https://academic.oup.com/annonc/article/29/12/2288/5126229
Catt S, Starkings R, Shilling V, Fallowfield L. Patient-reported outcome measures of the impact of cancer on patients' everyday lives: a systematic review. J Cancer Surviv [Internet]. 2017 Apr 10;11(2):211–32. Available from: http://link.springer.com/10.1007/s11764-016-0580-1
Vitry A, Nguyen T, Entwistle V, Roughead E. Regulatory withdrawal of medicines marketed with uncertain benefits: the bevacizumab case study. J Pharm Policy Pract [Internet]. 2015 Dec 19;8(1):25. Available from: http://www.joppp.org/content/8/1/25
Gabe J, Chamberlain K, Norris P, Dew K, Madden H, Hodgetts D. The debate about the funding of Herceptin: A case study of 'countervailing powers'. Soc Sci Med [Internet]. 2012 Dec;75(12):2353–61. Available from: http://linkinghub.elsevier.com/retrieve/pii/S0277953612006727
European Cancer Patient Coalition. Europe of Disparities [Internet]. [cited 2019 Jul 26]. Available from: http://www.ecpc.org/activities/policy-and-advocacy/policy-initiatives/europe-of-disparities
Mcmillan Cancer Support. We make change happen [Internet]. [cited 2019 Jul 26]. Available from: www.macmillan.org.uk/about-us/what-we-do/we-make-change-happen
Banks M. MEPs launch 'elections manifesto' in fight against cancer. The Parliament Magazine [Internet]. 2019 Jan 29; Available from: www.theparliamentmagazine.eu/articles/news/meps-launch-'elections-manifesto'-fight-against-cancer
The All Party Parliamentary Group on Cancer. Report of the All Party Parliamentary Group on Cancer's Inquiry into Inequalities in Cancer [Internet]. 2009. Available from: https://www.macmillan.org.uk/documents/getinvolved/campaigns/appg/britainagainstcancer2009/cancerinequalitiesreport.pdf
Gordon A, Gordon L. The Progeria Research Foundation: its remarkable journey from obscurity to treatment. Expert Opin Orphan Drugs [Internet]. 2014 Nov 30;2(11):1187–95. Available from: http://www.tandfonline.com/doi/full/10.1517/21678707.2014.970172
ALS Association. ALS Ice Bucket Challenge Commitments [Internet]. [cited 2019 Jul 22]. Available from: http://www.alsa.org/fight-als/ice-bucket-challenge-spending.html
AKU Society. DevelopAKUre [Internet]. [cited 2019 Jul 22]. Available from: www.developakure.eu

Parent Project Muscular Dystrophy. Research [Internet]. [cited 2019 Jul 22]. Available from: www.parentprojectmd.org/research

Findacure. Drug repurposing [Internet]. [cited 2019 Jul 22]. Available from: www.findacure.org.uk/drug-repurposing

NORD. Programs and Services [Internet]. [cited 2019 Jul 22]. Available from: http://rarediseases.org/about/what-we-do/programs-services

11

Pharmaceutical Policy and Practice Research: A Review of Studies in China

Caijun Yang, Amna Saeed, Khezar Hayat, Krizzia-Mae Lambojon, Ali Hassan Gillani, and Yu Fang

Global Pharmaceutical Policy

Medicines are one of the core elements for improving and maintaining people's health. No healthcare system can work effectively without the equitable access to quality-assured and affordable medicines (United Nations Development Group and United Nations 2003). However the drug prices have been increasing tremendously from the last few decades and are compromising equitable access. It is also noteworthy that the

C. Yang (✉) • A. Saeed • K.-M. Lambojon • A. H. Gillani • Y. Fang
Department of Pharmacy Administration and Clinical Pharmacy, School of Pharmacy, Xi'an Jiaotong University, Xi'an, China

Center for Drug Safety and Policy Research, Xian Jiaotong University, Xi'an, China

Shaanxi Center for Health Reform and Development Research, Xi'an, China
e-mail: yangcj@xjtu.edu.cn; yufang@xjtu.edu.cn

Z. Babar (ed.), *Global Pharmaceutical Policy*,
https://doi.org/10.1007/978-981-15-2724-1_11

increasing global pharmaceutical expenditure is making the drug pricing and financing difficult for almost all countries and has emerged as a major global challenge (Suh 2011). Moreover, the antimicrobial resistance demands immediate actions to ensure the proper use of antibiotics globally (Paphitou 2013)

To curb these issues, the World Health Organization (WHO) recommends the development and implementation of national pharmaceutical policy that should be in line with the overall healthcare framework of a particular region. It also serves as a legal framework to regulate the drug development, manufacture, pricing, selection of essential drugs, supply systems, drug financing, quality assurance, rational use, research, human resources, monitoring and evaluation (World Health Organization 2001). Most governments are now taking up, formulating and executing a national pharmaceutical policy that incorporates strategies to regulate the whole pharmaceutical sector, starting from the drug development to its rational use by the patients (Traulsen and Almarsdóttir 2005). Currently, more than 100 countries have developed their national pharmaceutical policies and the list is growing (Perehudoff et al. 2019). These policies are devised according to each country's healthcare needs and economic status. For instance, drug development requires ample funds, so it can be a priority for high-income countries, but for low- and middle-income countries, the case would be otherwise, due to the limited resources (Espin et al. 2011). Unfortunately, there is lack of evidence on effectiveness of all these

K. Hayat
Department of Pharmacy Administration and Clinical Pharmacy, School of Pharmacy, Xi'an Jiaotong University, Xi'an, China

Center for Drug Safety and Policy Research, Xian Jiaotong University, Xi'an, China

Shaanxi Center for Health Reform and Development Research, Xi'an, China

Institute of Pharmaceutical Sciences, University of Veterinary and Animal Science, Lahore, Pakistan
e-mail: khezar.hayat@uvas.edu.pk

policies, and there is a need as well as opportunity for researchers in this area (Acosta et al. 2014). We need to produce objective evidence to support and modify our current policies (Ritter 2009).

Pharmaceutical Policy in China

In the last three decades, the Chinese healthcare system had undergone tremendous changes. The government largely reduced its funding for public hospitals. The governmental funding constituted about 60% of hospital revenues in the 1980s, but it had fallen to 11% by 2009 (Wang et al. 2018). At the same time, public hospitals were allowed to earn a 15% mark-up on the sale of pharmaceutical products, which resulted in overprescribing of medicines to patients in the public hospitals. The problem of irrational use of medicines during this period was severe, and this also resulted in high healthcare expenditure for patients in China.

To improve the rational use of medicines and also to improve the availability and affordability of medicines, the National Essential Medicines Policy (NEMP) was launched as a part of health system reform by the Chinese government in 2009, along with Zero Mark-Up Policy as its matching policy (Jiang et al. 2015; Fang et al. 2013). A National Essential Medicine List (NEML) was issued in 2009, with 307 medicines at first. During the following years, the second edition of NEML with 520 medicines was issued in 2012 and the third edition with 685 medicines in 2018. All primary healthcare institutions were required to stock and dispense medicines on the National Essential Medicine List. The Zero Mark-Up Policy (ZMP) was introduced which required the healthcare institutions to sell medicines without mark-up, and to offset the losses in hospital revenues, the local government increased subsidies. Since the early of 2010, the ZMP was implemented in primary health institutions and all primary health institutions were covered by the end of 2011. The ZMP has been extended to all county hospitals in 2015, and in 2017 all the tertiary hospitals started to implement the ZMP.

The Genesis and Work of the Center of Drug Safety and Policy (CDSP) at Xi'an Jiaotong University

The Center of Drug Safety and Policy (CDSP), situated in Xi'an Jiaotong University (XJTU), founded in 2014 is working on pharmaceutical policy issues and providing the necessary evidence to see the shortcomings in the implementation of these policies. Many studies are conducted by CDSP-XJTU in China, using multiple methodologies to counteract the problems of drug inaccessibility, drug shortages, medicine misuse (especially antibiotics) and patient's non-adherence. Cooperating with renowned universities in the developed countries, i.e. Harvard University and the University of Minnesota, the CDSP affirms the position as a centre point in policy research in China. Also with the inauguration of a joint lab with developing countries, CDSP is promising to act as a hub in problem solving along with other countries in the One Belt One Road Initiative (Górski et al. 2017).

Access to Medicines

In developing countries, the expenditure on purchase of medicines may account for 50–90% of the non-personnel cost from the national healthcare budgets (Quick et al. 1997). About 90% of the population in low- and middle-income countries are paying out-of-pocket to get the medicines (Husereau and Cameron 2012). There is a need to develop better national policies and strategies for medicine pricing and procurement to ensure the availability and affordability of essential medicines (World Health Organization 2004). The major obstacles which hinder the governments in constructing comprehensive medicine pricing policies or assessing their impacts are numerous, such as difficulty in getting reliable data on the prices and availability of medicines (World Health Organization 2008). This also causes difficulty in evaluating whether the spending on medicines is comparable to other countries which are at similar stage of development. This section reports on the studies conducted by the Center of Drug Safety and Policy (CDSP), in Xi'an Jiaotong University (XJTU), China.

World Health Organization/Health Action International Standard Methodology

In order to monitor medicine prices and to help improve the access, the World Health Organization (WHO) and Health Action International (HAI) developed an evidence-based standardized methodology to measure prices, availability, affordability and price components of medicines. This allows the international comparisons and also to advocate to form appropriate national pricing policies and to monitor their impact. In this method the medicine procurement and patient prices (for both lowest-priced generics (LPGs) and originator brands (OBs)) are obtained and are compared with the international reference prices (IRPs). So, results are presented in the form of median price ratio (MPR), which is a ratio of local unit price to the unit IRP. MPR tells us how much the surveyed local median unit price is greater or less than the international reference unit price. WHO and HAI recommend the use of Management Sciences for Health (MSH) International Drug Price Indicator Guide as the source of IRPs. The MSH prices are net prices mostly obtained from non-profit suppliers to the developing countries and NGOs. These MSH reference prices are relatively low and offer a very useful standard to compare locally available medicines. The availability of medicines is presented in the form of percentage availability of a particular medicine at the day of the data collection. The affordability of medicines is reported in terms of number of days' wages required for the unskilled lowest-paid government worker to obtain the standard treatment for a selected medicine. The price components along the supply chain are also measured in order to have better understanding of the issues regarding medicine accessibility (World Health Organization 2008).

The Studies on Access to Medicines in China

Access to Essential Medicines

Jiang et al. conducted two cross-sectional surveys in Shaanxi Province in September 2010 and April 2012, as a measure to evaluate the medicine availability and prices during the initial years of health reform in China in which the key component was the implementation of NEMP (Jiang et al. 2015; Fang et al. 2013). Fang et al. compared these two surveys and measured the impact of health reform on medicine prices and availability employing the WHO/HAI methodology with some modifications. The mean availability in both public and private sector was noted to be very low compared with the ideal availability suggested by the WHO, i.e. more than 80%. A significant decrease in the availability of many surveyed essential medicines was noted in the two years (from 27.4% to 22.3% for LPGs, $p<0.0001$). The median government procurement prices for both OBs and LPGs were reduced in 2012 (difference −10.9%, $p=0.0004$, and −4.9%, $p=0.17$, respectively); however, the reduction in procurement prices of LPGs was insignificant. The MUPs for patients were significantly lower in 2012 for both OBs (−11.7%, $p=0.0019$) and LPGs (−5.2%, $p=0.0015$). So, it could be interpreted from the results that the early years of NEMP in Shaanxi, western China, had led to a reduction in medicine price; however, a point of concern is the significant reduction in availability of essential medicines specifically in primary care public hospitals. This indicated that the future policies must be directed towards improving medicine availability along with the reduction in medicine prices. This study also underscored the need for generation of evidence, using the data from both public and private sector healthcare outlets regarding medicine availability, prices and utilization to devise and modify future medicine policies (Fang et al. 2013).

Access to Paediatric Essential Medicines

In order to measure access to paediatric essential medicines, Wang et al. in Shaanxi Province, China, conducted a survey. The availability was poor in public and private sectors for OBs (10.8% and 27.3%) as well as LPGs (11.9% and 20.6%), respectively. The public procurement prices were 2.25 times the IRP for OBs and 0.52 times for LPGs. The patient prices in hospitals and retail pharmacies for OBs were 2.59 and 3.89 times the IRPs and for LPGs 0.93 and 1.25 times the IRPs. The standard treatments were found to be affordable, i.e. cost less than 1 days' wage of a lowest-paid government worker. The major contributor for the final prices of medicines was found to be the manufacturers' selling price. It was concluded that a national list of paediatric essential medicines must be launched by the government in this regard (Wang et al. 2018).

Access to Anti-Diabetic Medicines

As China has a large number of diabetes patients (Ogurtsova et al. 2017), recent studies published in 2019 by Yang et al. and Li et al. focused on evaluating the access to oral anti-diabetic medicines and insulin, respectively (Yang et al. 2019; Li et al. 2019). In 2015, Yang et al. measured the prices and availability of different strengths and dosage forms of eight oral diabetic medicines. The mean availabilities for both OBs and LPGs were poor in public sector hospitals (34.3% and 28.7%) as well as in private retail pharmacies (44% and 64%). The procurement prices for OBs and LPGs were 12.3 and 4.5 times the IRPs in public sector, while OBs and LPGs were procured at 10.2 and 2.8 times the IRPs in private sector. Treatment with OBs was found to be unaffordable (Yang et al. 2019). Li et al. surveyed the prices and availability of all insulin products in the market and five oral anti-diabetic medicines as comparators, in both public and private sector, in 2016. All insulin products were found to be available at all public sector outlets, while in private sector the availability was fairly high, i.e. 62.5% to 68.8%. But the prices of all products were quite high and ranged from 0.95 to 2.33 times the international reference prices (IRPs). All insulin products were found to be unaffordable. The largest price component was the manufacturers' selling price. So, it was concluded that the high prices are making the insulin inaccessible to the patients especially the ones who were poor. The authors emphasized on the need for either increased insurance compensation for the patients or to reduce the prices by negotiating with the manufacturers and suppliers (Li et al. 2019).

The Study on Access to Essential Medicines in Pakistan

A study was conducted to measure the access to essential medicines in Lahore, Pakistan, by Amna et al., using an adaptation of WHO/HAI methodology. The availability of originator brands (OBs) was reported to be poor in both public and private sector, i.e. 6.8% and 55%, respectively. The lowest-priced generics (LPGs) also showed poor availability in public (35.3%) and private sector (20.3%). Although the medicines were given free of charge to the patients at public sector, due to poor availability many patients purchase medicines from private sector. The treatment with OBs was found to be unaffordable while the treatment with LPGs was affordable. The prices of many OBs were found to be higher than IRPs; thus, the authors emphasized on forming a patient-friendly drug pricing policy (Saeed et al. 2019).

The Studies on Drug Shortages in China

Over the last few decades, drug shortages have become a complex global health problem affecting both developed and developing countries (Gray and Manasse 2012). China is also seriously affected by its drug shortage problems. By literature review, there were 148 drugs identified which were in shortage between 2006 and 2015, and most of them were cheap and essential medicines (Wu et al. 2016). Another evidence from Shaanxi Province, western China, reported that there were almost 100 drugs in short supply in only 20 hospitals (12 secondary hospitals and 8 tertiary hospitals) in 2016 (Yang et al. 2016). Five main determinants of drug shortages were detected by interview: too low prices, too low market demands, Good Manufacturing Practice (GMP) issues, materials issues and approval issues for imported drugs (Yang et al. 2016).

Among these drugs in shortage, the unavailability of emergency drugs can result in more severe consequences and therefore catch more governmental and social attention. An online survey involving 236 physicians working in emergency departments in Chinese secondary and tertiary hospitals in 2017 revealed that (1) more than half of the physicians (65.7%) experienced drug shortages at least once a month; (2) hospitals in the eastern and western regions of China had more emergency drugs in shortage than hospitals in central China, especially those big hospitals with many inpatient beds (>800); and (3) the shortage situation was more serious in secondary hospitals than in the tertiary hospitals (Yang et al. 2018).

To address the drug shortage problem, the Chinese government employed several pharmaceutical policies, among which is a new public medicine procurement policy (NPMPP), which was introduced in January 2015 (Xiong et al. 2019). Previously, each province in China had a medicine tender bidding center to select medicine manufacturers and to determine medicine prices for public health institutions using a "two-envelope" system, which usually prefers lowest price (Hu 2017). To win the tender, the manufacturers usually offered a very low price that would not change for a long time. In the NPMPP, as long as the manufacturers met the technical and quality requirements, these manufacturers could be the procurement sources for all the public hospitals (NHFPC 2015). This policy is only implemented for paediatrics medicines, gynaecological medicines, emergency medicines and some common low-priced medicines. By using interrupted time-series analysis, Hu et al. identified a statistically significant increase in the prices of emergency medicines and gynaecological medicines, but a statistically significant decrease in the prices of paediatrics medicines after the introduction of NPMPP (Hu et al. 2019).

The Impact of Zero Mark-Up Policy on Healthcare Expenditure in China

A study to measure the impact of Zero Mark-Up Policy (ZMP) was conducted by Yang et al. The study was an interrupted time-series analysis evaluating the impact of ZMP on hospitalization expenditure after reimbursement at primary healthcare settings in Shaanxi Province. Two key indicators were measured after the implementation of the ZMP, i.e.

monthly average hospitalization expenditures and monthly average hospitalization expenditures after reimbursement. A statistically significant decrease in the level and trend of both indicators was detected after the introduction of the policy. However, the hospitalization expenditure and hospitalization expenditure after reimbursement were still increasing (Yang et al. 2017).

Adherence

A randomized cluster trial evaluating the impact of short messages service (SMS) by the pharmacy students on hypertension medication adherence, which is expected to provide the promising outcomes for the future, was proposed (Zhai et al. 2019). Zhai et al. designed the trial to evaluate the change in the level of adherence (using MMAS-8 scale) and blood pressure in response to SMS, to be sent every third day, and personnel consultation, to be done every third month. The short messages included important instructive information, i.e. normal blood pressure level, hypertension complications, healthy diet, salt intake and antihypertensive medication schedule. The outcomes measured were change in medication adherence and mean blood pressure and proportion of patients reaching controlled blood pressure at month 3 and month 6. The process is expected to strengthen the practicability/applicability of providing cheap and up-to-date reminders to patients that will ultimately improve adherence.

Antibiotic Use Studies in China

Knowledge, Attitude and Practices Towards Antibiotics

Antibiotics were regarded as the cornerstone of modern medicines to cure numerous infectious diseases owing to their inherited miraculous effects. However, their effectiveness is declining exponentially due to the rapid emergence of resistance (Rice 2018). Approximately 700,000 to several million deaths are reported worldwide due to antimicrobial resistance (AMR) every year (O'Neill 2016). The situation is devastating across the globe, including developing countries such as China, Ethiopia and Pakistan, possibly due to the increasing access to antibiotics. It is estimated that as much as 2 million US people suffer infections from resistant bacteria, and 23,000 die each year (Centers for Disease Control and Prevention 2016). Developing countries are also facing the problem of AMR with higher intensity and magnitude due to their weaker healthcare system (Carlin et al. 2014).

The education and awareness of the general public could play a key role in curbing the issue. However, the misconceptions about the rational use of antibiotics are widespread in the community. For example, a study conducted by Dan Ye et al. on 1400 residents in three distinct regions (central, western and eastern) of China found serious gaps in knowledge and attitude towards antibiotic use (Ye et al. 2017). Moreover, it was also observed that a large number of respondents were also involved in self-medication with antibiotics. The similar findings were also highlighted by Ali Hassan Gillani et al. and Muhammad Majid Aziz et al. in their studies conducted in the Punjab province of Pakistan (Gillani et al. 2017; Aziz et al. 2018).

Dispensing of Antibiotics in Community Pharmacies in China

The community pharmacists are often the first point of contact to facilitate timely access to treatment for patients with their minor ailments. It was indicated in a multi-country survey that 93% of people received their most recently used antibiotics from a medical store or a pharmacy (World Health Organization 2015). This is very different from developed countries, including northern European and North American countries where the dispensing of antibiotics is strictly controlled by prescriptions (Morgan et al. 2011).

A study conducted by Jie Chang et al. on 256 community pharmacies in three cities of China found the unsatisfactory performance of pharmacy staff regarding the provision of advice and dispensing of antibiotics; also, in more than 50% of the surveyed pharmacies, antibiotics were sold without any prescription (Chang et al. 2017). There are numerous effective methods used to investigate the dispensing of antibiotics at community pharmacies, and the method of using simulated clients has gained much consideration in recent years (Chang et al. 2017; Zawahir et al. 2019; Zapata-Cachafeiro et al. 2018). Simulated client is a highly reliable and robust method to evaluate the quality of pharmaceutical care-related services (Fitzpatrick and Tumlinson 2017). A simulated client is a trained individual who visits a drug store or a pharmacy to enact a scenario that investigates the specific behaviour of the pharmacy staff, including the pharmacist (Watson et al. 2006).

Recently, a study was undertaken by Jie Chang et al. to determine the non-prescription sale of antibiotics in 221 counties located in six different provinces of China (Chang et al. 2019). The data was collected by using trained simulated clients in 2423 community pharmacies. Two distinct scenarios based on adult acute upper respiratory tract infection (URTI) and paediatric diarrhoea were used. Out of 4822 simulated interactions, antibiotics were obtained during 1169/2411 (48.5% [95% CI 46.5–50.5]) diarrhoea interactions and 1690/2411 (70.1% [68.2–71.9]) URTI interactions. This irrational practice was found to be more prevalent in central and western provinces and the rural areas of China. Moreover, an inverse relationship was noticed between the non-prescription antibiotic sale and the presence of an on-site pharmacist (odds ratio 0.66 [0.56–0.78], $p<0.0001$). The results of the current study are not encouraging, though China has planned to uproot the practice of selling antibiotics without a prescription nationwide before 2020. Multifaceted approaches, including public awareness and continuous training programmes, coupled with the regulatory interventions, are required to prevent the irrational use of antibiotics.

Conclusion

In view of the above research, it can be concluded that the pharmaceutical sector along with the healthcare system of China is going through tremendous changes. The researchers as well as the policy makers have identified the key challenges related to medicine use and access in China and also other countries along the One Belt One Road Initiative.

References

United Nations Development Group and United Nations. (2003). Indicators for monitoring the millennium development goals: definitions, rationale, concepts and sources (Vol. 95). United Nations Publications.

Suh, G.H. (2011). High medicine prices and poor affordability. *Current opinion in psychiatry*, 24(4):341–345.

Paphitou, N.I. (2013). Antimicrobial resistance: action to combat the rising microbial challenges. *International journal of antimicrobial agents*, 42:S25–S28.

World Health Organization. (2001). How to develop and implement a national drug policy. Geneva: World Health Organization.

Traulsen, J.M., Almarsdóttir, A.B. (2005). The argument for pharmaceutical policy. *Pharmacy World and Science*, 27(1): 7–12.

Perehudoff, S.K., Alexandrov, N.V., Hogerzeil, H.V. (2019). Access to essential medicines in 195 countries: A human rights approach to sustainable development. *Global public health*, 14(3): 431–444.

Espin, J., Rovira, J. de Labry, A.O. (2011). Review series on pharmaceutical pricing policies and interventions: working paper 1: *external reference pricing. WHO/HAI.*

Acosta, A., Ciapponi, A., Aaserud, M., Vietto, V., Austvoll-Dahlgren, A., Kösters, J.P et al. (2014). Pharmaceutical policies: effects of reference pricing, other pricing, and purchasing policies. *Cochrane Database of Systematic Reviews*, 10:CD005979.

Ritter, A. (2009). How do drug policy makers access research evidence? *International Journal of Drug Policy*, 20(1):70–75.

Wang, S., Zhu, J., Gao, Z., Wu, W., and Yao, L. (2018). Discussion on key drugs in shortage and their supply safeguard measures. *Chin. Pharm. Aff*, 8:1034–1042.

Jiang, M., Zhou, Z., Wu, L., Shen, Q., Lv, B., Wang, X., et al. (2015). Medicine prices, availability, and affordability in the Shaanxi Province in China: implications for the future. *International journal of clinical pharmacy*, 37(1), 12–17.

Fang, Y., Wagner, A.K., Yang, S., Jiang, M., Zhang, F., Ross-Degnan, D. (2013). Access to affordable medicines after health reform: evidence from two cross-sectional surveys in Shaanxi Province, western China. *The Lancet Global Health*, 1(4):e227–e237.

Górski, J., Chaisse, J, Chi, M. (2017). One Belt One Road Initiative ("OBOR"): Editorial. Transnational Dispute Management, 14(3). Available at SSRN: https://ssrn.com/abstract=3051785.

Quick, J.D., Hume, M.L., Rankin, J.R., O'Connor, R.W., Rankin, J.R., O'Connor, R. W. (1997). *Managing Drug Supply Management Sciences for Health.*

Husereau, D.R., & Cameron, C.G. (2012). Value-Based Pricing of Pharmaceuticals in Canada: Opportunities to Expand the Role of Health Technology Assessment? Canadian Health Services Research Foundation.

World Health Organization. (2004). WHO medicines strategy 2004–2007: countries at the core (No. WHO/EDM/2004.5). Geneva: World Health Organization.

World Health Organization. (2008). Measuring medicine prices, availability, affordability and price components (No. WHO/PSM/PAR/2008.3). Geneva: World Health Organization.

Ogurtsova, K., da Rocha Fernandes, J.D., Huang, Y., Linnenkamp, U., Guariguata, L., Cho, N.H., et al. (2017). IDF Diabetes Atlas: Global estimates for the prevalence of diabetes for 2015 and 2040. *Diabetes research and clinical practice*, 128:40–50.

Yang, C., Hu, S., Zhu, Y., Zhu, W., Li, Z., Fang, Y. (2019). Evaluating access to oral anti-diabetic medicines: A cross-sectional survey of prices, availability and affordability in Shaanxi Province, Western China. *PloS One*, 14(10): e0223769.

Li, Z., Feng, Q., Kabba, J.A., Yang, C., Chang, J., Jiang, M., et al. (2019). Prices, availability and affordability of insulin products: a cross-sectional survey in Shaanxi Province, western China. *Tropical Medicine & International Health*, 24(1):43–52.

Saeed A, Saeed H, Saleem Z, Fang Y, Babar Z-U-D. (2019). Evaluation of prices, availability and affordability of essential medicines in Lahore Division, Pakistan: A cross-sectional survey using WHO/HAI methodology. *PloS One*, 14(4): e0216122. https://doi.org/10.1371/journal.pone.0216122.

Gray A, Manasse HR Jr. (2012). Shortages of medicines: a complex global challenge. *Bulletin of World Health Organization*, 90(3): 158±158A.

Wu, L., Fang, Y., Yang, C., Shen, Q., Chang, J., Zhu, W., et al. (2016). A review of research on drug shortages in China. *Chin. Pharm. Aff*, 5:458–465.

Yang, C., Wu, L., Cai, W., Zhu, W., Shen, Q., Li, Z., et al. (2016). Current situation, determinants, and solutions to drug shortages in Shaanxi Province, China: a qualitative study. *PloS One*, 11(10): e0165183.

Yang, C., Cai, W., Li, Z., Page, A.T., Fang, Y. (2018). The current status and effects of emergency drug shortages in China: Perceptions of emergency department physicians. *PloS One*, 13(10): e0205238.

Xiong, K., Chen, H., Zhang, Z., and Xu, J. (2019). Feasibility demonstration and comparative study of "Two-Vote System" of pharmaceutical procurement of public medical institutions. *Chin. Hosp. Manage*, 2: 21–23.

Hu, S. (2017). The Theory and practice of "Two-Invoice System" in the drug procurement. *China Academic Journal Electronic Publishing House*, 4:8–10.

NHFPC. Notice on the procurement and supply of emergency medicine. Division of Drug Policy and Essential Drug Policy. Beijing: China's National Health and Family Planning Commission, 2015.

Hu, S., Chen, C., Yuan, S., Xue, F., Shi, L., Fang, Y., et al. (2019). The effects of a new public medicine procurement policy on medicine price in China: an interrupted time series analysis. *Frontiers in Pharmacology*, 10: 950.

Yang, C., Shen, Q., Cai, W., Zhu, W., Li, Z., Wu, L., et al. (2017). Impact of the zero-markup drug policy on hospitalisation expenditure in western rural China: an interrupted time series analysis. *Tropical Medicine & International Health*, *22*(2):180–186.

Zhai, P., Li, Q., Gillani, A.H., Hayat, K., Shi, L., Wang, S., et al. (2019). The impact of short message services and personal consultation by pharmacy students on medication adherence and blood pressure control: study protocol for a cluster randomized trial. *Patient Preference and Adherence*, 13:627.

Rice, L.B. (2018). Antimicrobial stewardship and antimicrobial resistance. *Medical Clinics*, *102*(5):805–818.

O'Neill, J. (2016). Tackling Drug-Resistant Infections Globally: Final Report and Recommendations. [cited 2019 December 1]; Available from: https://amr-review.org/sites/default/files/160525_Final%20paper_with%20cover.pdf

Centers for Disease Control and Prevention. Antibiotic/Antimicrobial Resistance. 2016 [Cited 2019 August 20]; Available from: https://www.cdc.gov/drugresistance/

Carlin, K., Lofmark, S., Blad, L. (2014). Swedish work on containment of antibiotic resistance. *Public Health Agency of Sweden: Stockholm, Sweden.*

Ye, D., Chang, J., Yang, C., Yan, K., Ji, W., Aziz, M.M., et al. (2017). How does the general public view antibiotic use in China? Result from a cross-sectional survey. *International Journal of Clinical Pharmacy*, 39(4): 927–934.

Gillani, A., Ji, W., Hussain, W., Imran, A., Chang, J., Yang, C. et al. (2017). Antibiotic self-medication among Non-Medical University Students in Punjab, Pakistan: a cross-sectional survey. *International Journal of Environmental Research and Public Health*, 14(10):1152.

Aziz, M.M., Masood, I., Yousaf, M., Saleem, H., Ye, D., Fang, Y. (2018). Pattern of medication selling and self-medication practices: A study from Punjab, Pakistan. *PloS One, 13*(3): e0194240.

World Health Organization. (2015). Antibiotic resistance: multi-country public awareness survey. [cited 2019 November 1]; Available from: Available at: http://apps.who.int/iris/bitstream/10665/194460/1/9789241509817_eng.pdf

Morgan, D.J., Okeke, I.N., Laxminarayan, R., Perencevich, E.N., Weisenberg, S. (2011). Non-prescription antimicrobial use worldwide: a systematic review. *The Lancet infectious diseases*, 11(9): 692–701.

Chang, J., Ye, D., Lv, B., Jiang, M., Zhu, S., Yan, K., et al. (2017). Sale of antibiotics without a prescription at community pharmacies in urban China: a multicentre cross-sectional survey. *Journal of Antimicrobial Chemotherapy, 72*(4):1235–1242.

Zawahir, S., Lekamwasam, S., Aslani, P. (2019). Antibiotic dispensing practice in community pharmacies: A simulated client study. *Research in Social and Administrative Pharmacy*, 15(5):584–590.

Zapata-Cachafeiro, M., Piñeiro-Lamas, M., Guinovart, M.C., López-Vázquez, P., Vázquez-Lago, J.M., & Figueiras, A. (2018). Magnitude and determinants of antibiotic dispensing without prescription in Spain: a simulated patient study. *Journal of Antimicrobial Chemotherapy*, 74(2):511–514.

Fitzpatrick, A., Tumlinson, K. (2017). Strategies for optimal implementation of simulated clients for measuring quality of care in low-and middle-income countries. *Global Health: Science and Practice*, 5(1):108–114.

Watson, M.C., Norris, P., Granas, A.G. (2006). A systematic review of the use of simulated patients and pharmacy practice research. *International Journal of Pharmacy Practice*, 14(2): 83–93.

Chang, J., Xu, S., Zhu, S., Li, Z., Yu, J., Zhang, Y., et al. (2019). Assessment of non-prescription antibiotic dispensing at community pharmacies in China with simulated clients: a mixed cross-sectional and longitudinal study. *The Lancet Infectious Diseases*, 19(12):1345–1354.

12

Access to Vaccines and Immunization Programme

Suthira Taychakhoonavudh

Introduction

Vaccines are among one of the most cost-effective health interventions known to man. The goal of vaccination is to protect humans against infectious diseases through training the human's immune system to quickly respond to microorganisms when it attacks the human body. With a long history of vaccination, smallpox has finally been eradicated from the world through systematic vaccination in 1980, and other diseases like polio are on its way to eradication (Henderson 2011; World Health Organization 2019a). The World Health Organization has estimated that immunization prevents an estimated 2.5 million child deaths annually (Maurice and Davey 2009).

According to WHO, there are vaccines which target more than 25 pathogens that are the cause of human diseases currently (World Health

S. Taychakhoonavudh (✉)
Social and Administrative Pharmacy Department, Faculty of Pharmaceutical Sciences, Chulalongkorn University, Bangkok, Thailand
e-mail: Suthira.T@Chula.ac.th

Z. Babar (ed.), *Global Pharmaceutical Policy*,
https://doi.org/10.1007/978-981-15-2724-1_12

Organization 2019b). It is reported that more than 132 vaccines are in the research and development from phase I to phase III clinical trials. These vaccines target 46 different pathogens (Angela and Shen 2018). The progress on immunization, however, is quite slow as before 1974, less than 5% of children were receiving a vaccine against six WHO target diseases including diphtheria, tetanus, whooping cough, polio, measles and tuberculosis during their first year of life (Keja et al. 1988). Access to vaccine especially in developing countries is thus a critical issue as the intervention itself has undoubtedly provided tremendous clinical and economic benefits. Subjects around the access to vaccine topics have been under the attention of international organizations as well as researchers around the world.

This chapter describes the unique characteristics of vaccines compared to other pharmaceutical products. Situation of access to vaccine and immunization as well as factors affecting vaccine uptake and policies and programmes addressing access to vaccine are explained. Current issues and challenges on access to vaccine and immunization including vaccine hesitancy and adolescent immunization are covered at the end of this chapter.

Why Vaccines are Different from Other Pharmaceutical Products?

Since the goal of vaccination is to train the human's immune system to recognize and respond to pathogens, most vaccines are agents that are similar to pathogens, for example, a weakened or killed version of the microorganisms. Vaccine is considered a biological product as the production of vaccine involves weakening or killing the pathogens or using recombinant technology to produce the vaccine. The vaccine thus can vary due to its production process from starting materials, the microorganism itself, the environmental condition of the microbial culture, the knowledge and experience of the manufacturing technician and the steps involved in the purification processes (Plotkin et al. 2017). This is different from the production of chemical drugs in which the production process is relatively well defined and uniform.

Before vaccine enters the market, manufacturers must demonstrate the safety, efficacy and quality of vaccine. The quality aspect of the vaccine intensifies the complexities of vaccine production since the methods used to analyse the quality of the vaccine often have high variability (Plotkin et al. 2017). Thus, when regulatory authorities approve the vaccine product, they do not approve only the vaccine product but also the processes through which the vaccine is produced (Mitchell et al. 1993; U.S. Food and Drug Administration 2018). Any changes made to the approved production process would result in the change in the quality, safety and efficacy of the final product, and as a result, regulatory authorities may need the manufacturer to conduct a clinical trial to validate this new process.

To add to the complexity, vaccine is a health intervention that is used in a healthy population. All of these combined are the major causes of vaccine supply shortage as found in the issue of the production of DTP-backboned combination vaccines commented by Vidor and colleagues (Vidor and Soubeyrand 2016). Thus, when the topic of access to vaccine is discussed, it always involves both the demand side and the supply side.

Measurement of Vaccination Coverage

Governments of countries around the world as well as international organizations put access to vaccine as one of their foci. It is important to have a timely and accurate measurement of vaccination coverage to evaluate the success of vaccination programme. The measurement of vaccination coverage can be as simple as how many children have received the vaccine as a numerator and how many children are eligible for vaccination as a denominator. However, the more critical issue regarding the measurement of vaccination coverage is the selection of the vaccine to be monitored. Since the vaccine schedule varies by region to region and country to country, the most commonly used measure to track global vaccination coverage is the coverage rate of diphtheria-tetanus-pertussis-containing vaccine (DTPCV) and measles-containing vaccine (MCV). Coverage rates of DTPCV and MCV are selected as the vaccines themselves are the common vaccines that should be administered in every region of the world. These vaccines are also among two of the first four from six vaccines that WHO aimed to have universal coverage (Keja et al. 1988).

The administration of DTPCV is generally three doses and mostly through routine immunization (RI). The high coverage of the first dose of diphtheria-tetanus-pertussis-containing vaccine (DTPCV1) suggests that the region or the country or the area has good access to primary healthcare facilities as well as population acceptance of vaccination (Cutts et al. 2016). The rate of DTPCV coverage between the first and third dose is usually compared and computed as a dropout rate to reflect the performance of country's healthcare system, for example, healthcare infrastructure including registry and surveillance of vaccination coverage system.

MCV coverage rate has a different aspect to monitor country's immunization programme since the administration of MCV is mostly through mass vaccination campaigns known as supplementary immunization activities (SIAs). SIAs usually involve the delivery of vaccine to target populations regardless of the person's previous vaccination status over a short period of time (Utazi et al. 2019). MCV coverage rate thus reflects the country's effort in disease control and elimination as well as how the country tackles the target populations who are missed by the routine vaccination programme (Utazi et al. 2019; Mbabazi et al. 2009).

Another aspect of monitoring coverage rate is to measure proportion of population that are fully immunized with the recommended vaccine or dropout rate. To fully stimulate the body's immune response towards the pathogen, most vaccines have to be administered several doses at different time frames. If not fully immunized, the duration of protection of the vaccine may be less than expected, and thus the person will still be susceptible to the targeted diseases. Normally, one specific vaccine dropout rate is measured; for example, the DTPCV1 to DTPCV3 dropout rate measures the proportion of the population that have received first dose of DTPCV and completed the third dose of DTPCV. This measure is usually considered as an indicator for vaccine delivery effectiveness (Mane 2015). A more recent measure of dropout rate recommended is the first dose of DTPCV to measles first dose dropout rate (DTPCV1-MCV1). This dropout measure is recommended since it measures dropout over a longer time interval between doses and could better reflect overall immunization programme effectiveness (Mane 2015).

Other measures of vaccination coverage include the missed opportunities to administer all vaccines scheduled at the same visit. This measure can be used to supplement the information regarding the country's immunization programme. When high proportion of population miss some vaccines that are scheduled at the same visit, this could indicate the supply shortage of some vaccines, the flaw in the children's vaccination record system as well as the acceptance of multiple vaccine administration (Sridhar et al. 2014).

Methods to Measure Vaccination Coverage

Even though vaccination coverage rate is in principle the number children who have received the vaccine divided by number of children who are eligible for vaccination, several methods have been proposed and used to measure vaccination coverage. Cutts and colleagues have summarized the methods mostly used to monitor coverage which include electronic vaccination registries, routine report of vaccinations delivered and community-based surveys (Cutts et al. 2016). An accurate measure of vaccination coverage is very important since it measures immunization programme effectiveness. When vaccination coverage is overestimated meaning that less numbers of children are being vaccinated than the reported number, an outbreak of the vaccine-preventable disease could be a case. In 2009, a national vaccination coverage of Burkina Faso, Africa, was estimated to be more than 95% of the population. However, in that year, a large measles outbreak occurred in Burkina Faso that resulted in 367 deaths, most of whom are unvaccinated children (Kidd et al. 2012). Thus, it is important to select the method to measure vaccination coverage that is appropriate to the context of the settings where vaccination coverage is measured.

The most complete and accurate method to monitor a real-time data on cumulative vaccination status of individual persons and populations is an electronic immunization registry. The registry itself can be used in conjunction with the vaccine supply and stock monitoring system. The challenges are instead the implementation of the system since it requires a good information technology and data structure as well as the budget and human resources to design, implement and maintain the system. The data structure not only includes data on vaccination status but also birth registry and person's unique identifier since these are the information needed to calculate coverage rate. The use of electronic vaccination registry is thus mostly reported in more developed countries, for example, immunization information systems (IISs) in the USA in which more than 94% of children aged 4 months through 5 years had ≥2 doses recorded in IISs (Murthy et al. 2017). More recent literatures have shown that the registry has been increasingly used in low- to middle-income countries like Brazil and Vietnam (Sato et al. 2018; Nguyen et al. 2017).

Many countries, however, still rely on routine report system of vaccinations delivered which is mostly paper-based. The number of children who are eligible for vaccination is mostly estimated and usually inaccurate especially at the local level. Use of paper-based routine report system is thus considered as unreliable since the records of individual vaccination status can be incomplete and mostly do not include vaccination done in private sector (Brown et al. 2014; Burton et al. 2009; Lim et al. 2008).

Another method mostly used by immunization programmes in many countries is survey of vaccination status of the population. The method is sometimes used in conjunction with paper-based routine report to triangulate the data from both sources. Since the measure relies on survey of the population, the reliability of the measure relies on the quality of the survey. The survey methods have been developed and used for more than 30 years from the time when many countries still have no baseline information on the immunization coverage. With the progress on the immunization, the sampling method employed by the survey has also been advanced. During the 1980s when the baseline information of immunization coverage is still not available, the assumption of 50% coverage or the spinning of a bottle on even ground in a central location in the village or town as a sampling method was deemed acceptable (World Health Organization 2005). As the immunization activities have progressed over the years, the use of vaccination coverage measure has changed to a more area-specific coverage rate as well as a root cause analysis of non-immunization. In order to do so, the cluster survey with probability sampling methods is now recommended by the World Health Organization (WHO) which includes the design of the survey, sample size calculation, analysis of the survey data and quality control of the data (Danovaro-Holliday et al. 2018).

Factors Affecting Access to Vaccines and Immunization Programme

When measuring access to vaccines and immunization, two main aspects of access are usually measured: the non-vaccinated and the under-vaccinated. An under-vaccinated child was defined as any child receiving at least one but not all recommended routine EPI vaccines while a non-vaccinated child was defined as one who has not received any EPI vaccines (Rainey et al. 2011).

The first dose of DTPCV coverage rate fundamentally reflects the non-vaccination rate of the population while the third dose of DTPCV coverage rate reflects the under-vaccination rate of the population. Many works have been done to explore what factor is associated with the non-vaccination and under-vaccination. Systematic review by Rainey and colleagues in 2009 has summarized reasons related to non-vaccination and under-vaccination of children in low- and middle-income countries from 202 studies conducted from 1999 to 2009. The main reasons for non-vaccination and under-vaccination can be categorized into four main causes: the immunization systems, family characteristics, parental attitudes and related knowledge and limitations or weaknesses in immunization-related communication and information. Another review of grey literatures by Favin et al. found similar factors that were related to non-vaccination and under-vaccination (Favin et al. 2012). Reasons linked to being non-vaccinated and under-vaccinated were, however, slightly different as the decision not to vaccinate the child and the decision not to fully vaccinate the child are different in context. It should also be noted that even though these factors were identified as a single factor, they are multi-factorial and could happen at the same time with different degrees (Xeuatvongsa et al. 2017).

For under-vaccination, the immunization systems are the most frequent factors found in the literatures which include access or distance to immunization services, missed opportunities due to lack of child's immunization, low health worker knowledge and cost for vaccinations. Family characteristics include socioeconomic status and education level that also play an important role of whether the child would be fully vaccinated. Parental attitudes and knowledge especially the benefits and importance of vaccine as well as how the healthcare workers communicate these benefits were also significant (Rainey et al. 2011; Favin et al. 2012).

Even though immunization systems were still the important factors linked to being completely non-vaccinated, parental attitudes and knowledge especially beliefs that are directly related to religious and cultural beliefs against vaccinations become the most cited cause of being completely non-vaccinated (Rainey et al. 2011; Favin et al. 2012). This suggests that reducing both direct and indirect costs related to immunization could increase access to vaccine to those who have financial barriers due to either vaccine or immunization service costs, time away from work or traveling costs. However, in those who decide not to vaccinate their child at all, this might directly be related to their personal beliefs that reducing financial barriers would not improve the access situation.

Policies and Programmes Aiming at Increasing Access to Vaccine and Immunization Services

The reasons for under-vaccination and non-vaccination are multi-factorial and thus require a complex intervention to address these barriers. Policies and programmes in the beginning have focused on making vaccine and immunization services to have universal coverage through donation and public funding. However, to make immunization programmes sustainable and strengthen the health system, the vaccine market should be under the attention of international organizations around the globe. Examples of key policies and programmes that have increased access to vaccine and immunization services are summarized.

Expanded Programme on Immunization (EPI) and National Immunization Programme

Situation of access to vaccine became an interest of health policy makers around the globe after the establishment of the Expanded Programme on Immunization (EPI). The programme was established in 1974 by the World Health Organization (WHO) whose aim is to increase uptake of vaccines against six major vaccine-preventable diseases including measles, diphtheria, pertussis, tetanus, poliomyelitis and tuberculosis around the globe by 1991. Before the programme was in place, less than 5% of the world's children were immunized against these six target diseases (Keja et al. 1988).

The establishment of the WHO's EPI was a game-changing policy in the immunization area. Even though the aim of the WHO's EPI is to achieve universal access to immunization, the programme's main activities are not limited to providing vaccine to countries in need but also to support technical and managerial functions necessary to routinely vaccinate children with a limited supply of vaccines. The WHO's EPI thus acts as a blueprint and makes recommendations for each country's national immunization programme. Therefore, the term country's national immunization programme (NIP) is sometimes used interchangeably with the Expanded Programme on Immunization (EPI). Apart from the six targeted diseases (diphtheria, measles, pertussis, poliomyelitis, tetanus and tuberculosis) which were the foci by the WHO's EPI in 1974, other new vaccines can be added to routine immunization schedule of each country independently (Keja et al. 1988). WHO's role is to make recommendations by providing global-level policies and technical guidance on what should be the national vaccine schedule. The decision-making authority is however on the national key decision-makers, for example, national immunization manager, chairs and members of national advisory committees on immunization.

A systematic review of national immunization policy making processes from 33 countries by Bryson found that decision-making processes and types of evidence used when making immunization policies vary from country to country. These evidences that were taken into account when making recommendations include burden of disease, economic evaluation results, feasibility of local vaccine production, recommendations by other countries, public perception regarding the vaccine and vaccine safety and effectiveness (Bryson et al. 2010). Since the information used to develop national immunization policies is complex, the establishment of National Immunization Technical Advisory Groups (NITAGs) in each country is recommended by WHO and emphasized in the Global Vaccine Action Plan (GVAP) (World Health Organization 2019c). National Immunization Technical Advisory Groups (NITAGs) are bodies composed of national experts including clinicians, epidemiologists, immunologists, health economists, infectious disease experts, microbiologists, nurses, paediatricians, public health experts and vaccine researchers as well as community members or insurance representatives (Bryson et al. 2010). NITAG's role is to guide the development of evidence-based national immunization policies by collecting, reviewing and assessing the current evidences of the vaccine of interest. It is also important that all of these processes are transparent and independent from any particular group. According to NITAG resource centre, from 190 countries, 124 countries reported the existence of NITAG while 82 of 124 meet all six of WHO's NITAG functionality criteria (NITAG Resource Center 2019).

Shen and colleagues have summarized the eight critical elements of routine immunization programmes which include (1) policy, standards and guidelines; (2) governance, organization and management; (3) human resources; (4) vaccine, cold chain and logistics management; (5) service delivery; (6) communication and community partnerships; (7) data generation and use; and (8) sustainable financing (Shen et al. 2014). Thus, the WHO's EPI has not only focused on making vaccine and immunization services available through donation and public funding but has also been working on health system strengthening to make access to immunization sustainable in the long run (Okwo-Bele and Cherian 2011). Health system strengthening activities done by WHO include training health personnel involved with EPI, improving infrastructure of the healthcare system (e.g. cold chain and vaccine logistics) and improving and ensuring the quality and safety of vaccine.

The Global Alliance for Vaccines and Immunisation (GAVI)

The immunization coverage statistics have shown progress on immunization as the coverage of DTPCV for the third dose has increased tremendously to 70% between the years 1990 and 2000 after the global implementation of EPI (Balasubramaniam 2014). However, this progress was ground to a halt as the coverage rate was hovering around this number with no increase. Immunization has become a spotlight among the country's leaders again in 2000 as a reduction of childhood mortality is in one of the Millennium Development Goals (MDGs). Eight Millennium Development Goals (MDGs) were committed by leaders of countries who are members of United Nations aiming at reducing poverty and improving human development by 2015, and MDG 4 calls for a two-third reduction of deaths of children under five years of age or under-five mortality rate.

The progress in global immunization coverage was also accelerated by the establishment of the Global Alliance for Vaccines and Immunisation (GAVI) in 2000. GAVI is a public-private partnership between major key stakeholders in immunization that included the industry, non-governmental organizations and foundations, academia, donor countries and key international organizations such as the United Nations Children's Fund (UNICEF), the World Health Organization (WHO) and the World Bank. With the initial funding from the Bill & Melinda Gates Foundation, GAVI works in the world's poorest countries whose aim is to increase equitable use of vaccine in these countries.

Countries with whom GAVI has been working with, for example, African and Southeast Asian regions, actually cover a high proportion of the world's population with growing economy making these countries a potential market for vaccine. Analysis by Makenga and colleagues revealed that, when targeting diseases almost exclusively in the African region, having a vaccine production facility for the region becomes feasible. Some common gaps in these countries include regulatory functionality gap, for example, the quality of control laboratories to test vaccine lots before release, technological gap that may need technology transfer from developed countries and more importantly political will from the government for the vaccine production in these countries to be a success (Makenga et al. 2019). Thus, GAVI's strategy does not only focus on introducing new vaccines to children in these countries (GAVI's vaccine goal in GAVI's strategic goal) but also expands their foci into health system strengthening (GAVI's health system goal), vaccine market shaping (GAVI's market shaping goal) and improving sustainability of the programme (GAVI's sustainability goal) (Storeng 2014). This is to ensure sustainability of high vaccination coverage especially after GAVI has withdrawn from these GAVI-supported countries (Gavi tVA 2017).

Global Vaccine Action Plan 2011–2020

The Global Vaccine Action Plan 2011–2020 (GVAP) is the most recent global movement towards the more equitable access to immunization. GVAP was endorsed by the World Health Assembly in 2012 whose goal is to reach ≥90% of national coverage for all vaccines in the country's routine immunization schedule by 2020.

The most recent report on global routine vaccination coverage in 2017 has shown that the global coverage of third dose of DTPCV, first dose of MCV and third dose of polio vaccine has remained stable at 84–85% since 2010. It was shown that some countries and regions have coverage rate of third dose of DTPCV reaching the GVAP 2020 target of >90% while almost 40% of the countries still remain below the target. Sixty-two percent of the children who were not vaccinated with the third dose of DTPCV were in ten countries. The trend is similar for coverage rate of first dose of MCV both globally and nationally. Targeted, context-specific strategies are the steps that should be a focus to reach GVAP 2020 goal. The coverage rates of other vaccines such as second dose of MCV, rotavirus vaccine, pneumococcal conjugate vaccine (PCV), rubella vaccine and *Haemophilus influenzae* type b (Hib) and hepatitis B (HepB) vaccine have also shown an increasing trend (VanderEnde et al. 2018).

Vaccine Hesitancy: A New Barrier to Access

With all the efforts being made for vaccine and immunization services to have universal coverage, most developed countries have a very high national childhood vaccination coverage rate. However, disease outbreaks of these vaccine-preventable diseases have been reported sporadically. In 2015, a measles outbreak in California in the USA has a total of 125 measles cases which originated from the Disneyland theme park. Almost half of these patients were unvaccinated due to several reasons including being too young to be vaccinated. However, the majority of the unvaccinated were intentionally unvaccinated because of personal beliefs (Zipprich et al. 2015). In the Netherlands, where MMRCV coverage rate is higher than 95%, several large measles epidemics occurred in 1992–1994, in 1999–2000 and in 2013–2014. The outbreaks mainly affected Orthodox Protestants who live in a geographically clustered population and refuse to be vaccinated (Woudenberg et al. 2017).

This refusal to be vaccinated is directly related to vaccine hesitancy which is defined by WHO as "a delay in acceptance or refusal of vaccines despite availability of vaccinations services" (Strategic Advisory Group of Experts (SAGE) on Immunization 2014). Vaccine hesitancy has been an issue for as long as vaccine has been used. The anti-vaccination movements are more powerful with the information exchange becoming easier through Internet and social media (Dubé et al. 2015a). It is, however, difficult to quantify the prevalence of vaccine consistency. WHO recently developed survey questions in order to improve the measurement of hesitancy, but the survey can provide only a rough estimate of the vaccine hesitancy problem (Larson et al. 2015).

As summarized in the previous section, parental attitudes and knowledge especially beliefs that are directly related to religious and cultural beliefs against vaccinations are the most important causes of being completely non-vaccinated (Rainey et al. 2011; Favin et al. 2012). These beliefs and perceptions surrounding the choice to vaccinate are context, time, place, programme and vaccine specific and require a complex and multi-dimensional approach to tackle the issue. WHO's SAGE working group has reviewed and provided the "3 Cs" model for determinants of vaccine hesitancy including confidence, complacency and convenience (Strategic Advisory Group of Experts (SAGE) on Immunization 2014).

In the model, confidence refers to trust in the efficacy and safety of vaccines, the reliability and competency of the delivery systems including healthcare services and professionals and the policy makers' motivation on the essential vaccines (Strategic Advisory Group of Experts (SAGE) on Immunization 2014). The most prominent cause of vaccine hesitancy is thus the nature of the vaccine product and immunization service itself. The unique characteristic of vaccine is that it is administered in healthy people and mostly administered in young children. The safety and quality of vaccine thus is very much a concern of parents, and perceived risks of vaccinating their children are greater than the actual risks. Salmon et al. have summarized perceived risks of vaccine that are directly related to vaccine hesitancy which include the inability of parents to control the risks of adverse reactions, the manmade nature of vaccines and the unpredictability of adverse reactions (Salmon et al. 2015). Historical controversies and vaccination scare also exacerbate vaccine refusal situation. Examples of these controversies are the association between the hepatitis B vaccine and multiple sclerosis in France that was found later on that there was no evidence of such an association and the well-known fraudulent association between the MMR vaccination and autism that is still referred by anti-vaccination groups today (François et al. 2005; Poland and Spier 2010). Vaccination complacency happens when the perceived risks of vaccine-preventable diseases are low (Strategic Advisory Group of Experts (SAGE) on Immunization 2014). Immunization programme success in the past is also the cause of vaccine complacency. With the progress in immunization, many parents have no experiences with those vaccine-preventable diseases and thus perceive low severity or low susceptibility of the disease (Smith et al. 2017). Lastly, vaccination convenience which includes vaccine and immunization service affordability, physical availability, geographical accessibility, language and health literacy of the person to understand the services would likely affect the decision to be vaccinated resulting in vaccine hesitancy (Strategic Advisory Group of Experts (SAGE) on Immunization 2014).

This "3Cs" model explains the root causes of vaccine hesitancy. However, the decision-making process of an individual is more complex and could be affected by many influential factors from contextual influences (influences arising due to historical, socio-cultural, environmental, health system/institutional, economic or political factors), individual and group influences (influences arising from personal perception of the vaccine or influences of the social/peer environment) and vaccine- or immunization-specific issues (influences directly related to vaccine or immunization service itself) (Strategic Advisory Group of Experts (SAGE) on Immunization 2014).

Mandatory Immunization: A New Approach to Increase Access to Vaccines

In the past, public health education campaigns are the main strategies used by public health professionals all over the world to increase access to vaccine. These public health education campaigns have been based on a "knowledge-deficit" approach assuming that individuals have incomplete information regarding the vaccine and immunization services and would change their mind if given the proper information. Decision-making process to vaccinate is far more complex and affected by many factors. A review of published reviews has found that there is no strong evidence to recommend any specific intervention to address vaccine hesitancy/refusal. It was found that many traditional educational tools (e.g. information pamphlets) had little or no impact on decision to be vaccinated (Dubé et al. 2015b). Instead, to strongly advocate a vaccination campaign may have negative unintended consequences from those already hesitant as found by Nyhan and colleagues (2014).

Mandatory immunization becomes appealing to health policy makers around the globe as a means to increase vaccine uptake. Mandatory immunization programmes have been implemented in many countries in which some are nationally implemented and some are implemented by state or local government. A review of vaccination policies in 31 European countries reveals that 11 countries have mandatory vaccination policies for at least one vaccine. The programmes however vary considerably by the level of enforcement (Bozzola et al. 2018). MacDonald and colleagues have summarized the mandatory immunization policy into five main types: (1) requiring immunization through law but anyone can opt out without penalty, (2) requiring immunization through law but anyone can opt out with personal or philosophical objection without penalty, (3) requiring parents to be educated about immunization and may opt out with personal or philosophical objection without penalty but requires specific notarization, (4) requiring immunization but can opt out with personal or philosophical objection that requires specific forms as well as penalty for noncompliance, and (5) requiring immunization with serious financial penalties or social restrictions, only allowing medical exemptions (MacDonald et al. 2018).

Even though mandatory immunization has been increasingly used by many countries, data on effectiveness of mandates is still unclear. Systematic review of the effect of immunization mandates on uptake of routine childhood immunizations has shown that immunization mandates generally led to increased short-term and long-term vaccine uptake. Studies included in this systematic review were, however, focused on middle school mandates in the USA (Lee and Robinson 2016). Mandatory immunization policy may also have negative aspects that health policy makers should take into account which include unintended consequences of mandates on the vaccines and government's compensation policy for adverse events following immunization (AEFIs) that were related to vaccination mandates. Otherwise it would be easier to extend the benefits of vaccination and services before considering mandating immunization.

Adolescent and Adult Vaccine: The New Challenges

The progress in global immunization to date has been surrounding around infant and childhood immunization. EPI's goal and mostly used vaccination coverage measures have focused on childhood vaccination coverage, for example, DTPCV coverage rate or MMR coverage rate. However, more adolescent (persons aged 10–19) and adult vaccines become available in the market, for example, human papillomavirus vaccine (HPV); tetanus, diphtheria and pertussis vaccine (Tdap); meningitis vaccine (meningococcal conjugate vaccine [MCV4]); herpes zoster vaccine (HZ); and seasonal influenza vaccine. These diseases that can be prevented in adolescents and adults have no less importance than vaccine-preventable diseases in infants and children. Adolescents are becoming more important as less infants and children are infected with these vaccine-preventable diseases; for example, pertussis incidence is highest in adolescents aged 11 to 18 years old (Broder et al. 2006).

The unique characteristic of adult vaccine is that immunization recommendations are usually for a specific population; for example, herpes zoster vaccine is recommended for adults aged 55 years and older. This does not include seasonal flu vaccine which is recommended to all adults with no contraindications (Kim et al. 2017).

In 2013, using National Health Interview Survey (NHIS) data, the US Centers for Disease Control and Prevention reported the coverage rate of adult vaccines in the USA to be low. Coverage for tetanus and diphtheria toxoid with acellular pertussis vaccine (Tdap) vaccination is 17.2% while coverage for human papillomavirus vaccination among males aged 19–26 years is as low as 5.9%. It was also found that there are racial/ethnic disparities in terms of access for routinely recommended adult vaccines (Williams et al. 2015).

Inadequate resources have been invested in immunizing adolescents and adults while the global population pattern is changing into ageing society and many more vaccines for adolescents and adults would become available in the market. The new challenge for controlling vaccine-preventable diseases is to plan on how to initiate immunization programmes for these age groups efficiently.

Conclusion

Since the first discovery of smallpox vaccine by Edward Jenner in 1796, the overall progress in immunization is promising as smallpox is finally eradicated while other diseases are on its path of being eliminated from the world. We have seen large humanitarian efforts from international organizations along with donor countries who work cooperatively to provide low-cost vaccines to individuals living in low-income countries. With several global movements described in this chapter, the situation of access to vaccines and immunization services in many low- to middle-income countries has shown promising progress. However, in order to maximize the benefits of vaccines, policy makers around the globe still need to overcome many challenges to make immunization a sustainable public health policy.

References

Henderson DA. The eradication of smallpox–an overview of the past, present, and future. Vaccine. 2011;29:D7–D9.

World Health Organization. Poliomyelitis Key facts: World Health Organization; 2019a Available from: https://www.who.int/en/news-room/fact-sheets/detail/poliomyelitis.

Maurice JM, Davey S. State of the World's Vaccines and Immunization: World Health Organization; 2009.

World Health Organization. Vaccines and diseases: World Health Organization; 2019b Available from: https://www.who.int/immunization/diseases/en/.

Angela K. Shen MTC. From the Analyst's Couch: Infectious disease vaccines: Nature Reviews Drug Discovery; 2018 Available from: https://www.nature.com/articles/d41573-018-00011-6.

Keja K, Chan C, Hayden G, Henderson RH. Expanded programme on immunization. World health statistics quarterly Rapport trimestriel de statistiques sanitaires mondiales. 1988;41(2):59–63.

Plotkin S, Robinson JM, Cunningham G, Iqbal R, Larsen S. The complexity and cost of vaccine manufacturing–an overview. Vaccine. 2017;35(33):4064–71.

Mitchell VS, Philipose NM, Sanford JP. The children's vaccine initiative: achieving the vision: National Academies Press; 1993.

U.S. Food and Drug Administration. Vaccine Product Approval Process: U.S. Food and Drug Administration; 2018 Available from: https://www.fda.gov/vaccines-blood-biologics/development-approval-process-cber/vaccine-product-approval-process.

Vidor E, Soubeyrand B. Manufacturing DTaP-based combination vaccines: industrial challenges around essential public health tools. Expert review of vaccines. 2016;15(12):1575–82.

Cutts FT, Claquin P, Danovaro-Holliday MC, Rhoda DA. Monitoring vaccination coverage: defining the role of surveys. Vaccine. 2016;34(35):4103–9.
Utazi CE, Thorley J, Alegana VA, Ferrari MJ, Takahashi S, Metcalf CJE, et al. Mapping vaccination coverage to explore the effects of delivery mechanisms and inform vaccination strategies. Nature communications. 2019;10(1):1633.
Mbabazi WB, Nanyunja M, Makumbi I, Braka F, Baliraine FN, Kisakye A, et al. Achieving measles control: lessons from the 2002–06 measles control strategy for Uganda. Health policy and planning. 2009;24(4):261–9.
Mane AB. Letter to Editor: Immunization Dropout Rates: Some Issues. Annals of medical and health sciences research. 2015;5(2):153.
Sridhar S, Maleq N, Guillermet E, Colombini A, Gessner BD. A systematic literature review of missed opportunities for immunization in low-and middle-income countries. Vaccine. 2014;32(51):6870–9.
Kidd S, Ouedraogo B, Kambire C, Kambou JL, McLean H, Kutty PK, et al. Measles outbreak in Burkina Faso, 2009: a case–control study to determine risk factors and estimate vaccine effectiveness. Vaccine. 2012;30(33):5000–8.
Murthy N, Rodgers L, Pabst L, Fiebelkorn AP, Ng T. Progress in childhood vaccination data in immunization information systems—United States, 2013–2016. MMWR Morbidity and mortality weekly report. 2017;66(43):1178.
Sato AS, Ferreira VDR, Tauil MDC, Costa ÂA, Inenami M, Rodrigues LC, et al. Monitoring vaccination coverage by electronic immunization registry in medium-sized city, Brazil. Revue d'Épidémiologie et de Santé Publique. 2018;66:S422.
Nguyen NT, Vu HM, Dao SD, Tran HT, Nguyen TXC. Digital immunization registry: evidence for the impact of mHealth on enhancing the immunization system and improving immunization coverage for children under one year old in Vietnam. Mhealth. 2017;3.
Brown DW, Burton AH, Feeney G, Gacic-Dobo M. Avoiding the will o' the wisp: challenges in measuring high levels of immunization coverage with precision. World Journal of Vaccines. 2014;4(03):97.
Burton A, Monasch R, Lautenbach B, Gacic-Dobo M, Neill M, Karimov R, et al. WHO and UNICEF estimates of national infant immunization coverage: methods and processes. Bulletin of the World Health Organization. 2009;87:535–41.
Lim SS, Stein DB, Charrow A, Murray CJ. Tracking progress towards universal childhood immunisation and the impact of global initiatives: a systematic

analysis of three-dose diphtheria, tetanus, and pertussis immunisation coverage. The Lancet. 2008;372(9655):2031–46.
World Health Organization. Immunization coverage cluster survey: Reference manual. Geneva: World Health Organization; 2005.
Danovaro-Holliday MC, Dansereau E, Rhoda DA, Brown DW, Cutts FT, Gacic-Dobo M. Collecting and using reliable vaccination coverage survey estimates: Summary and recommendations from the "Meeting to share lessons learnt from the roll-out of the updated WHO Vaccination Coverage Cluster Survey Reference Manual and to set an operational research agenda around vaccination coverage surveys", Geneva, 18–21 April 2017. Vaccine. 2018;36(34):5150–9.
Rainey JJ, Watkins M, Ryman TK, Sandhu P, Bo A, Banerjee K. Reasons related to non-vaccination and under-vaccination of children in low and middle income countries: findings from a systematic review of the published literature, 1999–2009. Vaccine. 2011;29(46):8215–21.
Favin M, Steinglass R, Fields R, Banerjee K, Sawhney M. Why children are not vaccinated: a review of the grey literature. International health. 2012;4(4):229–38.
Xeuatvongsa A, Hachiya M, Miyano S, Mizoue T, Kitamura T. Determination of factors affecting the vaccination status of children aged 12–35 months in Lao People's Democratic Republic. Heliyon. 2017;3(3):e00265.
Bryson M, Duclos P, Jolly A, Bryson J. A systematic review of national immunization policy making processes. Vaccine. 2010;28:A6–A12.
World Health Organization. Global Vaccine Action Plan 2011–2020: World Health Organization; 2019c Available from: https://www.who.int/immunization/global_vaccine_action_plan/GVAP_doc_2011_2020/en/.
NITAG Resource Center. National Immunization Technical Advisory Groups (NITAGs) Worldwide: NITAG Resource Center; 2019 Available from: http://www.nitag-resource.org/.
Shen AK, Fields R, McQuestion M. The future of routine immunization in the developing world: challenges and opportunities. Global Health: Science and Practice. 2014;2(4):381–94.
Okwo-Bele J-M, Cherian T. The expanded programme on immunization: a lasting legacy of smallpox eradication. Vaccine. 2011;29:D74–D9.
K V Balasubramaniam VS. Access to Vaccines and the Vaccine Industry - An Analysis. Journal of Vaccines & Vaccination. 2014;5(2).

Makenga G, Bonoli S, Montomoli E, Carrier T, Auerbach J. Vaccine Production in Africa: A Feasible Business Model for Capacity Building and Sustainable New Vaccine Introduction. Frontiers in public health. 2019;7:56.

Storeng KT. The GAVI Alliance and the 'Gates approach' to health system strengthening. Global public health. 2014;9(8):865–79.

Gavi tVA. Gavi Annual Progress Report 2017: Gavi, the Vaccine Alliance; 2017 Available from: http://gaviprogressreport.org/2017/.

VanderEnde K, Gacic-Dobo M, Diallo MS, Conklin LM, Wallace AS. Global Routine Vaccination Coverage – 2017. MMWR Morb Mortal Wkly Rep. 2018;67(45):1261–4.

Zipprich J, Winter K, Hacker J, Xia D, Watt J, Harriman K. Measles outbreak—California, December 2014–February 2015. MMWR Morbidity and mortality weekly report. 2015;64(6):153.

Woudenberg T, van Binnendijk RS, Sanders EA, Wallinga J, de Melker HE, Ruijs WL, et al. Large measles epidemic in the Netherlands, May 2013 to March 2014: changing epidemiology. Eurosurveillance. 2017;22(3).

Strategic Advisory Group of Experts (SAGE) on Immunization. Report of the SAGE Working Group on Vaccine Hesitancy World Health Organization; 2014 Available from: https://www.who.int/immunization/sage/meetings/2014/october/1_Report_WORKING_GROUP_vaccine_hesitancy_final.pdf.

Dubé E, Vivion M, MacDonald NE. Vaccine hesitancy, vaccine refusal and the anti-vaccine movement: influence, impact and implications. Expert review of vaccines. 2015a;14(1):99–117.

Larson HJ, Jarrett C, Schulz WS, Chaudhuri M, Zhou Y, Dube E, et al. Measuring vaccine hesitancy: the development of a survey tool. Vaccine. 2015;33(34):4165–75.

Salmon DA, Dudley MZ, Glanz JM, Omer SB. Vaccine hesitancy: causes, consequences, and a call to action. Vaccine. 2015;33:D66–D71.

François G, Duclos P, Margolis H, Lavanchy D, Siegrist C-A, Meheus A, et al. Vaccine safety controversies and the future of vaccination programs. The Pediatric infectious disease journal. 2005;24(11):953–61.

Poland GA, Spier R. Fear, misinformation, and innumerates: how the Wakefield paper, the press, and advocacy groups damaged the public health. Vaccine. 2010;28(12):2361.

Smith LE, Amlôt R, Weinman J, Yiend J, Rubin GJ. A systematic review of factors affecting vaccine uptake in young children. Vaccine. 2017;35(45):6059–69.

Dubé E, Gagnon D, MacDonald NE. Strategies intended to address vaccine hesitancy: Review of published reviews. Vaccine. 2015b;33(34):4191–203.

Nyhan B, Reifler J, Richey S, Freed GL. Effective messages in vaccine promotion: a randomized trial. Pediatrics. 2014;133(4):e835–e42.

Bozzola E, Spina G, Russo R, Bozzola M, Corsello G, Villani A. Mandatory vaccinations in European countries, undocumented information, false news and the impact on vaccination uptake: the position of the Italian pediatric society. Italian journal of pediatrics. 2018;44(1):67.

MacDonald NE, Harmon S, Dube E, Steenbeek A, Crowcroft N, Opel DJ, et al. Mandatory infant & childhood immunization: Rationales, issues and knowledge gaps. Vaccine. 2018.

Lee C, Robinson JL. Systematic review of the effect of immunization mandates on uptake of routine childhood immunizations. Journal of Infection. 2016;72(6):659–66.

Broder KR, Cortese MM, Iskander JK, Kretsinger K, Slade BA, Brown KH, et al. Preventing tetanus, diphtheria, and pertussis among adolescents; use of tetanus toxoid, reduced diphtheria toxoid and acellular pertussis vaccines: recommendations of the Advisory Committee on Immunization Practices (ACIP). 2006.

Kim DK, Riley LE, Harriman KH, Hunter P, Bridges CB. Advisory Committee on Immunization Practices recommended immunization schedule for adults aged 19 years or older—United States, 2017. MMWR Morbidity and mortality weekly report. 2017;66(5):136.

Williams WW, Lu P-J, O'Halloran A, Bridges CB, Kim DK, Pilishvili T, et al. Vaccination coverage among adults, excluding influenza vaccination—United States, 2013. MMWR Morbidity and mortality weekly report. 2015;64(4):95.

13

Global Antibiotics Use and Resistance

Mamoon Aldeyab, José-María López-Lozano, and Ian M. Gould

Antibiotic resistance is a major global threat to public health, due to the emergence and spread of multidrug-resistant (MDR) bacteria or "superbugs" (Davies and Davies 2010a). The decreased efficacy of surgical antibiotic prophylaxis, the emergence of pan-resistant microorganisms and the decreased investment in antibiotic development threaten many achievements of modern medicine (Dar et al. 2016; Teillant et al. 2015). Antibiotic resistance contributes to increasing morbidity and mortality, prolonged stay in hospital, loss of protection for patients undergoing operations and other medical procedures and significant increase in

M. Aldeyab (✉)
Department of Pharmacy, School of Applied Sciences, University of Huddersfield, Huddersfield, UK
e-mail: M.AlDeyab@hud.ac.uk

J.-M. López-Lozano
Research Group on Health Sciences Data Analysis, Universidad de Murcia, Murcia, Spain

I. M. Gould
Medical Microbiology Department, Aberdeen Royal Infirmary, Aberdeen, UK

Z. Babar (ed.), *Global Pharmaceutical Policy*,
https://doi.org/10.1007/978-981-15-2724-1_13

healthcare costs (Teillant et al. 2015; de Kraker et al. 2011; O'Neill 2016). In a review estimating the global economic cost of antimicrobial resistance by 2050, the burden of deaths from antimicrobial resistance could reach to10 million annually by 2050, resulting in a reduction of 2% to 3.5% in gross domestic product (GDP) at a cumulative cost to global economic output of 100 trillion USD (O'Neill 2016). It is important to note that any use of antibiotics, even if appropriate, may contribute to the development of resistance. However, inappropriate use of antibiotics may accelerate the development of antibiotic resistance resulting in losing current effective antibiotics more quickly. The overuse and misuse of antibiotics is facilitated by prescribing practices that vary significantly between, and within, countries. Reasons behind the latter vary between countries and are context dependent, including behavioural factors, enforcing of legislation to ban dispensing antibiotics without a prescription, education and level of awareness, developing and implementing appropriate antibiotic policies and non-existence of health insurance systems (Davies and Davies 2010a; O'Neill 2016; Goossens et al. 2005; Gould and Lawes 2016; Charani et al. 2011; Cole 2014).

Van Boeckel et al. (2014) assessed variations in antibiotic consumption using sales data for retail and hospital pharmacies from the IMS Health MIDAS database, between 2000 and 2010 in 71 countries (Van Boeckel et al. 2014). The results of this study showed an increase in consumption of antibiotic drugs by 36%, in Brazil, Russia, India, China and South Africa, and this accounted for 76% of global increase. In addition, increased consumption of carbapenems (45%) and polymyxins was also noted (13%) (Van Boeckel et al. 2014). Interestingly, the variation in antibiotic use was linked with antibiotic resistance with higher rates of antibiotic resistance observed in high-consuming countries (Goossens et al. 2005). In addition, with technological advancements, intercontinental travel has increased in volume and speed, and this facilitates the global spread of antimicrobial-resistant pathogens. It follows that countries should not act in isolation to tackle antibiotic resistance. Coordinated efforts by the international community to promote rational antibiotic use should be a priority. In response to the growing threat of antibiotic resistance, in May 2015, the World Health Assembly adopted a global action plan on antimicrobial resistance, with five objectives: (i) to improve awareness and understanding of antimicrobial resistance through effective communication, education and training; (ii) to strengthen the knowledge and evidence base through surveillance and research; (iii) to reduce the incidence of infection through effective sanitation, hygiene and infection prevention measures; (iv) to optimize the use of antimicrobial medicines in human and animal health; and (v) to develop the economic case for sustainable investment that takes account of the needs of all countries and to increase investment in new medicines, diagnostic tools, vaccines and other interventions (World Health Organization 2015).

Antibiotic use is one of the main drivers of antimicrobial resistance. The WHO published the results of antibiotic consumption from 65 countries and areas, contributing to our understanding of how antibiotics are used in these countries (World Health Organization 2018). The consumption data showed wide intra- and inter-regional variation in antibiotics use and the choice of antibiotics consumed. The overall consumption of antibiotics ranged from 4.4 to 64.4 defined daily doses (DDD) per 1000 inhabitants per day (World Health Organization 2018). In most countries amoxicillin and amoxicillin/clavulanic acid were the most frequently consumed antibiotics. These substances belong to the Model List of Essential Medicines, which includes antibiotics recommended as first- or second-line therapy for common infectious diseases, and according to WHO, these should be available in all countries (Sharland et al. 2019). In 49 countries, the Access category of antibiotics represent more than 50% of antibiotic consumption (World Health Organization 2018). Broad-spectrum antibiotics such as third-generation cephalosporins, quinolones and carbapenems are categorized as Watch antibiotics and should be used with caution because of their high potential to contribute towards the development of antimicrobial resistance and/or their side effects. The WHO report shows that the Watch category accounted for less than 20% of total antibiotic consumption in some countries, but more than 50% in others (World Health Organization 2018).

Antibiotics Use and Resistance

The links between antimicrobial usage in hospitals and antimicrobial resistance in hospital bacteria were proposed by McGowan (1983) as follows: (i) antimicrobial resistance is more prevalent in hospital bacterial strains than in strains from community-acquired cases; (ii) changes in antimicrobial usage lead to parallel changes in prevalence of resistance; (iii) during hospital outbreaks, patients with resistant strains are more likely to have received prior antibiotic therapy than patients infected or colonized with susceptible strains of the same organism; (iv) areas within hospitals having the highest usage of antimicrobials also have the highest rates of antimicrobial-resistant bacteria; and (v) increasing the duration of patient exposure to antimicrobials increases the likelihood of colonization with resistant organisms (Mcgowan 1983). McGowan suggested a biological model to explain the relationship between the proposed cause and effect. He stated that, as a result of using antibiotics extensively in hospitals, both patients and hospital employees are exposed to these drugs. Antimicrobial treatment with a specific drug can cause large modifications in the endogenous flora of an individual and select preferentially for microorganisms which are resistant to this drug (Mcgowan 1983).

Possible mechanisms by which antibiotics can create selection for resistance in the population have been reported by Lipsitch and Samore (2002). They suggested that treatment with antibiotics can modify the treated host's normal flora by eradicating the susceptible microorganisms, thus, increasing the patient's probability of being colonized with a resistant organism, during or shortly after treatment, if he/she is exposed to resistant organisms. Removing susceptible flora will result in reducing the competition between susceptible and resistant bacteria in favour of the latter, and this will increase the patients' receptiveness to acquire resistant strains. Another possible explanation for how antibiotic use increases antimicrobial resistance is by increasing the density of the resistant organism within a patient who already carries this organism at a lower density. This will enhance shedding of this organism and will result in an increased risk to other exposed patients (Lipsitch and Samore

2002). Many studies have related the acquisition of methicillin-resistant *Staphylococcus aureus* (MRSA) to the use of specific classes of antimicrobial therapy (Weber et al. 2003; LeBlanc et al. 2006; Mahamat et al. 2007; Monnet et al. 2004; Aldeyab et al. 2008; Baur et al. 2017). Interestingly, ciprofloxacin has been found to be excreted into sweat and across mucosal surfaces which might be colonized with MRSA (Hoiby et al. 1997). This provides MRSA with an ecologic privilege over other bacteria and promotes the spread of MRSA strains by eradication of susceptible microorganisms. The emergence of antibiotic-resistant bacterial strains is likely a result of already existing genetic mutations or due to the acquisition of genes carried on mobile plasmids (Levy and Marshall 2004; Davies and Davies 2010b). The use of cephalosporins, fluoroquinolones, aminoglycosides and tetracyclines has been reported in case-control studies and is associated with extended-spectrum β-lactamase (ESBL)-producing organisms (Colodner et al. 2004; Graffunder et al. 2005). The genes encoding for ESBL production are plasmid mediated, and other antibiotic resistance genes may also be carried on the same plasmid which results in resistance to multiple classes of antibiotic and co-selection of resistances (Rawat and Nair 2010). Therefore, the use of antibiotics other than beta-lactam agents will provide a selection pressure, resulting in the elimination of sensitive strains, thereby decreasing competition and allowing resistant strains to proliferate. Indeed fluoroquinolone antibiotics have been widely reported in several ecological studies to be associated with extended-spectrum β-lactamase (ESBL)-producing organisms (Vibet et al. 2015; Kaier et al. 2009; Vernaz et al. 2011; Aldeyab et al. 2012; Canton et al. 2008; Pitout and Laupland 2008).

Conserving the Effectiveness of Existing Antibiotics

Inappropriate antimicrobial use has been clearly shown to contribute to the selection and spread of drug-resistant microorganisms (Hecker et al. 2003; Gould 2008). Due to the selective pressure imposed by antibiotic agents over bacterial populations, antibiotic consumption has been linked to the increased prevalence of resistant bacterial infections (Levy and Marshall 2004; Davies and Davies 2010b; Lipsitch 2001; Marcusson et al. 2009; Andersson and Hughes 2010; Levy 1994; Davey et al. 2017). The rate of development of antibiotic non-susceptibility among organisms responsible for human infection is greater than the rate of antibiotic discovery and development. The rapid decrease in the number of new antibiotics approved has left the pipeline of antibiotic discovery dried up, highlighting that the "existing classes of antibiotics are probably the best we will ever have" (Laxminarayan et al. 2013; Cormican and Vellinga 2012). Even in the case of the development of a new antibiotic, the rapid evolution and development of antibiotic resistance will reduce its potential for sustained efficacy. Thus, conserving the effectiveness of existing antibiotics is a critical issue to be addressed.

Since the development of resistant infections is recognized as a multifactorial problem, guidelines on controlling healthcare-acquired infections emphasize the importance of the implementation of optimal infection control practices and the prudent use of antibiotics (Laxminarayan et al. 2013; Dellit et al. 2007; Muto et al. 2003). The core principles of infection control are effective and timely hand hygiene and maintenance of a clean environment.

Also, antibiotic stewardship programme aims to improve patient outcomes while reducing adverse effects associated with the antimicrobial use. This has proved to be effective in decreasing antimicrobial use and in reducing healthcare costs. These practices represent the standard of care for the patients.

Time-Series Analysis (TSA) and the Relationship Between Antibiotic Use and Resistance

Time-series analysis (TSA) techniques have been used to study the relationship between antibiotic use and resistance for over 20 years now (López-Lozano et al. 2000). The theory states that the resistance, measured over time and from an ecological perspective, is a stochastic phenomenon resulting from the dynamic interaction of several factors (e.g. antibiotic use, changes in the microbiome, infection control measures). Previously, analysis was based on a linear concept of the relationship between the trigger, e.g. antibiotic use, and the outcome, resistance, i.e. the more antibiotics were used, the more resistance would occur; this is regardless of the level or intensity of antimicrobial use.

Balancing the Drug-Resistance Equation

In a ground-breaking editorial published in 1994, Stuart Levy (1994) hypothesized that the relationship between intensity of antibiotic use and resistance might not be linear. Non-linear relationships are common in other biological systems but hadn't been considered in the context of antibiotic resistance up until then. Levy suggested that there might be a threshold of antibiotic use beyond which resistance would be triggered (Fig. 13.1).

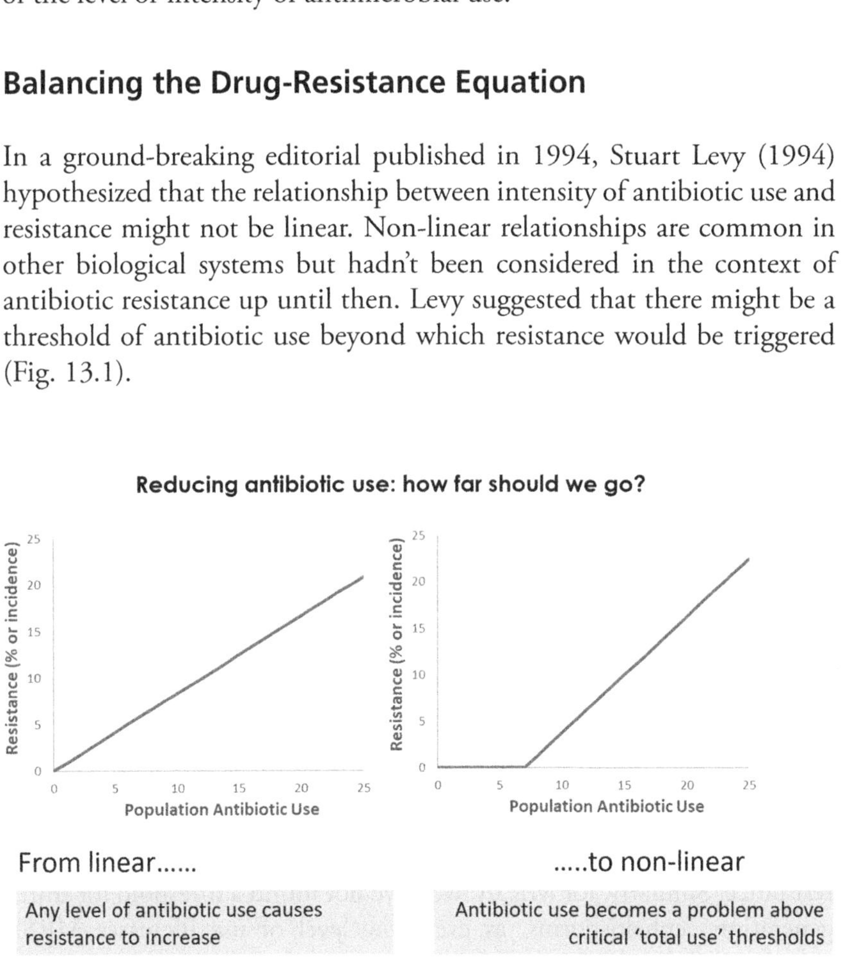

Fig. 13.1 Linear and non-linear relationships between antibiotic use and resistance

Thresholds

In the last few years, on the basis of Levy's 1994 hypothesis, we introduced statistical methods from the field of econometrics, suitable for the identification and estimation of non-linear models (López-Lozano et al. 2019; Lawes et al. 2015a, b, 2017). This methodology is known as multivariate adaptive regression splines (MARS) based on the separation of the data into sections or "regions" in which the ratio of the explanatory variables to the dependent variables changes and this allows the identification of the nodes in which the change occurs. This statistical approach has allowed us to detect multiple antibiotic use/resistance combinations in which, up to a certain threshold, no relationship is detected between the use of antibiotics and resistance, but beyond that threshold the relationship is positive.

A threshold is an estimate of the maximum use of any antibiotic in a population that can be used over a specific period without having resistance to that antibiotic. This can be converted into a maximum number of patients to be treated with the specific antibiotic in the population (e.g. a community or hospital, ward or unit). Each antibiotic has a threshold for individual resistance although this is likely to be variable depending on the microbe, use of other antibiotics and other factors still to be researched such as the patient population, the infection prevention and control (IPC) measures and the adaptability of the bacteria. All of these factors might alter individual threshold but more research is needed on this. Thresholds too have been found for other factors such as infection control parameters, e.g. pertaining to MRSA, alcohol hand rub use, admission screening, number of positive admissions for MRSA, bed numbers and length of stay, all of which displayed non-linear associations with MRSA prevalence. Ceiling effects too have been described, where, above a certain level of use, it does not lead to more resistance. Similarly, for MRSA, we have not found a threshold for third-generation cephalosporins, as even low level of use increases MRSA prevalence (López-Lozano et al. 2019).

Future Questions

If we were able to detect thresholds for all antibiotics used in a particular hospital, unit or community, we could establish a policy of use aimed at not exceeding those thresholds for each antibiotic in the hope that problematic resistance would remain at acceptable levels. This would be similar to establishing quotas (max number of treatable patients) in order to remain under the threshold, something akin to carbon credits to reduce CO_2 production. Detection of thresholds requires long time-series data sets, often of several years use and resistance and usually measured in monthly periods. Further research is needed on likely factors to influence specific thresholds, such as the population vulnerability (maybe lower in geriatric inpatients), molecular epidemiology (e.g. MRSA strain), intensity of IPC measures (which contributes to multivariate analyses) or epidemic phase of an outbreak strain (Fig. 13.2).

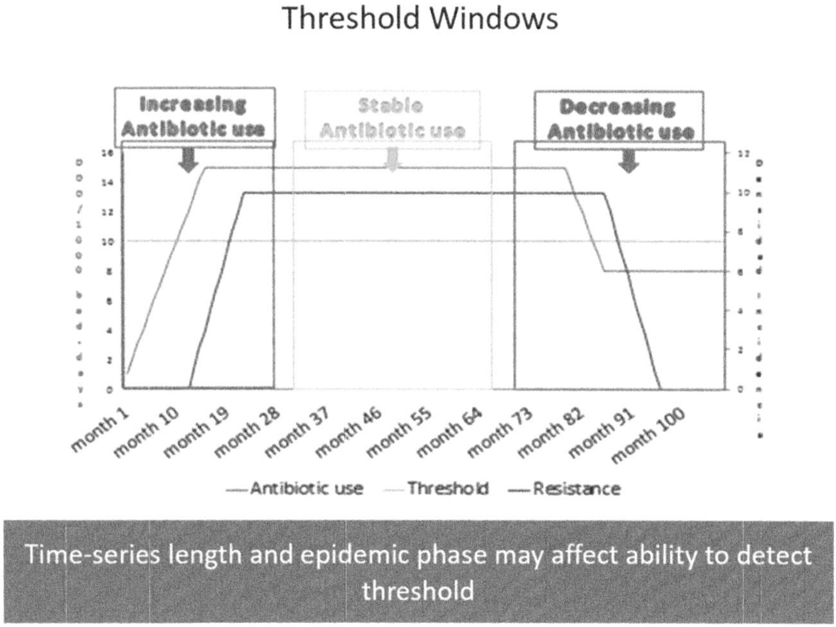

Fig. 13.2 Theoretical framework for the relationship between antibiotic use and resistance and the thresholds' concept

Acknowledgement This chapter is an extension of an APUA newsletter tribute to Stuart Levy, recently deceased, written by the authors (www.APUA.org).

References

Davies J, Davies D. Origins and evolution of antibiotic resistance. Microbiol Mol Biol Rev. 2010a;74:417–433.

Dar OA, Hasan R, Schlundt J, Harbarth S, Caleo G, Dar FK, Littmann J, Rweyemamu M, Buckley EJ, Shahid M, Kock R, Li HL, Giha H, Khan M, So AD, Bindayna KM, Kessel A, Pedersen HB, Permanand G, Zumla A, Røttingen JA, Heymann DL. Exploring the evidence base for national and regional policy interventions to combat resistance. Lancet. 2016; 387: 285–295

Teillant A Gandra S Barter D Morgan DJ Laxminarayan R. Potential burden of antibiotic resistance on surgery and cancer chemotherapy antibiotic prophylaxis in the USA: a literature review and modelling study. Lancet Infect Dis. 2015; 15: 1429–1437

de Kraker ME, Davey PG, Grundmann H; BURDEN study group. Mortality and hospital stay associated with resistant *Staphylococcus aureus* and *Escherichia coli* bacteremia: estimating the burden of antibiotic resistance in Europe. PLoS Med. 2011;8(10):e1001104.

O'Neill J. Tackling drug-resistant infections globally: final report and recommendations. 2016. Available at: https://amr-review.org/sites/default/files/160525_Final%20paper_with%20cover.pdf [Last accessed: December 2019].

Goossens H Ferech M Vander Stichele R Elseviers M ESAC Project Group. Outpatient antibiotic use in Europe and association with resistance: a cross-national database study. Lancet. 2005; 365: 579–587

Gould IM, Lawes T. Antibiotic stewardship: prescribing social norms. Lancet. 2016; 387:1699–701

Charani E, Edwards R, Sevdalis N, Alexandrou B, Sibley E, Mullett D, Franklin BD, Holmes A. Behavior change strategies to influence antimicrobial prescribing in acute care: a systematic review. Clin Infect Dis. 2011; 53: 651–62.

Cole A. GPs feel pressurised to prescribe unnecessary antibiotics, survey finds. BMJ. 2014; 349: 5238.

Van Boeckel TP, Gandra S, Ashok A, Caudron Q, Grenfell BT, Levin SA, Laxminarayan R. Global antibiotic consumption 2000 to 2010: an analysis of national pharmaceutical sales data. The Lancet Infectious Diseases 2014; 14(8): 742–750

Global action plan on antimicrobial resistance. World Health Organization 2015. Available at: https://apps.who.int/iris/bitstream/handle/10665/193736/9789241509763_eng.pdf?sequence=1 [Last accessed December 2019]

WHO report on surveillance of antibiotic consumption: 2016–2018 early implementation. Geneva: World Health Organization; 2018.

Sharland M, Gandra S, Huttner B, Moja L, Pulcini C, Zeng M, Mendelson M, Cappello B, Cooke G, Magrini N; EML Expert Committee and Antibiotic Working Group. Encouraging AWaRe-ness and discouraging inappropriate antibiotic use-the new 2019 Essential Medicines List becomes a global antibiotic stewardship tool. Lancet Infect Dis. 2019; 19:1278–1280.

Mcgowan JE JR. Antimicrobial resistance in hospital organisms and its relation to antibiotic use. *Reviews of Infectious Diseases* 1983;**5**:1033–48.

Lipsitch M, Samore MH. Antimicrobial use and antimicrobial resistance: a population perspective. Emerging Infectious Diseases 2002; 8:347–54.

Weber SG, Gold HS, Hooper DC, et al. Fluoroquinolones and the risk for methicillin-resistant *Staphylococcus aureus* in hospitalised patients. *Emerging Infectious Diseases* 2003;**9**:1415–22.

LeBlanc L, Pepin J, Toulouse K, et al. Fluoroquinolones and risk for methicillin-resistant *Staphylococcus aureus*, Canada. Emerging Infectious Diseases 2006; 12:1398–405.

Mahamat A, MacKenzie FM, Brooker K, et al. Impact of infection control interventions and antibiotic use on hospital MRSA: a multivariate interrupted time-series analysis. International Journal of Antimicrobial Agents 2007; 30:169–76.

Monnet DL, MacKenzie FM, López-Lozano JM, Beyaert A, Camacho M, Wilson R, Stuart D, Gould IM. Antimicrobial drug use and methicillin-resistant *Staphylococcus aureus*, Aberdeen, 1996–2000. Emerging Infectious Diseases 2004; 10:1432–41.

Aldeyab MA, Monnet DL, López-Lozano JM, Hughes CM, Scott MG, Kearney MP, Magee FA, McElnay JC. Modelling the impact of antibiotic use and infection control practices on the incidence of hospital-acquired methicillin-resistant *Staphylococcus aureus*: a time-series analysis. J Antimicrob Chemother. 2008; 62:593–600.

Baur D, Gladstone BP, Burkert F, Carrara E, Foschi F, Döbele S, Tacconelli E. Effect of antibiotic stewardship on the incidence of infection and colonisation with antibiotic-resistant bacteria and *Clostridium difficile* infection: a systematic review and meta-analysis. Lancet Infect Dis. 2017; 17:990–1001.

Hoiby N, Jarlov JO, Kemp M, et al. Excretion of ciprofloxacin in sweat and multiresistant *Staphylococcus epidermidis*. Lancet 1997; 349:167–9.
Levy SB, Marshall B. Antibacterial resistance worldwide: causes, challenges and responses. Nature Medicine 2004;10: S122–129
Davies J, Davies D. Origins and evolution of antibiotic resistance. Microbiology and Molecular Biology Reviews 2010b; 74: 417–433
Colodner R, Rock W, Chazan B, Keller N, Guy N, Sakran W, Raz R. Risk factors for the development of extended spectrum beta lactamase producing bacteria in non-hospitalised patients. European Journal of Clinical Microbiology and Infectious Disease 2004, 23: 163–167.
Graffunder EM, Preston KE, Evans AM, Venezia RA. Risk factors associated with extended spectrum beta-lactamase producing organisms in a tertiary care hospital. Journal of Antimicrobial Chemotherapy 2005; 56: 139–145.
Rawat D, Nair D. Extended spectrum beta lactamase in gram negative bacteria. Journal of Global Infectious Disease 2010; 2: 263–274.
Vibet MA, Roux J, Montassier C, Corvec S, Juvin ME, Ngohou C, Lepelletier D, Batard E. Systematic analysis of the relationship between antibiotic use and extended spectrum beta-lactamase resistance in *Enterobacteriaceae* in a French Hospital: a time series analysis. European Journal of Clinical Microbiology and Infectious Disease 2015; 34: 1957–1963.
Kaier K, Frank U, Hagist C, Conrad A, Meyer E. The impact of antimicrobial drug consumption and alcohol based hand rub use on the emergence and spread of extended spectrum β-lactamase-producing strains: a time series analysis. Journal of Antimicrobial Chemotherapy 2009; 63: 609–614.
Vernaz N, Huttner B, Muscionico D, Salomon JL, Bonnabry P, Lopez Lozano JM, Beyaert A, Schrenzel J, Harbarth S. Modelling the impact of antibiotic use on antibiotic resistant *Escherichia coli* using population based data from a large hospital and surrounding community. Journal of Antimicrobial Chemotherapy 2011; 66: 928–935.
Aldeyab MA, Harbarth S, Vernaz N, Kearney MP, Scott MG, Darwish Elhajji FW, Aldiab MA, McElnay JC. The impact of antibiotic use on the incidence and resistance pattern of extended spectrum beta-lactamase producing bacteria in primary and secondary healthcare settings. British Journal of Clinical Pharmacology 2012; 74: 171–179.
Canton R, Novais A, Valverde A, Machado E, Peixe L, Baquero F, Coque TM. Prevalence and spread of extended spectrum β lactamase producing *Enterobacteriaceae* in Europe. Clinical Microbiology and Infection 2008; 14(Suppl 1): 144–153.

Pitout JDD, Laupland KB. Extended Spectrum β-lactamase producing *Enterobacteriaceae* an emerging public health concern. Lancet Infectious Diseases 2008; 8:159166.

Hecker MT, Aron DC, Patel NP, Lehmann MK, Donskey CJ. Unnecessary use of antimicrobials in hospitalized patients: current patterns of misuse with an emphasis on the antianaerobic spectrum of activity. Arch Intern Med 2003; 163:972–8.

Gould IM. Antibiotic policies to control hospital-acquired infection. J Antimicrob Chemother 2008; 61:763–5

Lipsitch, M. The rise and fall of antimicrobial resistance. TRENDS in Microbiology 2001; 9: 438–444.

Marcusson LL, Frimoat-Møller N, Hughes D. Interplay in the selection of fluoroquinolone resistance and bacterial fitness. Plos Pathogens 2009; 8: DOI:https://doi.org/10.1371/journal.ppat.1000541.

Andersson DI, Hughes D. Antibiotic resistance and its cost: is it possible to reverse resistance? Nature Reviews Microbiology 2010; 8: 260–261.

Levy SB. Balancing the drug-resistance equation. Trends Microbiol. 1994; 2:341–2.

Davey P, Marwick CA, Scott CL, Charani E, McNeil K, Brown E, Gould IM, Ramsay CR, Michie S. Interventions to improve antibiotic prescribing practices for hospital inpatients. Cochrane Database Syst Rev 2017; 2:CD003543.

Laxminarayan R, Duse A, Wattal C, Zaidi AK, Wertheim HF, Sumpradit N, Vlieghe E, Hara GL, Gould IM, Goossens H, Greko C, So AD, Bigdeli M, Tomson G, Woodhouse W, Ombaka E, Peralta AQ, Qamar FN, Mir F, Kariuki S, Bhutta ZA, Coates A, Bergstrom R, Wright GD, Brown ED, Cars O. Antibiotic resistance-the need for global solutions. Antibiotic resistance-the need for global solutions. Lancet Infect Dis. 2013; 13:1057–98.

Cormican M, Vellinga A. Existing classes of antibiotics are probably the best we will ever have. BMJ 2012; 344:e3369.

Dellit TH, Owens RC, McGowan JE, Gerding DN, Weinstein RA, Burke JP, et al. Infectious Diseases Society of America and the Society for Healthcare Epidemiology of America Guidelines for Developing an Institutional Program to Enhance Antimicrobial Stewardship. *Clin Infect Dis.* 2007; 44(2):159–77.

Muto CA, Jernigan JA, Ostrowsky BE, *et al.* SHEA guideline for preventing nosocomial transmission of multidrug-resistant strains of *Staphylococcus aureus* and enterococcus. Infect Control Hosp Epidemiol 2003;**24**: 362–386.

López-Lozano JM et al. Modelling and forecasting antimicrobial resistance and its dynamic relationship to antimicrobial use: a time series analysis. Int J Antimicrob Agents. 2000;14:21–31

López-Lozano JM et al. A non-linear time-series analysis approach to identify thresholds in associations between population antibiotic use and rates of resistance. Nat Microbiol. 2019;4:1160–1172

Lawes T et al. Effect of a national 4C antibiotic stewardship intervention on the clinical and molecular epidemiology of *Clostridium difficile* infections in a region of Scotland: a non-linear time-series analysis. Lancet Infect Dis. 2017;17:194–206

Lawes T et al. Effects of national antibiotic stewardship and infection control strategies on hospital-associated and community-associated methicillin-resistant *Staphylococcus aureus* infections across a region of Scotland: a non-linear time-series study. Lancet Infect Dis. 2015a;15:1438–49

Lawes T et al. Turning the tide or riding the waves? Impacts of antibiotic stewardship and infection control on MRSA strain dynamics in a Scottish region over 16 years: non-linear time series analysis. BMJ Open. 2015b;5: e006596

14

Medicines Access, Use and Pharmaceutical Health System Issues: Reflections, Thoughts and Points to Consider

Zaheer-Ud-Din Babar and Shane L. Scahill

Prologue/Preface/Foreword

The following is a list of editorials that have been published over the past dozen years or so that we have been working together. But it's more than that, more than a list of front-end articles for a fledgling journal (*Southern Med Review*) and its contemporary, the *Journal of Pharmaceutical Policy and Practice*. As readers we often flick through a range of journals and read interesting editorials and viewpoints. It is not often we will sit down and read the editorials from one journal source and ponder the issues that have developed over time. This body of work together reflects a degree of

Z. Babar (✉)
Centre for Pharmaceutical Policy and Practice Research,
University of Huddersfield, Huddersfield, UK
e-mail: z.babar@hud.ac.uk

S. L. Scahill
School of Pharmacy, University of Auckland, Auckland, New Zealand

Z. Babar (ed.), *Global Pharmaceutical Policy*,
https://doi.org/10.1007/978-981-15-2724-1_14

forward thinking about some of the key issues that are presented to us as researchers and practitioners in the pharmaceutical policy and pharmacy practice space. It is good practice as researchers to look backwards as well as forwards! Has much changed, are these issues still there or have some of them been addressed and are resolved?

The papers are wide-ranging in this chapter. There are seven key editorials but they cover a number of key themes. The first would have to be *dissemination.* Prior to development of the *Southern Med Review* in 2008 and then the *Journal of Pharmaceutical Policy and Practice* several years later, there wasn't a publishing house that "really" provided a place for work from developing nations to be published. Of course now there is great interest (which is a positive thing) and mainstream pharmacy journals have associate editors dedicated to research from low- and middle-income countries.

The second word would need to be *comparison.* Several of the editorials fall into this domain. Comparing the systems, comparing the gaps and determining whether there is widening or closing of developed and developing nations when it comes to pharmaceutical policy and medicines optimization. Of course there is no point in this until the pharmaceutical systems in countries are mapped out and until the health system overall is strengthened to accommodate and improve the pharmaceutical systems.

The third word would be *borrowing.* There is room for nations to borrow from each other. The adoption of tools and theories upon which to base research and practice is a clear example. It is not all one way and there will be aspects of developing nation research and practice that high-income nations can think about more deeply and *learn from.* One area that comes to mind is the understanding of diverse cultural experiences within developing nations being wholly applied to ethnic minority populations within the context of developed nations…and there is an editorial on that!

Enjoy reading the interesting collection of editorials that this chapter brings. We hope that it stimulates ongoing thought and research in this rich and underserved domain of study.

Disseminating "Medicines Access and Use" Research

Citation Disseminating "Medicines Access and Use" Research, Southern Med Review.2008 Dec; 1(1):1

To improve medicines use as well as to build informed policies, appropriate medicine policy research is vital. However, only performing such research is not enough; publishing is the next step to disseminate the opinion to a wider audience. Nevertheless, publishing medicines use research has always been challenging in top-tier journals. Though to an extent, developed countries do manage the task with trained researchers—on the other hand, in developing countries, where the health systems are weak and the need to publish policy research is immense, the chore is an uphill task.

Factors which contribute to low volumes of publication from developing countries could be inexperienced researchers, poor quality of research as well as the "topics" out of scope of the well-established journals.

Therefore, the primary objective of this journal is to provide an alternative medium to researchers from developing countries (termed "the South") to showcase their ideas and research outputs to a global audience. The *Southern Med Review* will be publishing original research, commentaries, viewpoints and the development of clinical and social pharmacy across the globe.

In this issue, we are discussing the establishment of discipline of social pharmacy at Universiti Sains Malaysia—a premier discipline in Asia which has spurred pharmaceutical policy research in many developing countries. Two practice and policy articles, one from Nepal and the other from Pakistan, show the role of pharmacists in improving hospital pharmacy services in these countries. Articles of topical interest are also welcome from the Global North and under a section called "Innovative Approaches in Asia Pacific"; the relationship between studying organizational theory and improving community pharmacy services will be discussed.

It is interesting and encouraging to note that most of the contributors in this issue are doctoral students.

Mapping the Pharmaceutical Situation in Your Country: First Things First...

Citation Babar ZU, Scahill S. Mapping the pharmaceutical situation in your country: First things first... Southern med Review. 2009 Apr;2(1):1

Publishing the first edition of the *Southern Med Review* (SMR) was a milestone and the SMR is going from strength to strength. We gratefully appreciate the support we have received from *Pharmacy World and Science* (PWS) who invited us to write an editorial about the SMR.

Most of all though, thanks goes to you, the contributors, the readers and the members of the SMR Advisory Board, for providing a steadily growing pile of papers and constructive feedback about the contents and future direction of the journal. We have received papers about Central and Southeast Asia, the original focal area of the SMR. However, we are also very excited to have received submissions more latterly from Eastern Europe, the African continent and the Middle East. This widens the flavour of the SMR and allows the readership to understand and learn from those in other developing health systems. We have had contributions from researchers who are from developing countries and are currently residing in those countries. We have also received submissions from people whose origins are from developing countries but who are studying in the "Western world". Finally we have a number of researchers who originate from and who currently live in developed countries but whose passion for research lies with assisting the improvement of medicines use throughout the world. It is with this interesting mix of contribution and talent that we move forward with the SMR and develop the capacity to understand medicines policy research around the globe.

That brings us to a key question we wish to address in this editorial: What areas should researchers from developing countries focus on in order to improve the health systems within their countries? All too often, researchers from developing countries (whilst studying in the developed world) attempt to answer questions which are more applicable to "highly developed pharmacy systems" and may in fact have little relevance within their own countries. Undertaking research using the framework adopted by those working in advanced pharmacy systems does expose individuals to research processes and techniques. However, researchers' abilities in analysing their own pharmacy situations remain unknown. We believe that areas of research should closely align with the country's pharmaceutical problems. That could range from medicines pricing, generics and regulatory issues through to intellectual property rights and establishing basic pharmacy services such as pharmacovigilance programmes and drug information services.

At *Southern Med Review* we value this type of work and examples such as "Pharmacy in United Arab Emirates", "Community Pharmacy Practice in India "and "Pharmacovigilance in Nepal", all portraying basic problems of "medicines regulation and use", are published in the current issue. This reinforces the concept that there is a need to strengthen the "basic" pharmaceutical system before implementing advanced clinical pharmacy services in the developing world. In line with this discussion, we would like to gain the attention of the World Health Organization (WHO), the International Pharmaceutical Federation (FIP), Health Action International (HAI) and other organizations with a vested interest in development research to support initiatives of this nature, where researchers are trying to map "base pharmaceutical services".

We have received a number of commentaries providing an understanding of "medicines and health systems". Now we would also like to receive research papers which follow on from the issues outlined in these commentaries. As we move into the development of the next issue of the SMR, we are most happy to facilitate the dissemination of your valuable work. We hope that the SMR is of value to you and that it is making a difference to pharmaceutical policy research in the developing world. On that note, please keep those papers rolling in.

Community Pharmacy Practice in High and Low Income Countries: Commonalities, Differences and the Tension of Being "Retailer" Versus "Primary Health Care Provider"

Citation Scahill SL, Babar ZU. Community Pharmacy Practice in High and Low Income Countries: Commonalities, Differences and the Tension of Being "Retailer" Versus "Primary Health Care Provider". Southern Med Review (2010) 3; 2:1–2

High-Income Countries (The Developed World)

In the "high-income countries", there has been steady pressure from both health policy makers [1–4] and professional pharmacy associations [5–7] for pharmacy to take a greater role in the provision of services surrounding medicines use and to work more closely with other primary care providers such as nurses and doctors in the general practice setting. In this context, community pharmacy is expected to provide support for patients to improve adherence to prescription medicines, to help doctors rationalize their prescribing, through access to the doctor's clinical notes and vice versa. Pharmacists are deemed to be well positioned to deliver public health programmes such as weight management for chronic diseases like diabetes, swine and bird flu outbreaks, reducing illicit drug and alcohol use, alcohol consumption and so forth. Minor ailment programmes are expected to engage community pharmacists in more clinical activities whilst relieving general practice doctors and nurses from the burden of disease which can be supported by other primary care provider organizations like community pharmacy.

All of these changes, whether from policy makers or the profession itself, will require pharmacy organizations to "step up to the mark" and engage with other health professionals as well as funders and planners of primary healthcare services. Further, there is a need for health policy makers and funders and planners as well other healthcare professionals to be supportive of the approach the pharmacy needs to take when delivering extended services in the future [8]. This movement to include patient-centred clinical care as part of the pharmacy organizations' role is deemed "re-professionalization" [9]. This approach requires community pharmacy to continue functioning as a source and medicines supplier whilst extending some of its other roles. In the developed world this process is well regulated [10]. There are legislation, protocols, rules and service contracts regarding the provision of pharmaceutical services. Along with this, there is the requirement to undertake comprehensive post-registration continuing professional development. Despite this highly regulated environment, the tensions between being primarily a retailer and a primary care provider remain. Taking New Zealand as an example of a country in the developed world, these tensions remain a central issue in the community pharmacy sector. Pharmacists seem generally interested in adopting these new roles, but the pace at which they have been adopted and implemented has often been slower than expected. Experience suggests that there are significant barriers to changing and adopting a future vision which involves alignment with health policy (integration into primary care team) and the implementation of extended services which are patient-centred. Two of the identified barriers relate to the tension between retailer and care provider. The first is the way pharmacists view themselves and their activities, the way they think and act as well as the lack of a primary care practice model moving forward. Moving pharmacists from retailers to healthcare providers may be more difficult than is realized by the profession and policy makers. The second is pharmacists' relationship with funder stakeholders and the lack of remuneration for development and implementation of extended patient-centred services [11]. There are small levels of remuneration for the provision of some services over and above basic medicines sourcing, dispensing and distribution but this varies on a regional basis. The nationally set dispensing fee does not support widespread implementation and integration of these services, nor does the small pockets of regionally controlled money ring fenced by District Health Boards (DHBs). Therefore, it is the retailing side of the pharmacy business that subsidizes these extended services, by those pharmacy owners who chose to adopt them. The activities we are talking about include the sale of general and over-the-counter (OTC) medicines for minor ailments, companion sales of products in those patients on medicines for chronic diseases (e.g. sale of co-enzyme Q10 for patients on statin lipid-lowering medication) and the provision of complementary medicines.

The Low-Income Countries (The Developing World)

In many ways the context in which pharmacies provide services and the activities they undertake in the developing world are different from that previously outlined. What is common however is the tension between being a "retailer" and being an effective organization providing primary healthcare. In this issue of SMR Basak and Sathyanarayara report interesting findings from the region of Tamil Nadu in India. Looking from the perspective of the developed world, there are several striking aspects to this paper which highlight the opposing positions of retailer and healthcare provider. Firstly, medicines that are available only on prescription in the developed world are available over-the-counter. This has two potential effects: that of increased supplier-induced demand with pharmacies being "drug sellers" and the demand driven by customers who opt to self-medicate by obtaining prescription medicines based on their own knowledge and beliefs. This is highlighted by Hussain et al. in their paper in this issue of SMR which reports the medicines-seeking behaviour of people in various cities of Pakistan.

The second striking aspect reported in this paper is the lack of pharmacist attendance within pharmacy premises. It would be fair to suggest that as with pharmacy assistants in the developed world, "drug sellers" in countries like India are less qualified than their pharmacist counterparts. However, the difference is that in the "low-income countries" this scenario is coupled with the fact that prescription medicines are freely available OTC. As a result, medication is reduced to a commodity item, just like any other "retail item", and is reinforced by patients' beliefs and values about medicines as an available commodity.

Same broad issues, different contexts. Although we highlight that the "retailer"-"healthcare provider" paradox is common to both contexts, the drivers and barriers to the dominant retailer behaviour are clearly different. In the developed world the "business" of community pharmacy is, to a large extent, subsidizing any professional services provided (if they happen at all!!), and so the more patient-centred the pharmacy is with respect to medicines use, the less profitable it will be for the same sales levels. Further, the retailer culture of community pharmacy is solidly ingrained, and the shift to a true primary healthcare provider organization may be a difficult one for many pharmacies. In the developing world the retailer-healthcare provider tension is underpinned by a lack of regulation at the policy, legislation and provider levels. Trap et al. highlights the similar issues in the current version of the SMR highlighting that staff are often insufficiently trained, inappropriate sales practice is common, drug regulation is often not enforced and how medicines are stocked is not in line with good storage practices. Linked to all of these issues is the central aim in community pharmacy of keeping the patient safe whilst helping to improve primary care health outcomes. The guest editorial by Prof. Leufkens in this issue of SMR highlights the need for regulation of drug safety management to ensure good pharmacy practice. In a nutshell, for the developed world, the challenge lies with pharmacists moving towards the expectations of policy makers under a fully remunerated system which does not rely on retail sales subsidizing professional activities. For the developing world, the challenge lies with increased government regulation and substituting the less qualified staff with fully trained pharmacists.

References

1. Commonwealth Government (AUS). Compilation of the Fourth Community Pharmacy Agreement Between the Commonwealth of Australia and the Pharmacy Guild. Canberra, Australia (2005).
2. Dept of Health (UK). Pharmacy in England: Building on Strengths-Delivering the Future. London, UK (2008).
3. District Health Boards New Zealand (DHBNZ). National Framework for Pharmacist Services Wellington, New Zealand (2006).
4. Ministry of Health (NZ). Medicines New Zealand: Wellington, New Zealand (2007).
5. Canadian Pharmacists' Association. Blueprint for Pharmacy. Edmonton, Canada (2007).
6. Patel H. How the Pharmacy 2020 project is lighting the way for pharmacy's future. Pharm J;(279):131–132.
7. Pharmaceutical Society of New Zealand. Focus on the Future: Ten Year Vision for Pharmacists':2004–2014. Wellington (2004).
8. Scahill SL, Harrison J, Carswell P, Shaw J. Community pharmacy and health care policy: implications for the whole of primary care. NZ Med J, 2010;123(1317):41–51.
9. Gilbert L. Pharmacy's attempts to extend its roles: case study in South Africa. Social Science & Medicine 1998;47(2):153–164.

10. Bissell P, Morgall Traulsen J. Sociology and Pharmacy Practice.1st ed. London: Pharmaceutical Press (2005).
11. Scahill SL, Harrison J, Sheridan J. The ABC of New Zealand's Ten Year Vision for Pharmacists: Awareness, Barriers and Consultation. Intl J Pharm Pract, 2009;17(3):135–142.

Evidence Based Pharmaceutical Policy Research: Is It All Talk or Does It Contribute to Improving Health in Developing Countries?

Citation Babar ZU, Scahill SL. Evidence Based Pharmaceutical Policy Research: Is It All Talk or Does It Contribute to Improving Health in Developing Countries? Southern Med Review (2010) 3; 1:1–1

It is always said that the foundation to improving "medicines use" and developing a "health system" is to create reliable data—the hardcore evidence to explore and solve problems. The process of data gathering also has some other advantages; it provides an accurate picture of a country's pharmaceutical needs, serves as a training tool for researchers and increases the country's scientific output. However, naturally the main question we would be asking is whether the data has managed to serve its primary aim—to bring a positive change to people's lives. The answer to this question in many cases could be a "no" as policy implementation requires action, transparency and commitment. The problem with data gained from pharmaceutical policy research is that, if not properly used, its relevance diminishes rapidly. Also, however credible the evidence is, implementing policies requires political commitment. One such case study is World Health Organization/Health Action International research on medicines prices, availability and affordability. Examples from many developing countries [1, 2] show that no matter how robust the data is, stakeholders with vested interests are always willing to lay counterarguments [3–9]. Most often, the aim is to question the authenticity of data.

There is no problem in a scientific debate; however, very often during this disagreement process [3–9], the truth is lost and the public become confused with who is right and who is wrong. As a result, the opportunity to inform and build public opinion around a genuine public health issue vanishes.

The question then arises, what are developing countries gaining from this hardcore pharmaceutical evidence? In this scenario, would it not be more logical for them to focus on "hands-on clinical pharmacy activities" or "individualized pharmaceutical care" rather than investing on policy-based work? These hands-on activities could be better inhaler techniques, improving corticosteroid usage, monitoring adverse effects, medicines interaction reporting and managing medicines compliance. Would concentrating on these patient-related activities produce better "value for money" or even" value for time" in these countries? This is a rather provocative question, the answer to which is not an easy one; however, it certainly merits investigation. Either way, as a journal we advocate that there is a need to build a database which narrates the aims, objectives and most importantly *outcomes* of pharmaceutical policy-based projects—what is achieved and what is lost and whether the research has transformed into *action* or not.

Nevertheless, the *Southern Med Review* is a journal with a mission to support evidence-based pharmaceutical policy research, and in the current issue, two bibliometric reviews focusing on "policy and practice" have been published. Ritz et al. provide us with a bibliometric study of publication patterns in access to medicines research within the developing world.

The paper provides an understanding of the extent to which medicines policy research is being undertaken and helps to set a future research agenda. A letter to the editor by a pharmacy student published in the current issue also shows that our work is stimulating comparative thought and making a difference which is the primary objective of this journal.

With all of the above in mind, we welcome your contributions and look forward to a challenging yet rewarding 2010.

References

1. Babar ZU, Ibrahim M Izham M, Singh H, Bukhari NI, Creese A. (2007) Evaluating drug prices, availability, affordability, and price components: Implications for access to drugs in Malaysia. PLoS Med 4(3): 0466–0475
2. Prices, availability and affordability of medicines in Pakistan (2006). The Network for Consumer Protection, Islamabad, Pakistan. http://www.haiweb.org/medicineprices/surveys/200407PK/survey_report.pdf
3. Ministry mulls price control. The New Strait Times, 7th Jan 2007 Kuala Lumpur, Malaysia.
4. Access to medicines still good. The New Strait Times, 12th Feb 2007, Kuala Lumpur, Malaysia.
5. Cost of medicines: Study flawed because of assumptions. The New Strait Times, 3rd April 2007, Kuala Lumpur, Malaysia.
6. Drug price hike. Dawn 2nd Sep 2009, Karachi, Pakistan
7. Rationale behind drug prices. Dawn 26th Feb 2008, Karachi, Pakistan. http://www.dawn.com/2008/02/26/letted.htm#2
8. Drug price hike: industry's version. Dawn 26 Sep 2009, Karachi, Pakistan. http://www.dawn.com/wps/wcm/connect/dawncontent- library/dawn/the-newspaper/letters-to-the-editor/drugprice-hike-industrys-version-699
9. Drug prices: pharma industry's views. Dawn 7th Sep 2009, Karachi, Pakistan. http://www.dawn.com/wps/wcm/connect/dawn-content-library/dawn/the-newspaper/letters-to-theeditor/drug-prices-pharma-industrys-view-799

Social Pharmacy: Borrowing Tools and Theories the World Over

Citation Scahill SL, Babar ZU. Social Pharmacy: Borrowing Tools and Theories the World Over. Southern Med Review (2011) 4; 1:1. doi:https://doi.org/10.5655/smr.v4i1.78

There is no denying that challenges lay ahead for the discipline of social pharmacy. These challenges are both considerable and global, requiring the involvement of fraternities from both academia and practice. To date, high-income countries adopting the Western research paradigm have informed these challenges. They centre on improving practice, teaching and research through the application of knowledge and theories from other disciplines [1].

Beginning to think like those who trained outside of conventional pharmacy and applying accepted theoretical frameworks requires a shift in thought, along with considerable time and energy. Sustainable research streams within our emerging discipline of social pharmacy need to be structured upon what we need to know, but equally upon approaches that have gone before us by other disciplines. Since the mid-1960s the umbrella of academic pharmacy has developed from a predominantly science-based paradigm to include a much broader view of the world [2]. This has been achieved through the study of medicines in society and the term "social pharmacy" was coined.

Social pharmacy researchers based in the Western world have borrowed tools and theories from the social sciences including anthropology, sociology, history, economics and organizational science in order to answer complex questions relating to society and medicines [2]. Historically this occurred in the Nordic countries because Europe, in particular, faced up to the challenges of their ageing population [3–5]. Pharmacists were keen to study both medicines-seeking and medicines use behaviour and it all began from there. Elsewhere in high-income countries, it has taken a while; however, now it is happening and this demonstrates the coming of maturity within the profession, at least in academic terms.

In the same fashion we argue for the increased utility of social pharmacy in the context of low- and middle-income nations. This focus needs to be driven not only by academics residing in developing countries but also those academics within the high-income nations who have a passion, and are qualified, to explore broader "medicines use issues" through a different lens. A "North-South collaboration" is increasingly happening, as evidenced by the publications in this as well as previous issues of this journal. The *Southern Med Review* provides a sound platform for propagating this collaboration [6].

We argue that the benefits of social pharmacy research in the Global South are twofold. First, techniques borrowed from the social sciences could be applied to address fundamental questions. Second, it provides an impetus for countries in the Global South to view "medicines" in their totality, as part of the wider health system, rather than just "isolated chemical entities". Increasingly pharmacy schools in low-income countries are teaching social pharmacy concepts [7], and there is a greater call for the strengthening of social pharmacy before establishing clinical pharmacy practice [8].

We are cognizant that there are three main mechanisms by which the social pharmacy discipline can "spread the word" and "show the value" in the broadest sense. Teaching, research and partnering with or gaining support from significant non-governmental organizations (NGOs) such as the World Health Organization (WHO) are the main mechanisms cited in the literature [1]. Apart from teaching and learning of social pharmacy, more work needs to be undertaken to improve the other two mechanisms of internationalization of our discipline, research dissemination and development of partnerships.

References

1. Norris PT. Challenges facing social pharmacy. Research in Social and Administrative Pharmacy. 2009;5(3):195–196.
2. Bissell P, Morgall Traulsen J. Sociology and Pharmacy Practice. 1st ed. London: Pharmaceutical Press; 2005.
3. About Social Pharmacy, Faculty of Pharmacy, Universitetet I Oslo, Norway. Available at http://www.farmasi.uio.no/seksjoner/farmasoyt-isk/english.html. Accessed 23rd March 2011.
4. Department of Social Pharmacy, Faculty of Pharmacy, University of Kuopio, Finland. Available at http://www.uku.fi/farmasia/sofa/english/. Accessed 23rd March 2011.

5. Section for Social Pharmacy, Faculty of Pharmaceutical Sciences, University of Copenhagen, Denmark. Available at http://www.farma.ku.dk/index.php?id=181. Accessed 23 March 2011.
6. Babar Z, Beswick T. Southern Med Review: A New Forum to Publish "Local Pharmaceutical Policy in a Global Context". Pharmacy World & Science. 2009;31(2):143.
7. Clinical and Social Pharmacy, Faculty of Pharmaceutical Sciences, Kwame Nkrumah University of Science and Technology, Ghana. Available at http://www.knust.edu.gh/pages/sections.php?siteid=pharmacy&mid=607&sid=1827. Accessed 23rd March 2011.
8. Babar Z, Jamshed S. Social pharmacy strengthening clinical pharmacy: why pharmaceutical policy research is needed in Pakistan? Pharmacy World & Science. 2008;30(5):617.

Pharmacy Practice: Is the Gap Between the North and South Widening?

Citation Babar ZU, Vaughan C, Scahill S. Pharmacy Practice: Is the Gap Between the North and South widening? Southern Med Review (2012) 5; 1:1–2

The aim and objective of good pharmacy practice and optimal clinical pharmacy is to promote the appropriate use of medicines. However, the improvement in medicines use is very much dependent on health systems and has greatly benefited from the advances in science, technology and innovation and from those public policy measures, which support public health. Developed economies have been at the forefront of innovation, and as a result, their health systems have become stable and more advanced. The quality of service provision within pharmacy and across the system as a whole has contributed significantly to medicines-related patient care.

With the advantages of innovation and the changing pace of technology come changes in pharmacy practice which are transforming very quickly. This change is driven by influences within two domains. One is the development of new technologies in medicines, for example, better drug delivery methods or the use of robotics to dispense medicines. The other domain relates to the changes that are driven by demographics, disease prevalence, mortality rates and the ageing population.

An example of a policy change which has been influenced by the ageing population in the "North" is the expansion in roles of non-medical prescribers. Policy makers have been instrumental in shifting workloads in chronic care management to other healthcare professionals including pharmacists and nurses [1]. The opportunity for pharmacists to prescribe medicines independently or under the supervision of an experienced physician has released physician time and helped to meet the demand of an ageing population with diminishing numbers of doctors through facilitating improved access to care. One other example of change in Western developed countries is the argument that pharmacy practice must move away from "supply and distribution" as a main focus and should direct its attention to optimizing medicines-related health outcomes through clinical activity [1]. Pharmacists' time can then be better utilized within specialized clinical roles such as palliative care and care of the elderly [1].

The above-mentioned changes in developed economies have been policy-driven and designed after consideration of the opportunities to better utilize pharmacists' skills and to reconfigure services as applicable to the context of each country. In this editorial we pose the question "to what extent can such change be implemented in low- and middle-income countries and what might be the challenges to achieving this?" For example, there have been calls to promote pharmacist prescribing within developing countries. However, this does not equate to the developed world as the majority of pharmacies in low- and middle-income countries are manned by non-qualified personnel and prescription medicines can be purchased over-the-counter, without the need for a prescription.

Currently, under the Western developed model in the "North", non-pharmacist technicians are being utilized in order to release the pharmacist from more technical duties of procurement and supply, to undertake more clinically oriented services. Future developments in Western pharmacy practice may also include drug stores operated by non-pharmacists. However, in the South, where counterfeit medicines and assuring the quality of medicines are big challenges [2], placing pharmacists in procurement may have a positive impact on the successful supply and distribution of good-quality medicines [3]. In the South, "pharmacists within the pharmacy" as a concept has just started to emerge, and significant analysis and direction will be required in order for successful adoption of the Western concept.

The difference in emphasis and the practice of pharmacy in the North and South paint a stark contrast. The question we seek answers to is to what extent can the policy-driven and somewhat theoretical advances in pharmacy practice in the North be applied to the South? Authors in developed countries write about the potential for improvement in pharmacy practice at a global level; however, they fail to both realize and articulate the differences between the health systems and how pharmacy is positioned within these systems [4]. Returning to consider the two domains pertinent to change in the pharmacy sector and its practice, we believe that technological advances in drug delivery such as new methods of injecting vaccines and insulin could be safely implemented within developing countries. However, concepts such as pharmacist prescribing and the utilization of non-pharmacists in procurement and supply roles require careful regulation and planning to reduce the widening gap between pharmacy service provision in the North and South.

References

1. Shaw J. 20:20 Vision Focusing on the Future of Pharmacy Practice and Education. Life Long Learning Pharmacy Conference 29 July 2011, Rotorua, New Zealand.
2. WHO launches taskforce to fight counterfeit drugs. Bulletin of the World Health Organization. Volume 84, Number 9, September 2006, 685–764 available from http://www.who.int/bulletin/volumes/84/9/06-010906/en/

3. Rutta E, Senauer K, Johnson K et al. creating a new class of pharmaceutical services provider for underserved areas: the Tanzania accredited drug dispensing outlet experience. Progress in community health partnerships 2009;3:145–53.
4. Tsuyuki RT, Schindel TJ. Changing pharmacy practice: The leadership challenge. Can Pharm J 2008; 141: 174–80. http://www.cpjournal.ca/doi/pdf/10.3821/1913-701X(2008)141%5B174%3ACPPTLC%5D2.0.CO%3B2

Ethnicity, Migration and Minority Groups: Medicines Access and Use in High-Income Economies

Citation Scahill S. Vaughan C, Babar ZU. Ethnicity, Migration and Minority Groups: Medicines Access and Use in High-Income Economies. Southern Med Review (2012) 5; 2:1–2

In the previous SMR editorial, we highlighted in the broadest sense the widening gap between pharmacy practice activities in the Global North and South [1]. In this editorial we take the opportunity to think about the ethnic minorities residing in high-income countries. In many ways these groups are similar to populations in low-income countries.

The struggles that challenge health systems in developed countries with respect to innovative high-cost medicines are some of the challenges the Global South face when accessing essential medicines. Asthma is one such example in which access to essential medicines may not be a big problem in high-income countries but that compliance and optimal use may be similar to low-income countries, for some cohorts of the population.

When comparing North and South, one might expect all to be well in the developed world with regard to medicines access and use. This may not be the case, and populations such as Australian Aboriginals, Canadian Inuit, American Native Indians and many other ethnicities come to mind. Taking New Zealand as an example may help to extrapolate to the indigenous peoples previously outlined. Several cohort populations come to mind when thinking about potential disparities in access and health outcome. Firstly, the indigenous peoples of the land—the original owners and occupiers who settled from the Pacific in a pre-European era. In New Zealand these folk are the Maori people. For a number of complex and inter-related reasons, Maori die on average ten years younger than non-Maori, even within a developed healthcare system [2]. In general their presentation and access to healthcare services is at a lower rate than the Caucasian population. Availability of essential medicines has been addressed through the policies of the Pharmaceutical Management Agency of New Zealand (PHARMAC). However, Maori are over-represented in the lower socio-economic cohort of the New Zealand population, and so issues of medicines affordability and health literacy arise [3, 4]. Robust evaluation of affordability is yet to be undertaken across various lower socio-economic populations and/or high-need ethnic groups.

Another example is the people of the Pacific, those folk who migrated from Polynesian islands in the 1950s and continue to do so today. They are represented through a very large population grouping in the south of Auckland, New Zealand's largest city. There are now more peoples of Pacific island origin in Auckland than in the Pacific islands per se. The challenges with Pacific peoples are not dissimilar to Maori in that uptake of some health services is less than optimal and that much of the population falls into the high-need category in terms of socio-economic and healthcare [4].

The other important sub-groups are recent immigrants from countries in greater Asia, Middle East and Africa, to name a few. These populations have significant risk factors for the development of chronic diseases, and this is reflected in the high prevalence of cardiovascular disease and diabetes, to name two. Aside from the medical risk, there are misconceptions about the system and rules due to culture and language barriers, and as a result, the system relating to medicines is confusing. There are different perceptions with respect to quality of available medicines as well as variability in community pharmacy service provision to these communities. Financial barriers including lack of affordability, particularly for over-the-counter (OTC) therapies, have been reported [5]. All of these factors add to a complex picture of medicines use which may potentially impact on health outcomes for these subpopulations.

A New Zealand-based study conducted by Bassett-Clarke et al. (2012) also found ethno-cultural barriers with regard to medicines use [6]. They found that the conceptualization of medicine, self-medication and the seeking of further information varied amongst NZ European and Pacific peoples and Maori and folk from Asia especially South Asia.

We have taken New Zealand as our exemplar of some of the issues faced by ethnic minorities accessing and using pharmaceuticals. There are, however, many "like" examples including Hispanic and African races and the Hawaiian people of the United States (USA) [7, 8], Canadian Inuit [9], Australian Aboriginals [10] and Pakistanis in Scandinavia [11], to name a few. The European Union has created a huge melting pot of races and movement from Eastern European countries to the continent per se and there is huge potential for research in this area.

This is not an exhaustive list but, with common examples from high-income countries, it is fair to suggest that, for some populations, the gap between Global North and South may be less than we give credit for. In order to complement work in the Global South, we encourage authors to forward papers related to medicines policy and use in ethnic subpopulations and migrant groupings within high-income countries. It is expected that, by thinking about ethnic minorities and placing "culture" at the centre of social pharmacy practice and research, local and international disparities in access to and use of medicines, as well as pharmacy service provision, will be better addressed [12].

References

1. Babar, Z.-U.-D., Vaughan C, and Scahill S.L. Pharmacy practice: Is the gap between the North and South widening. Southern Med Review, 2012. 5(5): p. 1–2.
2. Smith, A.H. and N.E. Pearce. Determinants of differences in mortality between New Zealand Maoris and non-Maoris aged 15–64. The New Zealand medical journal, 1984. 97(750): p. 101–108.

3. Jatrana, S., P. Crampton, and P. Norris. Ethnic differences in access to prescription medication because of cost in New Zealand. Journal of Epidemiology and Community Health, 2011. 65(5): p. 454–460.
4. Norris, P., et al. Understanding of pharmacy-related terms among three ethnic groups in New Zealand. International Journal of Pharmacy Practice, 2001. 9(4): p. 269–274.
5. Babar, Z.-U.-D., et al. Migrant health in New Zealand: exploring issues concerning medicines access and use. Journal of Pharmaceutical Health Services Research: DOI: https://doi.org/10.1111/j.1759-8893.2012.00105.x
6. Bassett-Clarke, D., I. Krass, and B. Bajorek. Ethnic differences of medicines-taking in older adults: a cross cultural study in New Zealand. International Journal of Pharmacy Practice, 2012. 20(2): p. 90–98.
7. Young, H.N., et al. Pharmacists' provision of information to Spanish-speaking patients: A social cognitive approach. Research in Social and Administrative Pharmacy, 2013. 9(1): p. 4–12.
8. Jie, D., et al. The effects of health and treatment perceptions on the use of prescribed medication and home remedies among African American and White American hypertensives. Social Science and Medicine, 1996. 43(6): p. 903–917.
9. Newbold, K.B. Problems in Search of Solutions: Health and Canadian Aboriginals. Journal of Community Health, 1998. 23(1): p. 59–74.
10. Kowanko, I., et al. Better medication management for Aboriginal people with mental health disorders: a survey of providers. Australian Journal of Rural Health, 2004. 12(6): p. 253–257.
11. Håkonsen, H. and E.-L. Toverud, Special challenges for drug adherence following generic substitution in Pakistani immigrants living in Norway. European Journal of Clinical Pharmacology, 2011. 67(2): p. 193–201.
12. Scahill, S.L. Placing "culture" at the center of social pharmacy practice and research. Research in Social and Administrative Pharmacy, 2013. 9(1): p. 1–3.

The manufacturer's authorised representative in the EU is Springer Nature Customer Service Centre GmbH, Europaplatz 3, 69115 Heidelberg, Germany. If you have any concerns regarding our products, please contact ProductSafety@springernature.com

Printed and bound by CPI Group (UK) Ltd, Croydon, CR0 4YY
30/09/2026
02225460-0011